Long Term Care Facility Resident Assessment Instrument

User's Manual

James E. Allen, PhD, MSPH, CNHA is
Associate Professor of Health Policy and Administration
School of Public Health, 1105-C McGavran-Greenberg Hall
University of North Carolina at Chapel Hill
Chapel Hill, North Carolina, 27599-7400

The UNC-CH Long Term Care Administration Teaching Resources Program

This program makes available to students and course instructors relatively complete sets of materials for classroom use and for preparation for becoming a nursing home administrator.

Five key elements for this preparation are:

1. The text, *Nursing Home Administration*, 3rd. ed, Springer Publishing Company, 1997.

2. *Nursing Home Federal Requirements and Guidelines to Surveyors*, also by Springer Publishing Company, 3rd. ed., 1997 -- user friendly rendering of the Health Care Finance Administration's State Operations Manual, Provider Certification.

3. *The Licensing Exam Review Guide in Nursing Home Administration*, 3rd. ed., Springer Publishing Company, 1997 - 1,000 practice questions.

4. *Long Term Care Facility Resident Assessment Instrument User's Manual* for use with Version 2.0 of HCFA Minimum Data Set - the MDS and RAPs.

5. *The NAB Five-Step Administrator-in-Training Internship Program_* -available through the NAB.

Instructor's Guide -- 20 case studies plus several hundred questions for classroom use available to course instructors. Instructors: write to the author, James E. Allen.

Correspondence courses for licensure preparation - used by over a dozen state licensing boards.

For further information write to the above address, or call 919-966-7385 or fax 919-967-3438.

LONG TERM CARE FACILITY RESIDENT ASSESSMENT INSTRUMENT

User's Manual

for use with Version 2.0 of HCFA

Prepared by: James E. Allen, *MSPH, PhD, CNHA*

Minimum Data Set
Resident Assessment Protocols
and Utilization Guidelines
October, 1995

plus

HCFA's 249
Questions and Answers
August, 1996

Springer Publishing Company
New York

Springer Publishing Company, Inc.
536 Broadway
New York, NY 10012–3955

Cover design by Margaret Dunin
Acquisitions Editor: Bill Tucker

97 98 99 00 01 / 5 4 3 2 1

Library of Congress Cataloging-in Publication Data

Allen, James E. (James Elmore), 1935–
Long term care facility resident assessment instrument user's manual: for use with version 2.0 of HCFA minimum data set resident assessment protocols and utilization guidelines, October 1995, plus HCFA's 249 questions and answers, August 1996 / prepared by James E. Allen. 3rd ed. c 1977.
p. cm.
Companion v. to. Nursing home federal requirements and guidelines to surveyors / James E. Allen
Includes appendices.
Includes bibliographical references and index.
ISBN 0-8261-9900-3
1. Nursing home—United States—Medical records—Forms. 2. Nursing assessment—United States—Forms. 3. Long-term care facilities—United States —Medical records—Forms. 4. Geriatric nursing—United States—Forms. 5. United States. Health Care Financing Administration. I. Allen, James E. (James Elmore), 1935–Nursing home federal requirements and guidelines to surveyors. II. Title.
[DNLM: 1. Geriatric Assessment. 2. Medical Records, Problem-Oriented—Standards. 3. Long-Term Care—organization & administration—United States. 4. Nursing Home—United States—legislation. 5. Medicare—forms. 6. Medicaid—forms. WT 30 A427L 1997]
RA999.M43A44 1997
362. 1'6—dc21
DNLM/DLC
for Library of Congress 97-3056
CIP

Printed in the United States of America

TABLE OF CONTENTS

Chapter 1: Overview of the RAI

Chapter 2: Using the RAI: Statutory and Regulatory Requirements and Suggestions for Integration in Clinical Practice

Chapter 3: MDS Items

Chapter 4: Procedures for Completing the Resident Assessment Protocols (RAPs)

Chapter 5: Linking Assessment to Individualized Care Plans

Appendices

Index

Note to users

Springer's presentation of this working manual offers large print, easy to read MDS forms.

These HCFA guidelines on how to use the MDS to develop the residents' comprehensive care plans assist the facility staff to implement the federal requirements under OBRA (Nursing Home Reform Act of 1987).

The federal requirements and guidelines to surveyors, with a detailed index, are published by Springer as a companion volume to this User's Manual.

Use of Springer's two publications,

Nursing Home Federal Requirements and Guidelines to Surveyors and

Long Term Care Facility Resident Assessment Instrument User's Manual,

will, together, enable staff to both meet federal requirements and effectively implement the quality assurance program required for facilities which participate in Medicare and Medicaid.

Springer's version of federal requirements and guidelines to surveyors sets the standard as the most user-friendly rendering available, enabling staff to understand and better implement the federal requirements.

CHAPTER 1: OVERVIEW OF THE RAI

1.1 Overview of RAI Components

Providing care to residents of long term care facilities is complex and challenging work. It utilizes clinical competence, observational skills, and assessment expertise from all disciplines to develop individualized care plans. The Resident Assessment Instrument (RAI) helps facility staff to gather definitive information on a resident's strengths and needs which must be addressed in an individualized care plan. It also assists staff to evaluate goal achievement and revise care plans accordingly by enabling the facility to track changes in the resident's status. As the process of problem identification is integrated with sound clinical interventions, the care plan becomes each resident's unique path toward achieving or maintaining his or her highest practicable level of well-being.

The RAI helps facility staff to look at residents holistically — as individuals for whom quality of life and quality of care are mutually significant and necessary. Interdisciplinary use of the RAI promotes this very emphasis on quality of care and quality of life. Facilities have found that involving disciplines such as dietary, social work, physical therapy, occupational therapy, speech language pathology, pharmacy and activities in the RAI process has fostered a more holistic approach to resident care and strengthened team communication.

Persons generally enter a nursing facility due to functional status problems caused by physical deterioration, cognitive decline, or other related factors. The ability to manage independently has been limited to the extent that assistance or medical treatment is needed for residents to function or to live safely from day to day. All necessary resources and disciplines must be used to ensure that residents achieve the highest level of functioning possible (Quality of Care) and maintain their sense of individuality (Quality of Life). This is true for long stay residents, as well as the resident in a rehabilitative program anticipating return to a less restrictive environment.

Clinicians are generally taught a problem identification process as part of their professional education. For example, the nursing profession's problem identification model is called the nursing process, which consists of assessment, planning, implementation and evaluation. The RAI simply provides a structured, standardized approach for applying a problem identification process in long term care facilities. **The RAI should not, nor was it ever meant to be an additional burden for nursing facility staff.**

All good problem identification models have similar steps:

a.) **Assessment** - Taking stock of all observations, information and knowledge about a resident; understanding the resident's limitations and strengths; finding out who the resident is.

b.) **Decision-making** - Determining the severity, functional impact, and scope of a resident's problems; understanding the causes and relationships between a resident's problems; discovering the "whats" and "whys" of resident problems.

c.) **Care Planning** - Establishing a course of action that moves a resident toward a specific goal utilizing individual resident strengths and interdisciplinary expertise; crafting the "how" of resident care.

d.) **Implementation** - Putting that course of action (specific interventions on the care plan) into motion by staff knowledgeable about the resident care goals and approaches; carrying out the "how" and "when" of resident care.

e.) **Evaluation** - Critically reviewing care plan goals, interventions and implementation in terms of achieved resident outcomes and assessing the need to modify the care plan (i.e., change interventions) to adjust to changes in the resident's status, either improvement or decline.

This is how the problem identification process would look as a pathway. This manual will feature this pathway throughout and will highlight the point in the pathway that each chapter discusses.

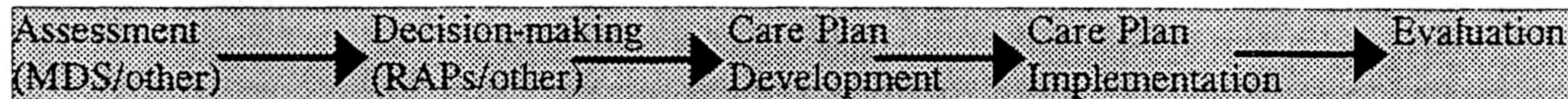

If you look at the RAI system as solution oriented and dynamic, it becomes a richly practical means of helping facility staff to gather and analyze information in order to improve a resident's quality of care and quality of life. In an already overburdened structure, the RAI offers a clear path toward utilizing all members of the interdisciplinary team in a proactive process. There is absolutely no reason to insert the RAI process as an added task or view it as another "layer" of labor.

The key to understanding the RAI process, and successfully using it, is believing that its structure is designed to enhance resident care and promote the quality of a resident's life. This occurs not only because it follows an interdisciplinary problem solving model but also because staff, across all shifts, are involved in its "hands on" approach. The result is a process that flows smoothly from one component to the next and allows for good communication and uncomplicated tracking of resident care. In short, it works!

Over the course of the years since the RAI has been implemented, facilities who have applied the RAI in the manner we have discussed have discovered that it works in the following ways:

Residents respond to individualized care. While we will discuss other positive responses to the RAI below, there is none more persuasive or powerful than good resident outcomes both in terms of a resident's quality of care and quality of life. Facility after facility has found that when the care plan reflects careful consideration of individual problems and causes, linked with appropriate resident specific approaches to care, residents have experienced goal achievement and either the level of functioning has improved or deteriorated at a slower rate. Facilities report that as individualized attention increases, resident satisfaction with quality of life is also increased.

Staff communication has become more effective. When staff are involved in a resident's ongoing assessment and have input into the determination and development of a resident's care plan, the commitment to and the understanding of that care plan is enhanced. All levels of staff, including nursing assistants, have a stake in the process. Knowledge gained from careful examination of possible causes and solutions of resident problems (i.e., from using the RAPs) challenges staff to hone the professional skills of their discipline as well as focus on the individuality of the resident and holistically consider how that individuality must be accommodated in the care plan.

Resident and family involvement in care has increased. There has been a dramatic increase in the frequency and nature of resident and family involvement in the care planning process. Input has been provided on individual resident strengths, problems, and preferences. Staff have a much better picture of the resident, and residents and families have a better understanding of the goals and processes of care.

Documentation has become clearer. When the approaches to achieving a specific goal are understood and distinct, the need for voluminous documentation diminishes. Likewise, when staff are communicating effectively among themselves with respect to resident care, repetitive documentation is not necessary and contradictory notes do not occur. In addition, new staff, consultants, or others who review records find that information documented about a resident is clearer and tracking care and outcomes is more easily accomplished.

It is the intent of this manual to offer clear guidance, through instruction and example, for the effective use of the RAI, and thereby help facilities achieve the benefits listed above.

In keeping with objectives set forth in the Institute of Medicine (IOM) study completed in 1986 that made recommendations to improve the quality of care in nursing homes, the RAI provides each resident with a standardized, comprehensive and reproducible assessment. It evaluates a resident's ability to perform daily life functions and identifies significant impairments in a resident's functional capacity. In essence, with an accurate RAI completed periodically, caregivers have a genuine and consistently recorded "look" at the resident and can attend to that resident's needs with realistic goals in hand.

With the consistent application of item definitions, the RAI ensures standardized communication both within the facility and between facilities (e.g., other long term care facilities or hospitals). Basically, when everyone is speaking the same language, the opportunity for misunderstanding or error is diminished considerably.

The RAI consists of three basic components; the **Minimum Data Set (MDS), Resident Assessment Protocols (RAPs)**, and **Utilization Guidelines** specified in State Operations Manual (SOM) Transmittal #272. All components are discussed in detail in this manual.

Utilization of the three components of the RAI yields information about a resident's functional status, strengths, weaknesses and preferences, and offers guidance on further assessment once problems have been identified. Each component flows naturally into the next as follows:

- **Minimum Data Set (MDS).** A core set of screening, clinical and functional status elements, including common definitions and coding categories, that forms the foundation of the comprehensive assessment for all residents of long term care facilities certified to participate in Medicare or Medicaid. The items in the MDS standardize communication about resident problems and conditions within facilities, between facilities, and between facilities and outside agencies. **A copy of the MDS Version 2.0 can be found at the end of this chapter, beginning on page 1-6 and Appendix B.**

- **Resident Assessment Protocols (RAPs).** A component of the utilization guidelines, the RAPs are structured, problem-oriented frameworks for organizing MDS information, and examining additional clinically relevant information about an individual. RAPs help identify social, medical and psychological problems and form the basis for individualized care planning.

- **Utilization Guidelines.** Instructions concerning when and how to use the RAI.

1.2 Overview of RAI Version 2.0 User's Manual

The manual layout is as follows:

Chapter 1 - Overview of the RAI

Chapter 2 - Using the RAI: Statutory and Regulatory Requirements and Suggestions for Integration in Clinical Practice

Chapter 3 - Completing the MDS: Item by Item Definitions and Instructions

Chapter 4 - Procedures for Completing the Resident Assessment Protocols (RAPs)

Chapter 5 - Linking Assessment to Individualized Care Plans

APPENDICES

Appendix A: State Agencies Responsible for Answering RAI Questions

Appendix B: MDS and Quarterly Review Forms for Version 2.0

Appendix C: Trigger Legend, RAP Summary Form and 18 RAPs for Version 2.0

Appendix D: Interviewing Techniques

Appendix E: Commonly Prescribed Medications by Category

Appendix F: Cognitive Performance Scale (CPS) Scoring Rules

Appendix G: Statutory and Regulatory Requirements for Long Term Care Facilities - Resident Assessment and Care Planning

Appendix H: RAI Background

Index

1.3 Suggestions for the Use of This Manual

This manual is designed to meet the needs of facility staff who are both skilled in the use of the RAI and staff who are just beginning to work with it.

For those who have had experience with the RAI, this manual will show you "what's new" about the RAI Version 2.0 and serve as a reference. While the MDS has changed, the process of completion and application has not. You will find the item by item section informative with respect to new items and items that have been refined or expanded. You will also find that the case studies and examples provide direction regarding "how to" complete the RAP review process and what kind of documentation is required.

If you are new to the RAI and its process, you will find this manual an invaluable companion. The following fundamental concepts associated with the RAI are interwoven as themes throughout this manual:

A. The resident is an individual with strengths, as well as functional limitations and health problems.

B. Possible causes for each problem area and guidance for further assessment and resolution or intervention are presented in the RAPs.

C. An <u>interdisciplinary</u> approach to resident care is vital — both in assessment and in developing the resident's care plan.

D. Good clinical practice requires solid, sound assessment.

In essence, this manual promotes a step-by-step system of assessing resident needs and functional status based on standardized definitions of items (the MDS). It then helps you think through possible reasons for and risk factors that contribute to a resident's clinical status (RAPs). This informative material offers the interdisciplinary team realistic approaches to resident care that are based on specific, individual characteristics.

Numeric Identifier_______________

MINIMUM DATA SET (MDS) — *VERSION 2.0*

FOR NURSING HOME RESIDENT ASSESSMENT AND CARE SCREENING

BASIC ASSESSMENT TRACKING FORM

SECTION AA. IDENTIFICATION INFORMATION

1.	RESIDENT NAME⊙	a. (First) b. (Middle Initial) c. (Last) d. (Jr/Sr)
2.	GENDER⊙	1. Male 2. Female
3.	BIRTHDATE⊙	Month — Day — Year
4.	RACE/⊙ ETHNICITY	1. American Indian/Alaskan Native 2. Asian/Pacific Islander 3. Black, not of Hispanic origin 4. Hispanic 5. White, not of Hispanic origin
5.	SOCIAL SECURITY⊙ AND MEDICARE NUMBERS⊙ [C in 1st box if non med. no.]	a. Social Security Number b. Medicare number (or comparable railroad insurance number)
6.	FACILITY PROVIDER NO.⊙	a. State No. b. Federal No.
7.	MEDICAID NO. ["+" *if pending, "N" if not a Medicaid recipient*] ⊙	
8.	REASONS FOR ASSESS-MENT	[Note—Other codes do not apply to this form] a. Primary reason for assessment 1. Admission assessment (required by day 14) 2. Annual assessment 3. Significant change in status assessment 4. Significant correction of prior assessment 5. Quarterly review assessment 0. *NONE OF ABOVE* **b. *Special codes for use with supplemental assessment types in Case Mix demonstration states or other states where required*** *1. 5 day assessment* *2. 30 day assessment* *3. 60 day assessment* *4. Quarterly assessment using full MDS form* *5. Readmission/return assessment* *6. Other state required assessment*
9.	SIGNATURES OF PERSONS COMPLETING THESE ITEMS:	

a. Signatures	Title	Date
b.		Date

GENERAL INSTRUCTIONS

Complete this information for submission with all full and quarterly assessments (Admission, Annual, Significant Change, State or Medicare required assessments, or Quarterly Reviews, etc.)

⊙ = Key items for computerized resident tracking

☐ = When box blank, must enter number or letter [a.] = When letter in box, check if condition applies

Resident ______________________ Numeric Identifier ______________________

MINIMUM DATA SET (MDS) — *VERSION 2.0*

FOR NURSING HOME RESIDENT ASSESSMENT AND CARE SCREENING

BACKGROUND (FACE SHEET) INFORMATION AT ADMISSION

SECTION AB. DEMOGRAPHIC INFORMATION

1.	DATE OF ENTRY	*Date the stay began. Note — Does not include readmission if record was closed at time of temporary discharge to hospital, etc. In such cases, use prior admission date* ☐☐ — ☐☐ — ☐☐☐☐ Month Day Year
2.	ADMITTED FROM (AT ENTRY)	1. Private home/apt. with no home health services 2. Private home/apt. with home health services 3. Board and care/assisted living/group home 4. Nursing home 5. Acute care hospital 6. Psychiatric hospital, MR/DD facility 7. Rehabilitation hospital 8. Other
3.	LIVED ALONE (PRIOR TO ENTRY)	0. No 1. Yes 2. In other facility
4.	ZIP CODE OF PRIOR PRIMARY RESIDENCE	☐☐☐☐☐
5.	RESIDENTIAL HISTORY 5 YEARS PRIOR TO ENTRY	*(**Check all settings** resident lived in during 5 years prior to date of entry given in item AB1 above)* Prior stay at this nursing home a. Stay in other nursing home b. Other residential facility—board and care home, assisted living, group home c. MH/psychiatric setting d. MR/DD setting e. *NONE OF ABOVE* f.
6.	LIFETIME OCCUPATION(S) [Put "/" between two occupations]	☐☐☐☐☐☐☐☐☐☐☐☐☐☐☐☐☐☐☐☐☐☐☐☐☐
7.	EDUCATION (*Highest Level Completed*)	1. No schooling 2. 8th grade/less 3. 9-11 grades 4. High school 5. Technical or trade school 6. Some college 7. Bachelor's degree 8. Graduate degree
8.	LANGUAGE	*(Code for correct response)* **a.** Primary Language 0. English 1. Spanish 2. French 3. Other **b. If other, specify** ☐☐☐☐☐☐☐☐☐☐
9.	MENTAL HEALTH HISTORY	Does resident's RECORD indicate any history of mental retardation, mental illness, or developmental disability problem? 0. No 1. Yes
10.	CONDITIONS RELATED TO MR/DD STATUS	*(**Check all conditions** that are related to MR/DD status that were manifested before age 22, and are likely to continue indefinitely)* Not applicable—no MR/DD (Skip to AB11) a. MR/DD with organic condition Down's syndrome b. Autism c. Epilepsy d. Other organic condition related to MR/DD e. MR/DD with no organic condition f.
11.	DATE BACKGROUND INFORMATION COMPLETED	☐☐ — ☐☐ — ☐☐☐☐ Month Day Year

SECTION AC. CUSTOMARY ROUTINE

1.	CUSTOMARY ROUTINE *(In year prior to DATE OF ENTRY to this nursing home, or year last in community if now being admitted from another nursing home)*	*(**Check all that apply.** If all information UNKNOWN, check last box only.)*	
		CYCLE OF DAILY EVENTS	
		Stays up late at night (e.g., after 9 pm)	a.
		Naps regularly during day (at least 1 hour)	b.
		Goes out 1+ days a week	c.
		Stays busy with hobbies, reading, or fixed daily routine	d.
		Spends most of time alone or watching TV	e.
		Moves independently indoors (with appliances, if used)	f.
		Use of tobacco products at least daily	g.
		NONE OF ABOVE	h.
		EATING PATTERNS	
		Distinct food preferences	i.
		Eats between meals all or most days	j.
		Use of alcoholic beverage(s) at least weekly	k.
		NONE OF ABOVE	l.
		ADL PATTERNS	
		In bedclothes much of day	m.
		Wakens to toilet all or most nights	n.
		Has irregular bowel movement pattern	o.
		Showers for bathing	p.
		Bathing in PM	q.
		NONE OF ABOVE	r.
		INVOLVEMENT PATTERNS	
		Daily contact with relatives/close friends	s.
		Usually attends church, temple, synagogue (etc.)	t.
		Finds strength in faith	u.
		Daily animal companion/presence	v.
		Involved in group activities	w.
		NONE OF ABOVE	x.
		UNKNOWN—Resident/family unable to provide information	y.

END

SECTION AD. FACE SHEET SIGNATURES

SIGNATURES OF PERSONS COMPLETING FACE SHEET:			
a. Signature of RN Assessment Coordinator			Date
b. Signatures	Title	Sections	Date
c.			Date
d.			Date
e.			Date
f.			Date
g.			Date

☐ = When box blank, must enter number or letter [a.] = When letter in box, check if condition applies

MINIMUM DATA SET (MDS) — *VERSION 2.0*
FOR NURSING HOME RESIDENT ASSESSMENT AND CARE SCREENING
FULL ASSESSMENT FORM

(Status in last 7 days, unless other time frame indicated)

SECTION A. IDENTIFICATION AND BACKGROUND INFORMATION

1.	RESIDENT NAME	a. (First) b. (Middle Initial) c. (Last) d. (Jr/Sr)
2.	ROOM NUMBER	
3.	ASSESS-MENT REFERENCE DATE	a. *Last day of MDS observation period* Month — Day — Year b. Original (0) or corrected copy of form (enter number of correction)
4a.	DATE OF REENTRY	**Date of reentry from most recent temporary discharge to a hospital in last 90 days (or since last assessment or admission if less than 90 days)** Month — Day — Year
5.	MARITAL STATUS	1. Never married 2. Married 3. Widowed 4. Separated 5. Divorced
6.	MEDICAL RECORD NO.	
7.	CURRENT PAYMENT SOURCES FOR N.H. STAY	(*Billing Office to indicate; **check all that apply in last 30 days***) Medicaid per diem a. Medicare per diem b. Medicare ancillary part A c. Medicare ancillary part B d. CHAMPUS per diem e. VA per diem f. Self or family pays for full per diem g. Medicaid resident liability or Medicare co-payment h. Private insurance per diem (including co-payment) i. Other per diem j.
8.	REASONS FOR ASSESS-MENT *[**Note—If this is a discharge or reentry assessment, only a limited subset of MDS items need be completed**]*	a. Primary reason for assessment 1. Admission assessment (required by day 14) 2. Annual assessment 3. Significant change in status assessment 4. Significant correction of prior assessment 5. Quarterly review assessment 6. Discharged—return not anticipated 7. Discharged—return anticipated 8. Discharged prior to completing initial assessment 9. Reentry 0. *NONE OF ABOVE* b. ***Special codes for use with supplemental assessment types in Case Mix demonstration states or other states where required*** *1. 5 day assessment* *2. 30 day assessment* *3. 60 day assessment* *4. Quarterly assessment using full MDS form* *5. Readmission/return assessment* *6. Other state required assessment*
9.	RESPONSI-BILITY/ LEGAL GUARDIAN	(***Check all that apply***) Legal guardian a. Other legal oversight b. Durable power of attorney/health care c. Durable power attorney/financial d. Family member responsible e. Patient responsible for self f. *NONE OF ABOVE* g.
10.	ADVANCED DIRECTIVES	(*For those items with supporting documentation in the medical record, **check all that apply***) Living will a. Do not resuscitate b. Do not hospitalize c. Organ donation d. Autopsy request e. Feeding restrictions f. Medication restrictions g. Other treatment restrictions h. *NONE OF ABOVE* i.

SECTION B. COGNITIVE PATTERNS

1.	COMATOSE	(*Persistent vegetative state/no discernible consciousness*) 0. No 1. Yes **(If yes, skip to Section G)**
2.	MEMORY	(*Recall of what was learned or known*) a. Short-term memory OK—seems/appears to recall after 5 minutes 0. Memory OK 1. Memory problem b. Long-term memory OK—seems/appears to recall long past 0. Memory OK 1. Memory problem
3.	MEMORY/ RECALL ABILITY	(***Check all that resident was normally able to recall during last 7 days***) Current season a. Location of own room b. Staff names/faces c. That he/she is in a nursing home d. *NONE OF ABOVE* are recalled e.
4.	COGNITIVE SKILLS FOR DAILY DECISION-MAKING	(*Made decisions regarding tasks of daily life*) 0. *INDEPENDENT*—decisions consistent/reasonable 1. *MODIFIED INDEPENDENCE*—some difficulty in new situations only 2. *MODERATELY IMPAIRED*—decisions poor; cues/supervision required 3. *SEVERELY IMPAIRED*—never/rarely made decisions
5.	INDICATORS OF DELIRIUM—PERIODIC DISOR-DERED THINKING/ AWARENESS	(*Code for behavior in the **last 7 days.***) ***[Note: Accurate assessment requires conversations with staff and family who have direct knowledge of resident's behavior over this time]*.** 0. Behavior not present 1. Behavior present, not of recent onset 2. Behavior present, over last 7 days appears different from resident's usual functioning (e.g., new onset or worsening) a. EASILY DISTRACTED—(e.g., difficulty paying attention; gets sidetracked) b. PERIODS OF ALTERED PERCEPTION OR AWARENESS OF SURROUNDINGS—(e.g., moves lips or talks to someone not present; believes he/she is somewhere else; confuses night and day) c. EPISODES OF DISORGANIZED SPEECH—(e.g., speech is incoherent, nonsensical, irrelevant, or rambling from subject to subject; loses train of thought) d. PERIODS OF RESTLESSNESS—(e.g., fidgeting or picking at skin, clothing, napkins, etc; frequent position changes; repetitive physical movements or calling out) e. PERIODS OF LETHARGY—(e.g., sluggishness; staring into space; difficult to arouse; little body movement) f. MENTAL FUNCTION VARIES OVER THE COURSE OF THE DAY—(e.g., sometimes better, sometimes worse; behaviors sometimes present, sometimes not)
6.	CHANGE IN COGNITIVE STATUS	Resident's cognitive status, skills, or abilities have changed as compared to status of **90 days ago** (or since last assessment if less than 90 days) 0. No change 1. Improved 2. Deteriorated

SECTION C. COMMUNICATION/HEARING PATTERNS

1.	HEARING	(*With hearing appliance, if used*) 0. *HEARS ADEQUATELY*—normal talk, TV, phone 1. *MINIMAL DIFFICULTY* when not in quiet setting 2. *HEARS IN SPECIAL SITUATIONS ONLY*—speaker has to adjust tonal quality and speak distinctly 3. *HIGHLY IMPAIRED*/absence of useful hearing
2.	COMMUNI-CATION DEVICES/ TECH-NIQUES	(***Check all that apply** during last 7 days*) Hearing aid, present and used a. Hearing aid, present and not used regularly b. Other receptive comm. techniques used (e.g., lip reading) c. *NONE OF ABOVE* d.
3.	MODES OF EXPRESSION	(***Check all used** by resident to make needs known*) Speech a. Writing messages to express or clarify needs b. American sign language or Braille c. Signs/gestures/sounds d. Communication board e. Other f. *NONE OF ABOVE* g.
4.	MAKING SELF UNDER-STOOD	(*Expressing information content—however able*) 0. *UNDERSTOOD* 1. *USUALLY UNDERSTOOD*—difficulty finding words or finishing thoughts 2. *SOMETIMES UNDERSTOOD*—ability is limited to making concrete requests 3. *RARELY/NEVER UNDERSTOOD*
5.	SPEECH CLARITY	(*Code for speech in the **last 7 days***) 0. *CLEAR SPEECH*—distinct, intelligible words 1. *UNCLEAR SPEECH*—slurred, mumbled words 2. *NO SPEECH*—absence of spoken words
6.	ABILITY TO UNDER-STAND OTHERS	(*Understanding verbal information content—however able*) 0. *UNDERSTANDS* 1. *USUALLY UNDERSTANDS*—may miss some part/intent of message 2. *SOMETIMES UNDERSTANDS*—responds adequately to simple, direct communication 3. *RARELY/NEVER UNDERSTANDS*
7.	CHANGE IN COMMUNI-CATION/ HEARING	Resident's ability to express, understand, or hear information has changed as compared to status of **90 days ago** (or since last assessment if less than 90 days) 0. No change 1. Improved 2. Deteriorated

☐ = When box blank, must enter number or letter

a. = When letter in box, check if condition applies

SECTION D. VISION PATTERNS

1.	VISION	(*Ability to see in adequate light and with glasses if used*) 0. *ADEQUATE*—sees fine detail, including regular print in newspapers/books 1. *IMPAIRED*—sees large print, but not regular print in newspapers/books 2. *MODERATELY IMPAIRED*—limited vision; not able to see newspaper headlines, but can identify objects 3. *HIGHLY IMPAIRED*—object identification in question, but eyes appear to follow objects 4. *SEVERELY IMPAIRED*—no vision or sees only light, colors, or shapes; eyes do not appear to follow objects	
2.	VISUAL LIMITATIONS/ DIFFICULTIES	Side vision problems—decreased peripheral vision (e.g., leaves food on one side of tray, difficulty traveling, bumps into people and objects, misjudges placement of chair when seating self)	a.
		Experiences any of following: sees halos or rings around lights; sees flashes of light; sees "curtains" over eyes	b.
		NONE OF ABOVE	c.
3.	VISUAL APPLIANCES	Glasses; contact lenses; magnifying glass 0. No 1. Yes	

SECTION E. MOOD AND BEHAVIOR PATTERNS

1.	INDICATORS OF DEPRES-SION, ANXIETY, SAD MOOD	(***Code for indicators observed in last 30 days, irrespective of the assumed cause***) 0. Indicator not exhibited in last 30 days 1. Indicator of this type exhibited up to five days a week 2. Indicator of this type exhibited daily or almost daily (6, 7 days a week)	
		VERBAL EXPRESSIONS OF DISTRESS	
		a. Resident made negative statements—e.g., "*Nothing matters; Would rather be dead; What's the use; Regrets having lived so long; Let me die*"	
		b. Repetitive questions—e.g., "*Where do I go; What do I do?*"	
		c. Repetitive verbalizations—e.g., calling out for help, ("*God help me*")	
		d. Persistent anger with self or others—e.g., easily annoyed, anger at placement in nursing home; anger at care received	
		e. Self deprecation—e.g., "*I am nothing; I am of no use to anyone*"	
		f. Expressions of what appear to be unrealistic fears—e.g., fear of being abandoned, left alone, being with others	
		g. Recurrent statements that something terrible is about to happen—e.g., believes he or she is about to die, have a heart attack	
		h. Repetitive health complaints—e.g., persistently seeks medical attention, obsessive concern with body functions	
		i. Repetitive anxious complaints/concerns (non-health related) e.g., persistently seeks attention/ reassurance regarding schedules, meals, laundry, clothing, relationship issues	
		SLEEP-CYCLE ISSUES	
		j. Unpleasant mood in morning	
		k. Insomnia/change in usual sleep pattern	
		SAD, APATHETIC, ANXIOUS APPEARANCE	
		l. Sad, pained, worried facial expressions—e.g., furrowed brows	
		m. Crying, tearfulness	
		n. Repetitive physical movements—e.g., pacing, hand wringing, restlessness, fidgeting, picking	
		LOSS OF INTEREST	
		o. Withdrawal from activities of interest—e.g., no interest in long standing activities or being with family/friends	
		p. Reduced social interaction	
2.	MOOD PERSIS-TENCE	**One or more indicators of depressed, sad or anxious mood were not easily altered by attempts to "cheer up", console, or reassure the resident over last 7 days** 0. No mood indicators 1. Indicators present, easily altered 2. Indicators present, not easily altered	
3.	CHANGE IN MOOD	Resident's mood status has changed as compared to status of **90 days ago** (or since last assessment if less then 90 days) 0. No change 1. Improved 2. Deteriorated	

			(A)	(B)
4.	BEHAVIORAL SYMPTOMS	(A) ***Behavioral symptom frequency in last 7 days*** 0. Behavior not exhibited in last 7 days 1. Behavior of this type occurred 1 to 3 days in last 7 days 2. Behavior of this type occurred 4 to 6 days, but less than daily 3. Behavior of this type occurred daily (B) ***Behavioral symptom alterability in last 7 days*** 0. Behavior not present OR behavior was easily altered 1. Behavior was not easily altered		
		a. WANDERING (moved with no rational purpose, seemingly oblivious to needs or safety)		
		b. VERBALLY ABUSIVE BEHAVIORAL SYMPTOMS (others were threatened, screamed at, cursed at)		
		c. PHYSICALLY ABUSIVE BEHAVIORAL SYMPTOMS (others were hit, shoved, scratched, sexually abused)		
		d. SOCIALLY INAPPROPRIATE/DISRUPTIVE BEHAVIORAL SYMPTOMS (made disruptive sounds, noisiness, screaming, self-abusive acts, sexual behavior or disrobing in public, smeared/threw food/feces, hoarding, rummaged through others' belongings)		
		e. RESISTS CARE (resisted taking medications/ injections, ADL assistance, or eating)		

5.	CHANGE IN BEHAVIORAL SYMPTOMS	Resident's behavior status has changed as compared to **status of 90 days ago** (or since last assessment if less than 90 days) 0. No change 1. Improved 2. Deteriorated	

SECTION F. PSYCHOSOCIAL WELL-BEING

1.	SENSE OF INITIATIVE/ INVOLVE-MENT	At ease interacting with others	a.
		At ease doing planned or structured activities	b.
		At ease doing self-initiated activities	c.
		Establishes own goals	d.
		Pursues involvement in life of facility (e.g., makes/keeps friends; involved in group activities; responds positively to new activities; assists at religious services)	e.
		Accepts invitations into most group activities	f.
		NONE OF ABOVE	g.
2.	UNSETTLED RELATION-SHIPS	Covert/open conflict with or repeated criticism of staff	a.
		Unhappy with roommate	b.
		Unhappy with residents other than roommate	c.
		Openly expresses conflict/anger with family/friends	d.
		Absence of personal contact with family/friends	e.
		Recent loss of close family member/friend	f.
		Does not adjust easily to change in routines	g.
		NONE OF ABOVE	h.
3.	PAST ROLES	Strong identification with past roles and life status	a.
		Expresses sadness/anger/empty feeling over lost roles/status	b.
		Resident perceives that daily routine (customary routine, activities) is very different from prior pattern in the community	c.
		NONE OF ABOVE	d.

SECTION G. PHYSICAL FUNCTIONING AND STRUCTURAL PROBLEMS

			(A) SELF-PERF	(B) SUPPORT
1.		(A) ADL SELF-PERFORMANCE—(***Code for resident's PERFORMANCE OVER ALL SHIFTS during last 7 days****—Not including setup*) 0. *INDEPENDENT*—No help or oversight —OR— Help/oversight provided only 1 or 2 times during last 7 days 1. SUPERVISION—Oversight, encouragement or cueing provided 3 or more times during last7 days —OR— Supervision (3 or more times) plus physical assistance provided only 1 or 2 times during last 7 days 2. *LIMITED ASSISTANCE*—Resident highly involved in activity; received physical help in guided maneuvering of limbs or other nonweight bearing assistance 3 or more times —OR—More help provided only 1 or 2 times during last 7 days 3. *EXTENSIVE ASSISTANCE*—While resident performed part of activity, over last 7-day period, help of following type(s) provided 3 or more times: — Weight-bearing support — Full staff performance during part (but not all) of last 7 days 4. *TOTAL DEPENDENCE*—Full staff performance of activity during entire 7 days 8. *ACTIVITY DID NOT OCCUR* during entire 7 days (B) ADL SUPPORT PROVIDED—(***Code for MOST SUPPORT PROVIDED OVER ALL SHIFTS during last 7 days; code regardless*** *of resident's self-performance classification*) 0. No setup or physical help from staff 1. Setup help only 2. One person physical assist 3. Two+ persons physical assist 8. ADL activity itself did not occur during entire 7 days		
a.	BED MOBILITY	How resident moves to and from lying position, turns side to side, and positions body while in bed		
b.	TRANSFER	How resident moves between surfaces—to/from: bed, chair, wheelchair, standing position (EXCLUDE to/from bath/toilet)		
c.	WALK IN ROOM	How resident walks between locations in his/her room		
d.	WALK IN CORRIDOR	How resident walks in corridor on unit		
e.	LOCOMO-TION ON UNIT	How resident moves between locations in his/her room and adjacent corridor on same floor. If in wheelchair, self-sufficiency once in chair		
f.	LOCOMO-TION OFF UNIT	How resident moves to and returns from off unit locations (e.g., areas set aside for dining, activities, or treatments). **If facility has only one floor,** how resident moves to and from distant areas on the floor. If in wheelchair, self-sufficiency once in chair		
g.	DRESSING	How resident puts on, fastens, and takes off all items of **street clothing**, including donning/removing prosthesis		
h.	EATING	How resident eats and drinks (regardless of skill). Includes intake of nourishment by other means (e.g., tube feeding, total parenteral nutrition)		
i.	TOILET USE	How resident uses the toilet room (or commode, bedpan, urinal); transfer on/off toilet, cleanses, changes pad, manages ostomy or catheter, adjusts clothes		
j.	PERSONAL HYGIENE	How resident maintains personal hygiene, including combing hair, brushing teeth, shaving, applying makeup, washing/drying face, hands, and perineum (EXCLUDE baths and showers)		

Resident ________________________________

2.	BATHING	How resident takes full-body bath/shower, sponge bath, and transfers in/out of tub/shower (EXCLUDE washing of back and hair.) **Code for most dependent** *in self-performance and support.* (A) BATHING SELF-PERFORMANCE codes appear below 0. Independent—No help provided 1. Supervision—Oversight help only 2. Physical help limited to transfer only 3. Physical help in part of bathing activity 4. Total dependence 8. Activity itself did not occur during entire 7 days *(Bathing support codes are as defined in Item 1, code B above)*	(A)	(B)
3.	TEST FOR BALANCE (see training manual)	*(Code for ability during test in the last 7 days)* 0. Maintained position as required in test 1. Unsteady, but able to rebalance self without physical support 2. Partial physical support during test; or stands (sits) but does not follow directions for test 3. Not able to attempt test without physical help a. Balance while standing b. Balance while sitting—position, trunk control		
4.	FUNCTIONAL LIMITATION IN RANGE OF MOTION (see training manual)	*(Code for limitations during* ***last 7 days*** *that interfered with daily functions or placed resident at risk of injury)* (A) *RANGE OF MOTION* — 0. No limitation; 1. Limitation on one side; 2. Limitation on both sides (B) *VOLUNTARY MOVEMENT* — 0. No loss; 1. Partial loss; 2. Full loss a. Neck b. Arm—Including shoulder or elbow c. Hand—Including wrist or fingers d. Leg—Including hip or knee e. Foot—Including ankle or toes f. Other limitation or loss	(A)	(B)
5.	MODES OF LOCOMOTION	***(Check all that apply*** *during* ***last 7 days)*** Cane/walker/crutch — a. Wheeled self — b. Other person wheeled — c. Wheelchair primary mode of locomotion — d. *NONE OF ABOVE* — e.		
6.	MODES OF TRANSFER	***(Check all that apply*** *during* ***last 7 days)*** Bedfast all or most of time — a. Bed rails used for bed mobility or transfer — b. Lifted manually — c. Lifted mechanically — d. Transfer aid (e.g., slide board, trapeze, cane, walker, brace) — e. *NONE OF ABOVE* — f.		
7.	TASK SEGMENTATION	Some or all of ADL activities were broken into subtasks during **last 7 days** so that resident could perform them 0. No 1. Yes		
8.	ADL FUNCTIONAL REHABILITATION POTENTIAL	Resident believes he/she is capable of increased independence in at least some ADLs — a. Direct care staff believe resident is capable of increased independence in at least some ADLs — b. Resident able to perform tasks/activity but is very slow — c. Difference in ADL Self-Performance or ADL Support, comparing mornings to evenings — d. *NONE OF ABOVE* — e.		
9.	CHANGE IN ADL FUNCTION	Resident's ADL self-performance status has changed as compared to status of **90 days ago** (or since last assessment if less than 90 days) 0. No change 1. Improved 2. Deteriorated		

SECTION H. CONTINENCE IN LAST 14 DAYS

1.	CONTINENCE SELF-CONTROL CATEGORIES ***(Code for resident's PERFORMANCE OVER ALL SHIFTS)*** 0. *CONTINENT*—Complete control *[includes use of indwelling urinary catheter or ostomy device that does not leak urine or stool]* 1. *USUALLY CONTINENT*—BLADDER, incontinent episodes once a week or less; BOWEL, less than weekly 2. *OCCASIONALLY INCONTINENT*—BLADDER, 2 or more times a week but not daily; BOWEL, once a week 3. *FREQUENTLY INCONTINENT*—BLADDER, tended to be incontinent daily, but some control present (e.g., on day shift); BOWEL, 2-3 times a week 4. *INCONTINENT*—Had inadequate control BLADDER, multiple daily episodes; BOWEL, all (or almost all) of the time		
a.	BOWEL CONTINENCE	Control of bowel movement, with appliance or bowel continence programs, if employed	
b.	BLADDER CONTINENCE	Control of urinary bladder function (if dribbles, volume insufficient to soak through underpants), with appliances (e.g., foley) or continence programs, if employed	
2.	BOWEL ELIMINATION PATTERN	Bowel elimination pattern regular—at least one movement every three days — a. Constipation — b. Diarrhea — c. Fecal impaction — d. *NONE OF ABOVE* — e.	

Numeric Identifier ________________________________

3.	APPLIANCES AND PROGRAMS	Any scheduled toileting plan — a. Bladder retraining program — b. External (condom) catheter — c. Indwelling catheter — d. Intermittent catheter — e. Did not use toilet room/commode/urinal — f. Pads/briefs used — g. Enemas/irrigation — h. Ostomy present — i. *NONE OF ABOVE* — j.	
4.	CHANGE IN URINARY CONTINENCE	Resident's urinary continence has changed as compared to status of **90 days ago** (or since last assessment if less than 90 days) 0. No change 1. Improved 2. Deteriorated	

SECTION I. DISEASE DIAGNOSES

Check only those diseases that have a relationship to current ADL status, cognitive status, mood and behavior status, medical treatments, nursing monitoring, or risk of death. (Do not list inactive diagnoses)

1.	DISEASES	***(If none apply, CHECK the NONE OF ABOVE box)*** **ENDOCRINE/METABOLIC/NUTRITIONAL** Diabetes mellitus — a. Hyperthyroidism — b. Hypothyroidism — c. **HEART/CIRCULATION** Arteriosclerotic heart disease (ASHD) — d. Cardiac dysrhythmias — e. Congestive heart failure — f. Deep vein thrombosis — g. Hypertension — h. Hypotension — i. Peripheral vascular disease — j. Other cardiovascular disease — k. **MUSCULOSKELETAL** Arthritis — l. Hip fracture — m. Missing limb (e.g., amputation) — n. Osteoporosis — o. Pathological bone fracture — p. **NEUROLOGICAL** Alzheimer's disease — q. Aphasia — r. Cerebral palsy — s. Cerebrovascular accident (stroke) — t. Dementia other than Alzheimer's disease — u. Hemiplegia/Hemiparesis — v. Multiple sclerosis — w. Paraplegia — x. Parkinson's disease — y. Quadriplegia — z. Seizure disorder — aa. Transient ischemic attack (TIA) — bb. Traumatic brain injury — cc. **PSYCHIATRIC/MOOD** Anxiety disorder — dd. Depression — ee. Manic depression (bipolar disease) — ff. Schizophrenia — gg. **PULMONARY** Asthma — hh. Emphysema/COPD — ii. **SENSORY** Cataracts — jj. Diabetic retinopathy — kk. Glaucoma — ll. Macular degeneration — mm. **OTHER** Allergies — nn. Anemia — oo. Cancer — pp. Renal failure — qq. *NONE OF ABOVE* — rr.	
2.	INFECTIONS	***(If none apply, CHECK the NONE OF ABOVE box)*** Antibiotic resistant infection (e.g., Methicillin resistant staph) — a. Clostridium difficile (c. diff.) — b. Conjunctivitis — c. HIV infection — d. Pneumonia — e. Respiratory infection — f. Septicemia — g. Sexually transmitted diseases — h. Tuberculosis — i. Urinary tract infection in last 30 days — j. Viral hepatitis — k. Wound infection — l. NONE OF ABOVE — m.	
3.	OTHER CURRENT OR MORE DETAILED DIAGNOSES AND ICD-9 CODES	a. ________________ b. ________________ c. ________________ d. ________________ e. ________________	

SECTION J. HEALTH CONDITIONS

1.	PROBLEM CONDITIONS	***(Check all problems present in last 7 days*** *unless other time frame is indicated)* **INDICATORS OF FLUID STATUS** Weight gain or loss of 3 or more pounds within a 7 day period — a. Inability to lie flat due to shortness of breath — b. Dehydrated; output exceeds input — c. Insufficient fluid; did NOT consume all/almost all liquids provided during **last 3 days** — d. **OTHER** Delusions — e. Dizziness/Vertigo — f. Edema — g. Fever — h. Hallucinations — i. Internal bleeding — j. Recurrent lung aspirations in **last 90 days** — k. Shortness of breath — l. Syncope (fainting) — m. Unsteady gait — n. Vomiting — o. *NONE OF ABOVE* — p.	

Resident ______________________

2.	PAIN SYMPTOMS	(*Code the **highest level of pain** present in the **last 7 days***) a. **FREQUENCY** with which resident complains or shows evidence of pain 0. No pain (***skip to J4***) 1. Pain less than daily 2. Pain daily b. **INTENSITY** of pain 1. Mild pain 2. Moderate pain 3. Times when pain is horrible or excruciating
3.	PAIN SITE	(*If pain present, **check all sites** that apply in **last 7 days***) Back pain a. Bone pain b. Chest pain while doing usual activities c. Headache d. Hip pain e. Incisional pain f. Joint pain (other than hip) g. Soft tissue pain (e.g., lesion, muscle) h. Stomach pain i. Other j.
4.	ACCIDENTS	(***Check all that apply***) Fell in **past 30 days** a. Fell in **past 31-180 days** b. Hip fracture in **last 180 days** c. Other fracture in **last 180 days** d. *NONE OF ABOVE* e.
5.	STABILITY OF CONDITIONS	Conditions/diseases make resident's cognitive, ADL, mood or behavior patterns unstable—(fluctuating, precarious, or deteriorating) a. Resident experiencing an acute episode or a flare-up of a recurrent or chronic-problem b. End-stage disease, 6 or fewer months to live c. *NONE OF ABOVE* d.

SECTION K. ORAL/NUTRITIONAL STATUS

1.	ORAL PROBLEMS	Chewing problem a. Swallowing problem b. Mouth pain c. *NONE OF ABOVE* d.
2.	HEIGHT AND WEIGHT	*Record **(a.) height in inches** and **(b.) weight in pounds**. Base weight on most recent measure in **last 30 days**; measure weight consistently in accord with standard facility practice—e.g., in a.m. after voiding, before meal, with shoes off, and in nightclothes* a. HT (in.) b. WT (lb.)
3.	WEIGHT CHANGE	a. **Weight loss**—5 % or more in **last 30 days**; or 10 % or more in **last 180 days** 0. No 1. Yes b. **Weight gain**—5 % or more in **last 30 days**; or 10 % or more in **last 180 days** 0. No 1. Yes
4.	NUTRITIONAL PROBLEMS	Complains about the taste of many foods a. Regular or repetitive complaints of hunger b. Leaves 25% or more of food uneaten at most meals c. *NONE OF ABOVE* d.
5.	NUTRITIONAL APPROACHES	(***Check all that apply in last 7 days***) Parenteral/IV a. Feeding tube b. Mechanically altered diet c. Syringe (oral feeding) d. Therapeutic diet e. Dietary supplement between meals f. Plate guard, stabilized built-up utensil, etc. g. On a planned weight change program h. *NONE OF ABOVE* i.
6.	PARENTERAL OR ENTERAL INTAKE	(***Skip to Section L if neither 5a nor 5b is checked***) a. Code the proportion of **total calories** the resident received through parenteral or tube feedings in the **last 7 days** 0. None 1. 1% to 25% 2. 26% to 50% 3. 51% to 75% 4. 76% to 100% b. Code the average **fluid** intake per day by IV or tube in **last 7 days** 0. None 1. 1 to 500 cc/day 2. 501 to 1000 cc/day 3. 1001 to 1500 cc/day 4. 1501 to 2000 cc/day 5. 2001 or more cc/day

SECTION L. ORAL/DENTAL STATUS

1.	ORAL STATUS AND DISEASE PREVENTION	Debris (soft, easily movable substances) present in mouth prior to going to bed at night a. Has dentures or removable bridge b. Some/all natural teeth lost—does not have or does not use dentures (or partial plates) c. Broken, loose, or carious teeth d. Inflamed gums (gingiva); swollen or bleeding gums; oral abcesses; ulcers or rashes e. Daily cleaning of teeth/dentures or daily mouth care—by resident or staff f. *NONE OF ABOVE* g.

Numeric Identifier ______________________

SECTION M. SKIN CONDITION

1.	ULCERS (Due to any cause)	(*Record the number of ulcers at each ulcer stage—regardless of cause. If none present at a stage, record "0" (zero). Code all that apply during **last 7 days**. Code 9 = 9 or more.) **[Requires full body exam.]*** Number at Stage a. Stage 1. A persistent area of skin redness (without a break in the skin) that does not disappear when pressure is relieved. b. Stage 2. A partial thickness loss of skin layers that presents clinically as an abrasion, blister, or shallow crater. c. Stage 3. A full thickness of skin is lost, exposing the subcutaneous tissues - presents as a deep crater with or without undermining adjacent tissue. d. Stage 4. A full thickness of skin and subcutaneous tissue is lost, exposing muscle or bone.
2.	TYPE OF ULCER	(*For each type of ulcer, **code for the highest stage in the last 7 days** using scale in item M1—i.e., 0=none; stages 1, 2, 3, 4*) a. Pressure ulcer—any lesion caused by pressure resulting in damage of underlying tissue b. Stasis ulcer—open lesion caused by poor circulation in the lower extremities
3.	HISTORY OF RESOLVED ULCERS	Resident had an ulcer that was resolved or cured in **LAST 90 DAYS** 0. No 1. Yes
4.	OTHER SKIN PROBLEMS OR LESIONS PRESENT	(***Check all that apply** during **last 7 days***) Abrasions, bruises a. Burns (second or third degree) b. Open lesions other than ulcers, rashes, cuts (e.g., cancer lesions) c. Rashes—e.g., intertrigo, eczema, drug rash, heat rash, herpes zoster d. Skin desensitized to pain or pressure e. Skin tears or cuts (other than surgery) f. Surgical wounds g. *NONE OF ABOVE* h.
5.	SKIN TREATMENTS	(***Check all that apply** during **last 7 days***) Pressure relieving device(s) for chair a. Pressure relieving device(s) for bed b. Turning/repositioning program c. Nutrition or hydration intervention to manage skin problems d. Ulcer care e. Surgical wound care f. Application of dressings (with or without topical medications) other than to feet g. Application of ointments/medications (other than to feet) h. Other preventative or protective skin care (other than to feet) i. *NONE OF ABOVE* j.
6.	FOOT PROBLEMS AND CARE	(***Check all that apply** during **last 7 days***) Resident has one or more foot problems—e.g., corns, callouses, bunions, hammer toes, overlapping toes, pain, structural problems a. Infection of the foot—e.g., cellulitis, purulent drainage b. Open lesions on the foot c. Nails/calluses trimmed during **last 90 days** d. Received preventative or protective foot care (e.g., used special shoes, inserts, pads, toe separators) e. Application of dressings (with or without topical medications) f. *NONE OF ABOVE* g.

SECTION N. ACTIVITY PURSUIT PATTERNS

1.	TIME AWAKE	(***Check appropriate time periods over last 7 days***) Resident awake all or most of time (i.e., naps no more than one hour per time period) in the: Morning a. Afternoon b. Evening c. *NONE OF ABOVE* d.
		(If resident is comatose, skip to Section O)
2.	AVERAGE TIME INVOLVED IN ACTIVITIES	(**When awake and not receiving treatments or ADL care**) 0. Most—more than 2/3 of time 1. Some—from 1/3 to 2/3 of time 2. Little—less than 1/3 of time 3. None
3.	PREFERRED ACTIVITY SETTINGS	(***Check all settings** in which activities are preferred*) Own room a. Day/activity room b. Inside NH/off unit c. Outside facility d. *NONE OF ABOVE* e.
4.	GENERAL ACTIVITY PREFERENCES (adapted to resident's current abilities)	(***Check all PREFERENCES** whether or not activity is currently available to resident*) Cards/other games a. Crafts/arts b. Exercise/sports c. Music d. Reading/writing e. Spiritual/religious activities f. Trips/shopping g. Walking/wheeling outdoors h. Watching TV i. Gardening or plants j. Talking or conversing k. Helping others l. *NONE OF ABOVE* m.

Resident ______________________ Numeric Identifier ______________________

5.	PREFERS CHANGE IN DAILY ROUTINE	*Code for resident preferences in daily routines* 0. No change 1. Slight change 2. Major change	
		a. Type of activities in which resident is currently involved	
		b. Extent of resident involvement in activities	

SECTION O. MEDICATIONS

1.	NUMBER OF MEDICATIONS	***(Record the number of different medications used in the last 7 days; enter "0" if none used)***	
2.	NEW MEDICATIONS	*(Resident currently receiving medications that were initiated during the **last 90 days**)* 0. No 1. Yes	
3.	INJECTIONS	***(Record the number of DAYS** injections of any type received during **the last 7 days; enter "0" if none used)***	
4.	DAYS RECEIVED THE FOLLOWING MEDICATION	***(Record the number of DAYS during last 7 days; enter "0" if not** used. Note—enter "1" for long-acting meds used less than weekly)*	
		a. Antipsychotic	
		b. Antianxiety	
		c. Antidepressant	
		d. Hypnotic	
		e. Diuretic	

SECTION P. SPECIAL TREATMENTS AND PROCEDURES

1. SPECIAL TREATMENTS, PROCEDURES, AND PROGRAMS

a. **SPECIAL CARE—*Check*** *treatments or programs received during* ***the last 14 days***

TREATMENTS			
Chemotherapy	a.	Ventilator or respirator	l.
Dialysis	b.	**PROGRAMS**	
IV medication	c.	Alcohol/drug treatment program	m.
Intake/output	d.	Alzheimer's/dementia special care unit	n.
Monitoring acute medical condition	e.	Hospice care	o.
Ostomy care	f.	Pediatric unit	p.
Oxygen therapy	g.	Respite care	q.
Radiation	h.	Training in skills required to return to the community (e.g., taking medications, house work, shopping, transportation, ADLs)	r.
Suctioning	i.		
Tracheostomy care	j.		
Transfusions	k.	*NONE OF ABOVE*	s.

b. **THERAPIES** - *Record the number of days and total minutes each of the following therapies was administered (for at least 15 minutes a day) in the **last 7 calendar days** (Enter 0 if none or less than 15 min. daily)*
[Note—count only post admission therapies]
(A) = **# of days** administered for **15 minutes or more**
(B) = **total # of minutes** provided in **last 7 days**

	DAYS (A)	MIN (B)
a. Speech - language pathology and audiology services		
b. Occupational therapy		
c. Physical therapy		
d. Respiratory therapy		
e. Psychological therapy (by any licensed mental health professional)		

2. INTERVENTION PROGRAMS FOR MOOD, BEHAVIOR, COGNITIVE LOSS

(Check all interventions or strategies used in last 7 days—no matter where received)

Special behavior symptom evaluation program	a.
Evaluation by a licensed mental health specialist in **last 90 days**	b.
Group therapy	c.
Resident-specific deliberate changes in the environment to address mood/behavior patterns—e.g., providing bureau in which to rummage	d.
Reorientation—e.g., cueing	e.
NONE OF ABOVE	f.

3. NURSING REHABILITATION/ RESTORATIVE CARE

*Record the NUMBER OF DAYS each of the following rehabilitation or restorative techniques or practices was **provided to the resident for more than or equal to 15 minutes per day in the last 7 days** (Enter 0 if none or less than 15 min. daily.)*

a. Range of motion (passive)		f. Walking	
b. Range of motion (active)		g. Dressing or grooming	
c. Splint or brace assistance		h. Eating or swallowing	
TRAINING AND SKILL PRACTICE IN:		i. Amputation/prosthesis care	
d. Bed mobility		j. Communication	
e. Transfer		k. Other	

4.	DEVICES AND RESTRAINTS	*(Use the following codes for **last 7 days**:)* 0. Not used 1. Used less than daily 2. Used daily	
		Bed rails	
		a. —Full bed rails on all open sides of bed	
		b. —Other types of side rails used (e.g., half rail, one side)	
		c. Trunk restraint	
		d. Limb restraint	
		e. Chair prevents rising	
5.	HOSPITAL STAY(S)	Record number of times resident was admitted to hospital with an overnight stay **in last 90 days** (or since last assessment if less than 90 days). *(Enter 0 if no hospital admissions)*	
6.	EMERGENCY ROOM (ER) VISIT(S)	Record number of times resident visited ER without an overnight stay **in last 90 days** (or since last assessment if less than 90 days). *(Enter 0 if no ER visits)*	
7.	PHYSICIAN VISITS	In the **LAST 14 DAYS** (or since admission if less than 14 days in facility) how many days has the physician (or authorized assistant or practitioner) examined the resident? *(Enter 0 if none)*	
8.	PHYSICIAN ORDERS	In the **LAST 14 DAYS** (or since admission if less than 14 days in facility) how many days has the physician (or authorized assistant or practitioner) changed the resident's orders? *Do not include order renewals without change. (Enter 0 if none)*	
9.	ABNORMAL LAB VALUES	Has the resident had any abnormal lab values during the **last 90 days** (or since admission)? 0. No 1. Yes	

SECTION Q. DISCHARGE POTENTIAL AND OVERALL STATUS

1.	DISCHARGE POTENTIAL	a. Resident expresses/indicates preference to return to the community 0. No 1. Yes	
		b. Resident has a support person who is positive towards discharge 0. No 1. Yes	
		c. Stay projected to be of a short duration— discharge projected within **90 days** (do not include expected discharge due to death) 0. No 1. Within 30 days 2. Within 31-90 days 3. Discharge status uncertain	
2.	OVERALL CHANGE IN CARE NEEDS	Resident's overall self sufficiency has changed significantly as compared to status of **90 days ago** (or since last assessment if less than 90 days) 0. No change 1. Improved—receives fewer supports, needs less restrictive level of care 2. Deteriorated—receives more support	

SECTION R. ASSESSMENT INFORMATION

1.	PARTICIPATION IN ASSESSMENT	a. Resident	0. No	1. Yes		
		b. Family	0. No	1. Yes	2. No family	
		c. Significant other	0. No	1. Yes	2. None	

2. SIGNATURES OF PERSONS COMPLETING THE ASSESSMENT:

a. Signature of RN Assessment Coordinator (sign on above line)

b. Date RN Assessment Coordinator signed as complete ☐☐ — ☐☐ — ☐☐☐☐
Month Day Year

c. Other Signatures	Title	Sections	Date
d.			Date
e.			Date
f.			Date
g.			Date
h.			Date

Resident ______________________ Numeric Identifier ______________________

SECTION T. SUPPLEMENT—CASE MIX DEMO

1.	SPECIAL TREAT-MENTS AND PROCE-DURES	**a. RECREATION THERAPY**—*Enter number of days and total minutes of recreation therapy administered* (***for at least 15 minutes a day***) *in the* ***last 7 days*** (*Enter 0 if none*) (A) = **# of days** administered for 15 minutes or more (B) = **total # of minutes** provided in last 7 days	DAYS (A) / MIN (B)
		Skip unless this is a Medicare 5 day or initial admission assessment.	
		b. ORDERED THERAPIES—*Has physician ordered any of following therapies to begin in FIRST 14 days of stay—physical therapy, occupational therapy, or speech pathology service?* 0. No 1. Yes	
		If not ordered, skip to item 2	
		c. Through day 15, provide an estimate of the number of days when at least 1 therapy service can be expected to have been delivered.	
		d. Through day 15, provide an estimate of the number of therapy minutes (across the therapies) that can be expected to be delivered?	
2.	WALKING WHEN MOST SELF SUFFICIENT	***Complete item 2 if ADL self-performance score for TRANSFER (G.1.b.A) is 0,1,2, or 3 AND at least one of the following are present:*** • Resident received physical therapy involving gait training (P.1.b.c) • Physical therapy was ordered for the resident involving gait training (T.2.b) • Resident received nursing rehabilitation for walking (P.3.f) • Physical therapy involving walking has been discontinued within the past 180 days ***Skip to item 3 if resident did not walk in last 7 days*** ***(FOR FOLLOWING FIVE ITEMS, BASE CODING ON THE EPISODE WHEN THE RESIDENT WALKED THE FARTHEST WITHOUT SITTING DOWN. INCLUDE WALKING DURING REHABILITATION SESSIONS.)***	
		a. **Furthest distance walked** without sitting down during this episode. 0. 150+ feet 1. 51-149 feet 2. 26-50 feet 3. 10-25 feet 4. Less than 10 feet	
		b. **Time walked** without sitting down during this episode. 0. 1-2 minutes 1. 3-4 minutes 2. 5-10 minutes 3. 11-15 minutes 4. 16-30 minutes 5. 31+ minutes	
		c. **Self-Performance in walking** during this episode. 0. *INDEPENDENT*—No help or oversight 1. *SUPERVISION*—Oversight, encouragement or cueing provided 2. *LIMITED ASSISTANCE*—Resident highly involved in walking; received physical help in guided maneuvering of limbs or other nonweight bearing assistance 3. *EXTENSIVE ASSISTANCE*—Resident received weight bearing assistance while walking	
		d. **Walking support provided** associated with this episode (code regardless of resident's self-performance classification). 0. No setup or physical help from staff 1. Setup help only 2. One person physical assist 3. Two+ persons physical assist	
		e. **Parallel bars** used by resident in association with this episode. 0. No 1. Yes	
3.	CASE MIX GROUP	**Medicare** ☐☐☐☐☐ **State** ☐☐☐☐☐	

SECTION U. MEDICATIONS—CASE MIX DEMO

List all medications that the resident **received** during the last 7 days. Include scheduled medications that are used regularly, but less than weekly .

1. **Medication Name and Dose Ordered.** Record the name of the medication and dose ordered.
2. **Route of Administration (RA).** Code the Route of Administration using the following list:

   1=by mouth (PO)
   2=sub lingual (SL)
   3=intramuscular (IM)
   4=intravenous (IV)
   5=subcutaneous (SQ)
   6=rectal (R)
   7=topical
   8=inhalation
   9=enteral tube
   10=other

3. **Frequency.** Code the number of times per day, week, or month the medication is administered using the following list:

PR=(PRN) as necessary
1H=(QH) every hour
2H=(Q2H) every two hours
3H=(Q3H) every three hours
4H=(Q4H) every four hours
6H=(Q6H) every six hours
8H=(Q8H) every eight hours
1D=(QD or HS) once daily
2D=(BID) two times daily (includes every 12 hrs)
3D=(TID) three times daily
4D=(QID) four times daily
5D=five times daily
1W=(Q week) once each wk
2W=two times every week
3W=three times every week
QO=every other day
4W=4 times each week
5W=five times each week
6W=six times each week
1M=(Q month) once every month
2M=twice every month
C=continuous
O=other

4. **Amount Administered (AA).** Record the number of tablets, capsules, suppositories, or liquid (any route) **per dose** administered to the resident. Code 999 for topicals, eye drops, inhalants and oral medications that need to be dissolved in water..

5. **PRN-number of days (PRN-n).** If the frequency code for the medication is "PR", record the number of times during the last 7 days each PRN medication was given. Code STAT medications as PRNs given once.

6. **NDC Codes.** Enter the National Drug Code for each medication given. Be sure to enter the correct NDC code for the drug name, strength , and form. The NDC code must match the drug dispensed by the pharmacy.

1. Medication Name and Dose Ordered	2. RA	3. Freq	4. AA	5. PRN-n	6. NDC Codes

CHAPTER 2: USING THE RAI: STATUTORY AND REGULATORY REQUIREMENTS AND SUGGESTIONS FOR INTEGRATION IN CLINICAL PRACTICE

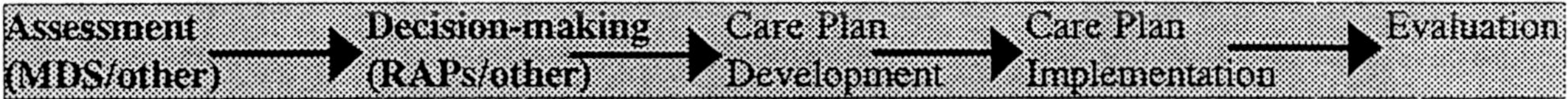

This chapter presents the regulatory basis for the RAI and discusses how the RAI process can be implemented procedurally in the course of clinical practice with facility residents. Some of the procedures are required by statutory law, Federal regulation or HCFA utilization guidelines, while others are recommended based on sound experience of facilities that have used the RAI process successfully.

2.1 Statutory and Regulatory Basis for the RAI

The statutory authority[1] for the Minimum Data Set (MDS) and the Resident Assessment Instrument (RAI) is found in section 1819 (f)(6)(A-B) for Medicare and 1919 (f)(6)(A-B) for Medicaid in the Social Security Act, as amended by the Omnibus Budget Reconciliation Act of 1987 (OBRA 1987). These sections of the Social Security Act required the Secretary of the Department of Health and Human Services (the Secretary) to specify a minimum data set of core elements to use in conducting comprehensive assessments. It furthermore required the Secretary to designate one or more resident assessment instruments based on the minimum data set. The Secretary designated Version 2.0 of the RAI in the State Operations Manual Transmittal #272, issued April 1995.

Federal requirements[1] at 42 CFR 483.20 (b)(1)(i) -- (F272) require that facilities use an RAI that has been specified by the State. This assessment system provides a comprehensive, accurate, standardized, reproducible assessment of each long term care facility resident's functional capabilities and helps staff to identify health problems.

2.2 Content of the RAI

All State RAIs include at least the Health Care Financing Administration's (HCFA's):

- **MDS**
- **Triggers**
- **Resident Assessment Protocols (RAPS)**
- **Utilization Guidelines**

---

[1]For further information regarding the statutory basis for the RAI, see Appendix G.

Some States have added items to the core MDS that must be completed for each resident when an RAI comprehensive assessment is required. Thus, while the basic MDS form (as included in this manual) is the standard foundation for States, you may find that other items have been added at the end of the form (i.e., Sections S, T, or U) in your State.

Additionally, States must specify a Quarterly Assessment Form for use by facilities that includes at least the items on the HCFA-designated form. **(See Section 2.4 and Appendix B of this manual for a list of the items.)** Several States have also expanded the list of MDS items that must be documented on the resident's Quarterly Assessment.

HCFA's approval of a State's RAI covers the core items included on the instrument, the working and sequence of those items, and all definitions and instructions for the RAI. HCFA's approval of the RAI does not include characteristics related to formatting (e.g., print type, color coding, or changes such as printing triggers on the assessment form).

If allowed by the State, facilities may have some flexibility in form design (e.g., print type, color, shading, integrating triggers) or use a computer generated printout of the RAI as long as the State can ensure that the facility's RAI form in the resident's record accurately and completely represents the State's RAI as approved by HCFA in accordance with 42 CFR 483.20 (b). This applies to either pre-printed forms or computer generated printouts. States also have the prerogative of requiring facilities to use the State form. Facilities may insert additional items within automated assessment programs but must be able to "extract" and print the MDS in a manner that replicates the State's RAI (i.e., using the exact wording and sequencing of items as is found on the State RAI). Facility assessment systems must always be based on the MDS (i.e., both item terminology and definitions).

Additional information about State specification of the RAI, variations in format and HCFA approval of alternative State instruments can be found in Sections 4145.1 - 4145.6 of the HCFA State Operations Manual, Transmittal #272 issued April 1995.

To fulfill Federal requirements at 42 CFR 483.20, each time a comprehensive assessment is required, long term care facilities must complete:

- The **MDS**, plus any additional **core items that make up the State RAI**;
- The **RAP Summary form**, on which facilities must indicate which RAPs have been triggered, the location of information gathered during the RAP review process, and the final care planning decision; and
- **Documentation of clinical information** (e.g., assessment information) from the RAP review to assist in care planning and follow-up.

The following is a schematic of the overall **RAI framework**:

MDS + TRIGGERS + RAPS --------------------------> COMPREHENSIVE ASSESSMENT
(UTILIZATION GUIDELINES)

The **MDS** consists of a core set of screening and assessment elements, including common definitions and coding categories, that forms the foundation of the comprehensive assessment.

The **triggers** are specific resident responses for one or a combination of MDS elements. The triggers identify residents who either have or are at risk for developing specific functional problems and require further evaluation using Resident Assessment Protocols (RAPs) designated within the State specified RAI. MDS item responses that define triggers are specified in each RAP and on the Trigger Legend form. Turn to the RAPs (in Appendix C) to review these items and the accompanying RAP Guidelines. Once you are familiar with the RAP triggers and guidelines, the Trigger Legend form serves as a useful summary of all RAP triggers. Note that the symbols on this form have been changed and the process streamlined. The **Trigger Legend** summarizes which MDS item responses trigger individual RAPs and has been designed as a helpful tool for facilities if they choose to use it. **It is a worksheet, not a required form**, and does not need to be maintained in each resident's clinical record.

The **RAPs** provide structured, problem-oriented frameworks for organizing MDS information, and additional clinically relevant information about an individual's health problems or functional status. What are the problems that require immediate attention? What risk factors are important? Are there issues that might cause you to proceed in an unconventional manner for the RAP in question? Clinical staff are responsible for answering questions such as these. The information from the MDS and RAPs forms the basis for individualized care planning.

The **Utilization Guidelines** are instructions concerning when and how to use the RAI. The Utilization Guidelines for Version 2.0 of the RAI were published by HCFA in the State Operations Manual[2] Transmittal #272, and are discussed more extensively in this User's Manual.

The individual resident's care plan must be evaluated and revised, if appropriate, each time an RAI comprehensive assessment is completed. Facilities may either make changes on the original care plan or develop a new care plan.

Additional information relevant to a resident's status, but not necessarily included on the RAI, may be documented in the resident's active record. This documentation should include progress notes or facility specific flowsheets.

---

[2]The SOM is a reference only; it is not necessary for effective use of the RAI. The SOM can be ordered from the National Technical Information Service (NTIS); PB# 95-950007; $27; (703) 487-4650.

2.3 Applicability of RAI to Facility Residents

The requirements for resident assessment found at 42 CFR 483.20 are applicable to all residents in certified long term care facilities. The requirements are applicable regardless of age, diagnosis, length of stay or payment category.

An RAI must be completed for any resident residing in the facility **longer than 14 days**, including:

- All residents of Medicare (Title 18) skilled nursing facilities or Medicaid (Title 19) nursing facilities. This includes **distinct part** certified SNFs or NFs and certified SNFs or NFs in hospitals, regardless of payment source.

- Hospice Residents. When a SNF or NF is the hospice patient's residence for purposes of the hospice benefit, the facility must comply with the requirements for participation in Medicare or Medicaid. This means the hospice resident must be assessed using the RAI, have a care plan and be provided with the services required under the plan of care. This can be achieved through cooperation between the hospice and long term care facility staff with the consent of the resident. In these situations, the hospice team may participate in completing the RAI.

- Short term stay or respite residents. An RAI must be completed for any individual residing more than 14 days on a unit of a facility that is certified as a long term care facility for participation in the Medicare or Medicaid programs.

  Given the nature of short stay or respite admissions, staff members may not have access to all information required to complete some MDS items prior to the resident's discharge (e.g., the physician may not be available, or the family may not be able to provide information on the resident's Customary Routine.) In that case the "no-information" convention should be used. ("NA" or "circled" dash - **See Section 2.7 for more information.**) For respite residents who come in and out of the facility on a relatively frequent basis and readmission can be expected, the resident may be discharged to "extended" leave status. This status does not require reassessment each time the resident returns to the facility unless a significant change in the resident's status has occurred in the intervening period.

- Special populations (e.g. pediatric or residents with a psychiatric diagnosis). Certified facilities are required to complete an RAI for all residents who reside in the facility, regardless of age or diagnosis.

An RAI is not required for:

- SNF residents residing in a Medicare certified "swing-bed" hospital. The requirement for a comprehensive assessment is not incorporated in the long term care requirements for "swing-bed" hospitals at 42 CFR 482.66.

- Individuals residing in non-certified units of long term care facilities or licensed only facilities. This does not preclude a State from mandating the RAI for residents who live in these units.

2.4 Types of RAI Assessments and Timing of Assessments

Although the RAI assessments discussed in the following section must occur at specific times by Federal regulation, a facility's obligation to meet each resident's needs through ongoing assessment is not neatly confined to these mandated time frames. Likewise, completion of the RAI in the prescribed time frame does not necessarily fulfill a facility's obligation to perform a comprehensive assessment. Facilities are responsible for assessing areas that are relevant to individual residents regardless of whether these areas are included in the RAI.

Comprehensive RAI assessments require completion of the MDS and review of triggered RAPs, followed by development or review of the comprehensive care plan within 7 days of completion of the RAI. The following table summarizes the different types of Federally mandated assessments:

TYPE OF ASSESSMENT	TIMING OF ASSESSMENT	REGULATORY REQUIREMENT HCFA "F" TAG
Admission (Initial) Assessment	Must be completed by 14th day of resident's stay.	42 CFR 483.20 (b)(4)(i)/F 273
Annual Reassessment	Must be completed within 12 months of most recent full assessment.	42 CFR 483.20 (b)(4)(v)/F 275
Significant Change in Status Reassessment	Must be completed by the end of the 14th calendar day following determination that a significant change has occurred.	42 CFR 483.20 (b)(4)(iv)/F 274
Quarterly Assessment	Set of MDS items, mandated by State (contains at least HCFA established subset of MDS items). Must be completed no less frequently than once every 3 months.	42 CFR 483.20 (b)(5)/F 276

ADMISSION (INITIAL) ASSESSMENTS

The admission or initial assessment for a new resident must be completed by the end of the **14th calendar day following admission to the facility if this is the resident's first stay in the facility or if the resident returns to the facility after being discharged with no expectation of return.** The 14 day calculation does include weekends. When calculating when the RAI is due, the day of admission is counted as day "0". For example, if a resident is admitted at 8:30 a.m. on Wednesday, a completed RAI is required by the end of the day Wednesday, two weeks after admission. If a resident dies or is discharged within 14 days of admission, then whatever portions of the RAI that have been completed must be maintained in the resident's discharge record.[3] In closing the record, the facility **may** wish to note why the RAI was not completed. (MDS items that were not completed prior to the day of death or discharge are left blank. [Sections AA, AD (if relevant), and R are signed.] - **See Section 2.5 regarding necessary signatures.**)

The interdisciplinary team may start and complete the initial assessment at any time prior to the end of the 14th day. If desired by the facility, the MDS could be completed in entirety on the day of admission. However, this requires the staff to rely on resident and family reporting of information and transfer documentation to a large degree as a source of information on the resident's status during the time periods used to code each MDS item, as opposed to allowing a period for facility observation. Facilities may find early completion of the MDS and RAPs particularly beneficial for individuals with short lengths of stay, when the assessment and care planning process is often accelerated.

EXAMPLES

Miss A. is admitted on Friday, September 1. Staff establish the Assessment Reference Date as September 8, which means that September 8 is the final day of the observation period for all MDS items (i.e., count back 7 days to determine the period of observation for 7 day items, count back 14 days for 14 day items, and so on). As this is an initial assessment, staff must rely on the resident and family's verbal history and transfer documentation accompanying Miss. A. to complete items requiring longer than a 7 day period of observation. Staff complete the MDS by September 12 (note that the Assessment Reference Date (A3a) does not need to be the same as the Date RN Assessment Coordinator Signed as Complete (R2b). Staff take an additional 3 days to assess the resident using triggered RAPs and to complete all related documentation, which is noted

[3] The RAI is considered part of the resident's clinical record and is treated as such by the RAI Utilization Guidelines, e.g., portions of the RAI that are "started" must be saved.

as a date field that accompanies the signature of the RN Coordinator for the RAP Assessment Process on the RAP Summary form (VB2).

Miss L. is admitted on Monday morning. Staff review the admitting documentation, talk with the physician, and have a brief conversation with her on that day. More information is gathered from the resident and her sister over the next 7 days. In this case, the Assessment Reference Date (A3a) is set as Tuesday of the following week, and observations by all relevant team members are completed as of that date. The MDS and RAPs are completed on Wednesday of that week, nine days after admission, with Wednesday being the date the RN Assessment Coordinator signs off on the MDS (R2b). In this case, Wednesday is also the day the RN Coordinator signs the RAP Summary form as complete (VB2).

If a resident goes to the hospital and returns during the 14 day assessment period and most of the initial assessment was completed prior to the hospitalization, then the facility may wish to continue with the original assessment, provided the resident did not have a significant change in status. Otherwise the assessment should be reinitiated and completed within 14 days after readmission from the hospital. The portion of the resident's record that was previously completed should be stored on the resident's record with a notation that the assessment was reinitiated because the resident was hospitalized.

Good clinical practice dictates that some MDS items be assessed within the first hours after admission although not necessarily documented at that time (e.g., nutritional status and needs). Other MDS items can best be observed with the passage of time (e.g., resident or staff interaction patterns). The resident's needs will dictate the order and manner in which the interdisciplinary team proceeds throughout the assessment. For example, if a new resident is admitted short of breath and hypotensive, it is imperative to conduct an assessment of the resident's acute cardiorespiratory needs. Likewise, a new resident who is angry with his or her family for admitting him or her to the nursing home, and is actively grieving over losses, will benefit from an early assessment of Customary Routine, Psychosocial Well-Being, and Depression, Anxiety, Sad Mood MDS items.

ANNUAL REASSESSMENTS

The annual RAI reassessment must be completed **within 12 months of the most recent full assessment**. The annual reassessment may be initiated at any point prior to the end of the 1-year follow-up date, but must be completed by the end of the 365th calendar day after the most recent full RAI assessment (i.e., the date the RN Coordinator has certified the completion of the assessment on the RAP Summary form under VB2). If a significant change reassessment is completed in the interim, the clock "restarts," with the next assessment due within 365 days of the significant change reassessment. Routinely scheduled RAI assessments may be scheduled early if a facility wants to stagger due dates for assessments.

SIGNIFICANT CHANGE IN STATUS ASSESSMENTS

Facilities have an ongoing responsibility to assess resident status and intervene to assist the resident to meet his or her highest practicable level of physical, mental, and psychosocial well-being. If interdisciplinary team members identify a significant change (either improvement or decline) in a resident's condition they should share this information with the resident's physician, who they may consult about the permanency of change. The facility's medical director may also be consulted when differences of opinion about a resident's status occur among team members.

Document the initial identification of a significant change in terms of the resident's clinical status in the progress notes. Complete a full comprehensive assessment as soon as needed to provide appropriate care to the individual, but in no case, later than 14 days of determining a significant change has occurred.

A "**significant change**" is defined as a major change in the resident's status that:

1. **Is not self-limiting**
2. **Impacts on more than one area of the resident's health status; and**
3. **Requires interdisciplinary review or revision of the care plan.**

A condition is defined as "self-limiting" when the condition will normally resolve itself without further intervention or by staff implementing standard disease related clinical interventions. For example, normally a 5% unplanned weight loss would trigger a "significant change" reassessment. **(See GUIDELINES FOR DETERMINING CHANGE IN RESIDENT STATUS below.)** However, if a resident had the flu and experienced nausea and diarrhea for a week, a 5% weight loss may be an expected outcome. In this situation, staff should monitor the resident's status and attempt various interventions to rectify the immediate weight loss. If the resident did not become dehydrated and started to regain weight after the symptoms subsided, a comprehensive assessment would not be required. The amount of time that would be appropriate for a facility to monitor a resident depends on the clinical situation and severity of symptoms experienced by the resident. Generally, if the condition has not resolved within approximately 2 weeks, staff should begin a comprehensive RAI assessment. This time frame is not meant to be prescriptive, but rather should be driven by clinical judgment and the resident's needs.

Other conditions may not be permanent but would have such an impact on the resident's overall status that they would require a comprehensive assessment and care plan revision. For example, a hip fracture may be viewed as a transient condition but it would generally have a major impact on the resident's functional status in more than one area (e.g., ambulation, toileting, elimination patterns, activity patterns). Changes in the resident's condition that would affect the resident's functional capacity and day to day routine should be investigated in a holistic manner through the

RAI reassessment. Therefore, concepts associated with significant change are "major" or "appears to be permanent" but a change does not need to be both major and permanent.

A significant change assessment is appropriate if there is a consistent pattern of changes, with either two or more areas of decline, or two or more areas of improvement. This may include two changes within a particular domain (e.g., two areas of ADL decline or improvement). Any determination about whether a resident has experienced a significant change in status is a clinical decision.

GUIDELINES FOR DETERMINING SIGNIFICANT CHANGE IN RESIDENT STATUS. (Please note this is not an exhaustive list.)

Decline:

- Resident's decision making changes from 0 or 1 to 2 or 3 for B4 of the MDS;
- Emergence of sad or anxious mood pattern as a problem that is not easily altered (E2 of the MDS);
- Increase in the number of areas where Behavioral Symptoms are coded as "not easily altered" (i.e., an increase in the number of code "1"s for E4B of the MDS);
- Any decline in an ADL physical functioning area where a resident is newly coded as 3, 4, or 8 (Extensive assistance, Total dependency, Activity did not occur) for G1A of the MDS;
- Resident's incontinence pattern changes from 0 or 1 to 2, 3 or 4 (H1a or b of the MDS), or there was placement of an indwelling catheter (H3d of the MDS);
- Emergence of unplanned weight loss problem (5% change in 30 days or 10% change in 180 days) (K3a of the MDS);
- Emergence of a pressure ulcer at Stage II or higher, when no ulcers were previously present at Stage II or higher (M2a of the MDS);
- Resident begins to use trunk restraint or a chair that prevents rising when it was not used before (P4c and e of the MDS);
- Overall deterioration of resident's condition; resident receives more support (e.g., in ADLs or decision-making) (item Q2 = 2 on the MDS);
- Emergence of a condition or disease in which a resident is judged to be unstable (item J5a on the MDS).

> **EXAMPLE**
>
> Mr. T. no longer responds to verbal requests to alter his screaming behavior. It now occurs daily and has neither lessened on its own nor responded to treatment. He is also starting to resist his daily care, pushing staff away from him as they attempt to assist with his ADLs. This is a significant change and reassessment is required since there has been a deterioration in the behavioral symptoms to the point where it is occurring daily and new approaches are needed to alter the behavior. Mr. T.'s behavioral symptoms could have many causes, and reassessment will provide an opportunity for staff to consider illness, medication reactions, environmental stress, and other possible sources of Mr. T.'s disruptive behavior.

Improvement

- Any improvement in an ADL physical functioning area where a resident is newly coded as 0, 1, or 2 when previously scored as a 3, 4, or 8 (G1A of the MDS);
- Decrease in the number of areas where Behavioral Symptoms or Sad or Anxious Mood are coded as "not easily altered" (E2 and E4B of the MDS);
- Resident's decision-making changes from 2 or 3 to 0 or 1 (B4 of the MDS);
- Resident's incontinence pattern changes from 2, 3, or 4 to 0 or 1 (H1a or b of the MDS);
- Overall improvement of resident's condition; resident receives fewer supports (item Q2 = 1 on the MDS).

> **EXAMPLE**
>
> Mrs. G. has been in the facility for 5 weeks, following an 8 week acute hospitalization. On admission she was very frail, had trouble thinking, was confused, and had many behavioral complications. The course of treatment led to steady improvement and she is now stable. She is no longer confused or agitated. All concerned - the resident, her family, and staff - agree that she has made remarkable progress. A reassessment is required at this time. The resident is not the person she was at admission; her initial problems have resolved. Reassessment will permit the interdisciplinary team to review her needs and plan a new course of care for the future.

While a facility may choose to perform more frequent comprehensive assessments than mandated by HCFA, **reassessments are not required for minor or temporary variations in resident status. However, staff must note these transient changes in the resident's status in the resident's record and implement necessary clinical interventions**, even though a reassessment is not required. In these cases the resident's condition is expected to return to baseline within a short period of time, such as 1-2 weeks.

GUIDELINES FOR WHEN A CHANGE IN RESIDENT STATUS IS NOT SIGNIFICANT (Please note this is not an exhaustive list)

- Discrete and easily reversible cause(s) documented in the resident's record and for which the interdisciplinary team can initiate corrective action (e.g., an anticipated side effect of introducing a psychoactive medication while attempting to establish a clinically effective dose level. Tapering and monitoring of dosage would not require a significant change reassessment).

- Short-term acute illness such as a mild fever secondary to a cold from which the interdisciplinary team expects the resident to fully recover.

- Well-established, predictable cyclical patterns of clinical signs and symptoms associated with previously diagnosed conditions (e.g., depressive symptoms in a resident previously diagnosed with bipolar disease would not precipitate a significant change assessment).

- Instances in which the resident continues to make steady progress under the current course of care. Reassessment is required only when the condition has stabilized.

- Instances in which the resident has stabilized but is expected to be discharged in the immediate future. The facility has engaged in discharge planning with the resident and family, and a comprehensive reassessment is not necessary to facilitate discharge planning.

- In an end-stage disease status, a full reassessment is optional, depending on a clinical determination of whether the resident would benefit from it. The facility is still responsible for providing necessary care and services to assist the resident to achieve his or her highest practicable well-being. However, provided that the facility identifies and responds to problems and needs associated with the terminal condition, a comprehensive re-assessment is not necessarily indicated. (Documented at item J5c on the resident's most current MDS.)

EXAMPLES

Mr. M. has been in this facility for two and one-half years. He has been a favorite of staff and other residents and his daughter has been an active volunteer on the unit. Mr. M. is now in the end stage of his course of chronic dementia — diagnosed as probable Alzheimer's. He experiences recurrent pneumonias and swallowing difficulties, his prognosis is guarded, and family are fully aware of his status. He is on a special dementia unit, staff have detailed palliative care protocols for all such end stage residents, and there has been active involvement of his daughter in the care planning process. As changes have occurred, staff have responded in a timely, appropriate manner. In this case, Mr. M.'s care is of a high quality, and as his physical state has declined, there is no need for staff to complete a new MDS assessment for this bedbound, highly dependent terminal resident.

Mrs. K. came into the facility with identifiable problems and has steadily responded to treatment. Her condition has improved over time and plateaued. She will be discharged within 5 days. The initial RAI helped to set goals and start care. Care was modified as necessary to ensure continued improvement. The interdisciplinary team's treatment response reversed the causes of the resident's condition. A reassessment need not be completed in view of the imminent discharge. **Remember, facilities have 14 days to complete a reassessment once the resident's condition has stabilized, and if Mrs. K. is discharged within this period, a new assessment is not required. If the resident's discharge plans change or if she is not discharged, a reassessment is required by the end of the allotted 14 day period.**

Mrs. P., too, has responded to care. Unlike Mrs. K., however, she continues to improve. Her discharge date has not been specified. She is benefiting from her care and full restoration of her functional abilities seems possible. In this case, treatment is focused appropriately, progress is being made, staff are on top of the situation, and there is nothing to be gained by requiring an MDS reassessment at this time. However, if her condition were to stabilize and her discharge was not imminent, a reassessment would be in order.

ASSESSMENTS ON RETURN STAY/READMISSION

If a facility has discharged a resident without the expectation that the resident would return, then the returning resident is considered a **new admission** (return stay) and would require an initial admission RAI comprehensive assessment including Sections AB (Demographic Information) and AC (Customary Routine) within **14 days of admission**.

If a resident returns to a facility following a temporary absence for hospitalization or therapeutic leave, it is considered a **readmission**. Facilities are not required to assess a resident if they are readmitted, unless a significant change in the resident's condition has occurred. In these situations follow the procedures for significant change assessments. **(See SIGNIFICANT CHANGE IN STATUS ASSESSMENTS above.)** It is not necessary to complete Sections AB (Demographic

Information) or AC (Customary Routine) of the MDS if this information has previously been collected and entered into the resident's record.

QUARTERLY ASSESSMENTS

The Quarterly Assessment is used to track resident status between comprehensive assessments, and to ensure monitoring of critical indicators of the gradual onset of significant changes in resident status. At a minimum, **three quarterly reviews and one full assessment are required in each 12 month period.**

Although a review of **key mandated items is required in each 3 month period**, facilities may vary or stagger their schedules (e.g., a facility may choose to review all residents in February, May, August and November, while another facility may choose to stagger their quarterly assessments for residents by reviewing some in January, others in February and the remainder in March, with the first group reviewed again in April).

The resident's status must be assessed for each of the **key mandated items of the Quarterly Assessment using the State-specified form.** There is now a mandated form from HCFA,[4] which must be used for all quarterly assessments, unless your State has specified another form. In conducting Quarterly Assessments, facilities must also assess any additional items required for use by the State. Based on the Quarterly Assessment, the resident's care plan is revised if necessary. Once Federal or State computerization requirements are effective, facilities must complete Section AA, Identification Information on the Basic Assessment Tracking form, as well as the items listed in the table below:

[4]HCFA's Quarterly Assessment Form is found in Appendix B. A three-page optional Quarterly Assessment Form for use in RUGs-III payment systems may be required by your State (also in Appendix B).

KEY MANDATED MDS ITEMS FOR QUARTERLY ASSESSMENT

Section A: Identification and Background Information

Item 1 - Resident Name
Item 2 - Room Number
Item 3a - Assessment Reference Date
Item 4a - Date of Reentry
Item 6 - Medical Record Number

Section B: Cognitive Patterns

Item 1 - Comatose
Item 2 - Memory
Item 4 - Cognitive Skills for Daily Decision-making
Item 5 - Indicators of Delirium--Periodic Disordered Thinking/Awareness

Section C: Communication/Hearing Patterns

Item 4 - Making Self Understood
Item 6 - Ability to Understand Others

Section E: Mood and Behavior Patterns

Item 1 - Indicators of Depression, Anxiety, Sad Mood
Item 2 - Mood Persistence
Item 4 - Behavioral Symptoms

Section G: Physical Functioning and Structural Problems

Item 1 - ADL Self-Performance
Item 2 - Bathing
Item 4 - Functional Limitation in Range of Motion
Items 6a, b and f - Modes of Transfer

Section H: Continence in Last 14 Days

Item 1 - Continence Self-Control
Item 2d and e - Bowel Elimination Pattern
Items 3a, b, c, d, i and j - Appliances and Programs

Section I: Disease Diagnoses

Items 2j and m - Infections

Item 3 - Other Current Diagnoses and ICD-9 Codes

(Note only those diseases diagnosed in the last 90 days that have a relationship to current ADL status, cognitive status, mood and behavior status, medical treatments, nursing monitoring or risk of death.)

Section J: Health Conditions

Items 1c, i, and p - Problem Conditions

Item 2 - Pain Symptoms

Item 4 - Accidents

Item 5 - Stability of Conditions

Section K: Oral/Nutritional Status

Item 3 - Weight Change

Items 5b, h, and i - Nutritional Approaches

Section M: Skin Condition

Item 1 - Ulcers

Item 2 - Type of Ulcer

Section N: Activity Pursuit Patterns

Item 1 - Time Awake

Item 2 - Average Time Involved in Activities

Section O: Medications

Item 1 - Number of Medications

Item 4 - Days Received the Following Medications

Section P: Special Treatments and Procedures

Item 4 - Devices and Restraints

Section Q: Discharge Potential

Item 2 - Overall Change in Care Needs

Section R: Assessment/Discharge Information

Item 2 - Signatures of Persons Completing the Assessment

2.5 Completion of the RAI Assessment and Certification of Accuracy and Completeness

PARTICIPANTS IN THE ASSESSMENT PROCESS

Federal regulations[5] require that the RAI assessment must be conducted or coordinated with the appropriate participation of health professionals. Although not required, completion of the RAI is best accomplished by an interdisciplinary team that includes facility staff with varied clinical backgrounds. Such a team brings their combined experience and knowledge together for a better understanding of the strengths, needs and preferences of each resident to ensure the best possible quality of care and quality of life. In general, participation by all relevant interdisciplinary team members will encourage more active and appropriate assessment and care planning processes.

Facilities have flexibility in determining who should participate in the assessment process as long as it is accurately conducted. A facility may assign responsibility for completing the RAI to a number of qualified staff members. In most cases, participants in the assessment process are licensed health professionals. It is the facility's responsibility to ensure that all participants in the assessment process have the requisite knowledge to complete an accurate and comprehensive assessment.

The RAI must be conducted or coordinated by an RN who signs and certifies the completion of the assessment[6]. If a facility does not have an RN on its staff (i.e., has an RN waiver granted under 42 CFR 483.30 (c) or (d) -- F354) it must still provide an RN to complete the RAI. This requirement can be met by hiring an RN specifically for this purpose. In this situation, the LPN responsible for the care of the resident should participate in the resident assessment process and the development of the resident's care plan.

The attending physician is also an important participant in the RAI process. The facility needs the physician's evaluation and orders for the resident's immediate care as well as for a variety of treatments and laboratory tests. Furthermore, the attending physician may provide valuable input on sections of the MDS and RAPs and is a member of the mandated interdisciplinary team that prepares the resident's comprehensive care plan.

While some aspects of the assessment process are dictated by regulation, much flexibility remains for facilities to determine how to integrate the RAI into their day-to-day operations. For example, facilities should develop their own policies and procedures to accomplish the following:

---

[5] 42 CFR 483.20 (c)(1)(i)--(F 278)

[6] 42 CFR 483.20 (e)(1)(ii)--(F 278)

- Train facility staff on the circumstances that require a comprehensive assessment and the staff that should be involved.

- Assign responsibility for completing sections of the MDS to staff who have clinical knowledge about the resident, such as staff nurses, attending physicians, social workers, activities specialists, physical, occupational, or speech therapists, dietitians and pharmacists.

- Assure that residents and their families are actively involved in the information sharing and decision-making processes.

- Assure that the insights of all non-licensed persons who regularly provide direct care to the resident (e.g., nursing assistants, activity aides, volunteers) are included in the assessment process.

- Assure that key clinical personnel on all shifts (including nursing assistants) are knowledgeable about the information found in the resident's most current assessment and report changes in the resident's status that may affect the accuracy of this information or the need to perform a significant change reassessment.

- Instruct staff on how to integrate MDS information with existing facility resident assessment and care planning practices.

CERTIFYING ACCURACY AND COMPLETENESS

Each individual team member who completes a portion of the assessment must sign and certify its accuracy.[7] Each interdisciplinary team member who completes a portion of the MDS assessment signs, dates, and indicates the portion of the assessment he or she completed. The RN Coordinator is required to sign to certify that the MDS is complete.[8] The RN Coordinator must not sign and attest to completion of the assessment until all other individual team members participating in the assessment have finished their portions of the MDS. If the RN does all of the MDS, then the nurse alone would sign and be responsible for certifying accuracy and completeness.

The RN Coordinator must also sign the RAP Summary form to signify completion of the RAI assessment. For the admission assessment, the RN Coordinator must sign and date the RAP Summary form within 14 days of the resident's admission to the facility. There is no Federal requirement that each individual team member completing a RAP sign and date the RAP Summary form to certify its accuracy. It is assumed that other team members' documentation for a RAP will be signed wherever it appears in the clinical record. However, if desired, individual team

---

[7] 42 CFR 483.20 (c)(2)--(F 278)

[8] 42 CFR 483.20 (c)(1)(ii)--(F 278)

members may indicate which RAP(s) they completed, list their credentials, and the date it was completed by signing the form wherever there is room to do so in a legible manner.

It is never permissible to certify or backdate RAI forms for another individual on the interdisciplinary team. If an individual who completed a portion of the MDS is not available to sign it, then another team member should review the information and sign the form. Facilities should establish a policy regarding accountability for the RAI when these situations occur.

The staff member entering the care planning decision information must also sign and date the RAP Summary form (VB3 and 4). The facility has 7 days after completing the assessment to complete the care plan. The date for entering of the care plan information may be up to 7 days after the RAPs are completed (i.e., the date on which the RN coordinator signed the RAP Summary form to indicate completion of the RAP assessment process - VB2).

REPRODUCTION OF THE RAI IN THE RESIDENT'S RECORD AND MAINTENANCE OF THE RAI

Facilities are required to produce a hard copy of each RAI (including the MDS and RAP Summary form) conducted on admission, after a significant change in the resident's status, at least annually, as well as intervening quarterly assessments.

Facilities are required to maintain **15 months** of assessment data in the resident's active clinical record according to HCFA policy. **This includes all MDS forms, RAP Summary forms and Quarterly Assessment Forms as required during the previous 15 month period.** Assessment data need not be stored in one binder. Rather, facilities may choose to maintain assessment and care planning information in a separate binder or kardex system, as long as the information is kept in a centralized location and is accessible to all professional staff members (including consultants) who need to review the information in order to provide care to the resident. After the 15 month period, RAI information may be thinned from the clinical record and stored in the medical records department, provided that it is easily retrievable if requested by clinical staff or State agency surveyors.

The 15 month period for maintaining assessment data does not restart with each readmission to the facility. In some cases when a resident is out of the facility for a short period (i.e., hospitalization), the facility must close the record because of bed hold policies. When the resident then returns to the facility and is "readmitted", the facility must open a new record. The facility may copy the previous RAI and transfer a copy to the new record. In this case, the facility should also copy the previous 15 months of assessment data and place it on the new record. Facilities may develop their own specific policies regarding how to handle readmissions, but the 15 month requirement for maintenance of the RAI data does not restart with each new admission.

If a facility has an electronic clinical record (i.e., does not maintain any paper records), the facility does not need to maintain a hard copy of the RAI, if the system meets the following minimum criteria:

- The system must maintain 15 months' worth of assessment data according to HCFA policy and must be able to print all assessments for that period upon request;
- The facility must have a back-up system to prevent data loss or damage;
- The information must always be readily available and accessible to staff and surveyors; and
- The system must comply with HCFA requirements for safeguarding the confidentiality of clinical records.[9]

2.6 Sources of Information for Completion of the RAI

The process for performing an accurate and comprehensive assessment requires that information about residents be gathered from multiple sources. It is the role of the individual interdisciplinary team members completing the assessment to validate the information obtained from the resident, resident's family, or other health care team members through observation, interviewing, reviewing lab results, and so forth to ensure accuracy. Similarly, information in the resident's record is validated by interacting with the resident and direct care staff.

The following sources of information must be used in completing the RAI. Although not required, the review sequence for the assessment process generally follows the order below:

- **Review of the resident's record.** Depending on whether the assessment is an admission or follow-up assessment, the review could include: preadmission, admission or transfer notes; current plan of care; recent physician notes or orders; documentation of services currently provided; results of recent diagnostic or other test procedures; monthly nursing summary notes and medical consultations for the previous 60 day period; and a record of medications administered for the prior 30 day period.
- **Communication with and observation of the resident.**
- **Communication with direct-care staff** (e.g., nursing assistants, activity aides) from all shifts.
- **Communication with licensed professionals** (from all disciplines) who have recently observed, evaluated, or treated the resident. Communication can be based on discussion or licensed staff can be asked to document their impressions of the resident.
- **Communication with the resident's physician.**

---

[9] See confidentiality requirements at 42 CFR 483.75 (n)(4)(i-iii) --F516

- **Communication with the resident's family**. Not all residents will have family. For some residents, family members may be unavailable or the resident may request that you not contact them. Where the family is not involved, someone else may be very close to the resident, and the resident may wish that this person be contacted.

REVIEW OF THE RESIDENT'S RECORD

The resident's record provides a starting point in the assessment process to review information about the resident in written staff notes across all shifts over multiple days. Starting with the resident's record, however, does not indicate that it is the most critical source of information, but only a convenient source.

At admission, record review includes an examination of notes written in the first 2 weeks (assuming the full 14 day period is used to complete the assessment), documentation that came with the resident at admission, facility intake forms (e.g., social service notes), and any preadmission test results including copies of the MDS and RAPs from another nursing home if the resident was transferred. Obviously, transcribing the previous facility's MDS is inappropriate.

Subsequent reassessments should focus on recorded information from earlier MDS assessments and quarterly assessments, written information from the previous 3 month period, and notes made during the prior 30 day period.

The following are important considerations when reviewing the resident's record:

- **Review the information documented in the record, keeping in mind the required MDS definitions.** Make sure that assumptions based on the record are compatible with MDS definitions (e.g., resident self-performance is evaluated with appliances if used, such as locomotion with a walker; similarly, according to the MDS, a resident, who stays "dry" with a catheter may be considered continent).

- **Make sure that the information taken from the record covers the same observation period as that specified by the MDS items.** The MDS refers to specific time frames for each item; for example ADL status is based on resident performance over a 7 day period. To ensure uniformity, the MDS has an Assessment Reference Date (A3a) that establishes a common reference end-point for all items. **Consequently, it is necessary to pay careful attention to the notes regarding time frames for each section of the MDS and also to the Item- by Item instructions in Chapter 3.**

- **Be aware of discrepancies and view the record information as preliminary only.** Clarify and validate all such information during the assessment process. Be alert to information in the record that is not consistent with verbal information or physical assessment findings. Discuss discrepancies with other interdisciplinary team members (e.g., nurses, social workers, therapists). The extent to which the record can be relied upon for information will depend on the comprehensiveness of the record system. Note what information the record usually contains (e.g., current service notes, care plans, flow sheets, medication sheets); where different types of information are maintained in the clinical record; and more importantly, what information is missing.

- **Where information in the record is sufficiently detailed and conforms to MDS descriptions and time periods, complete the MDS items.** A few MDS items can be completed in full from information found in the record. Comprehensive and accurate assessment of most items, however, requires information from other sources (i.e., the resident, the resident's family, and facility staff). **Where information is incomplete or contradictory, make a note of the issues in question.** This note can help plan contacts with the resident, facility staff and resident's family. There is no requirement that such a note be maintained as part of the resident's permanent record; it is a work tool only.

- **As you observe, talk with, and discuss the resident with other staff members, verify the accuracy of what you learned from reviewing the record.**

COMMUNICATION WITH AND OBSERVATION OF THE RESIDENT

The resident is a primary source of information and may be the only source of information for many items (e.g., customary routine, activity preferences, vision, hearing, identification with past roles, and, in some instances, problem conditions). Many MDS items will not be documented elsewhere in the clinical record, and the completed MDS may ultimately be the single source of documentation about these issues.

Become familiar with the MDS items to make communication and observation of the resident an ongoing everyday activity in the facility. For example, an RN can observe and interact with a resident when medications are given, during meals, or when the resident comes to ask a question. Interaction with the resident may be a crucial factor in confirming staff judgments of resident problems. **Weigh what the resident says, and what is observed about the resident against other information obtained from the resident record and facility staff.**

To be most efficient, organize a framework for how to interview and observe the resident. Allow flexibility to accommodate the resident. Carefully listen and observe the resident to get guidance as to how to pursue the necessary information gathering. Try to interact with the resident, even if the resident may have difficulty responding. The degree and character of the difficulty in responding, as well as nonverbal responses (e.g., fearfulness) provide important information. Sensitive staff judgment is necessary in gathering information. **(See Appendix D for further information on "Interviewing Techniques".)**

COMMUNICATION WITH DIRECT CARE STAFF

Direct care staff (e.g., nursing assistants and activity aides) have daily, intimate contact with residents and are often the most reliable source of information about the resident. Direct care staff talk with and listen to the resident. They observe and assist the resident's performance of ADLs and involvement in activities. They observe the resident's physical, cognitive and psychosocial status daily during all shifts, seven days a week. Key considerations when communicating with direct care staff are:

- **Be sure to speak with a person who has first-hand knowledge of the resident.** Plan for sufficient time to talk with direct care staff person(s).

- **Start by asking about the resident's performance on ADLs and activities.** What can the resident do without assistance? What do staff members do for the resident? What might the resident be able to do that he or she is not doing now? Continue by asking about communication and memory skills, body control, activity preferences, and the presence of mood or other behavioral symptoms.

- **Talk with direct care staff across all shifts, if possible.** The information from other shifts may be obtained in other ways as well (e.g., from change-of-shift reports if direct care staff comments are included).

(See Appendix D for further information on "Interviewing Techniques".)

COMMUNICATION WITH LICENSED PROFESSIONALS

Licensed practical nurses (LPNs), RNs, social workers, activities professionals, occupational therapists, physical therapists, speech therapists, pharmacists, and other professionals who have observed, evaluated, or treated the resident should be interviewed about their knowledge of resident capabilities, performance patterns and problems. Their special expertise will enhance the accuracy and comprehensiveness of the resident assessment.

COMMUNICATION WITH THE RESIDENT'S PHYSICIAN

The physician's role is central to the overall management and outcome of resident care. The MDS assessment process should include a review of the physician's examination of the resident, plan of care, hospital discharge plan, goals of care, and medication and treatment orders. At the **Quarterly Assessments and Annual assessments**, review the most recent physician orders and notes. Also, review the MDS with the resident's attending physician to share and validate pertinent information. If there is difficulty obtaining information or input for the assessment from the attending physician (or transferring institution), the facility's medical director should be asked to intervene.

COMMUNICATION WITH THE RESIDENT'S FAMILY

The resident's family (or person closest to the resident) can be a valuable source of information about the resident's health history, history of strengths and problems in various functional areas, and customary routine prior to first nursing home admission. Using this source obviously depends on the presence of family members, their willingness to participate, and the resident's preferences. In most instances, family will not be the sole source of information but will supplement information from other sources. The RAI assessment process provides an excellent opportunity for caregivers to develop trusting, working relationships with the resident and family.

2.7 Completing the MDS Form - Coding and Correction of Errors

Utilizing appropriate information gathered from all of the areas discussed in **Section 2.6** above, the individual completing the assessment is required to make a best judgment about each item in each section of the MDS form. <u>The MDS is part of the medical record and should always be typed or prepared in ink.</u>

CODING CONVENTIONS

The following table specifies the coding conventions to be used when preparing the MDS form:

MDS CODING CONVENTIONS

- **Each section of the MDS contains one or more items labeled sequentially.** For instance, the third item in Section B (Memory/Recall Ability) is labeled "B3", the second item in Section E (Mood Persistence) is labeled "E2".

- **Use the following coding conventions to enter information on the MDS form:**

  Use a check mark for white boxes with lower case letters, if specified condition is met; otherwise these boxes remain blank (e.g., N4, General Activity Preferences - boxes a. - m.).

  Use a numeric response (a number or preassigned value) for blank white boxes (e.g., H1a, Bowel Incontinence.)

  Darkly shaded areas remain blank; they are on the form to set off boxes visually.

- **The convention of entering "0"**: In assigning values for items that have an ordered set of responses (e.g., from independent to dependent), zero ("0") is used universally to indicate the lack of a problem or that the resident is self-sufficient. For example, a resident whose ADL codes are almost all coded "0" is a self-sufficient resident; the resident whose ADLs have no "0" codes indicates a resident that receives help from others.

- **USE PRINTED CAPITAL LETTERS to respond to items that require an open-ended response.** Print legibly (e.g., for "Lifetime Occupations", a line is provided to fill in the resident's previous occupation(s)).

- **Dates** - Where recording month, day, and year, enter two digits for the month and the day, but four digits for the year. For example, the third day of January in the year 1996 is recorded as :

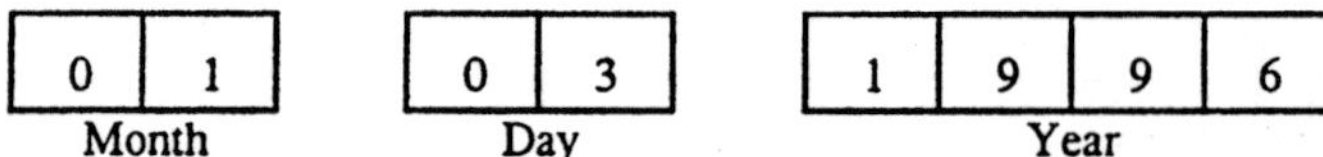

- **The standard no-information code is either a "circled" dash or an "NA".** This code indicates that all available sources of information have been exhausted; that is the information is not available, and despite exhaustive probing, it remains unavailable. Although the "circled dash" was originally conceived for use on computerized versions of the MDS, it is also the recommended method of coding on manual forms to "set-off" these responses on the forms.

- **NONE OF ABOVE is a response item to several items** (e.g., I2, Infections, box m). **Check this item where none of the responses apply; it should not be used to signify lack of information about the item.**

- **"Skip" Patterns - There are a few instances where scoring on one item will govern how scoring is completed for one or more additional items.** The instructions direct the assessor to "skip" over the next item (or several items) and go on to another (e.g., B1, Comatose, directs the assessor to "skip" to Section G. if B1 is answered "1" - "Yes". **The intervening items from B2 - F3 would not be scored.** If B1 was recorded as "0" - "No", then the assessor would continue with item B2.).

  A useful technique for visually checking the proper use of the "skip" pattern instructions is to circle the "skip" instructions before going to the next appropriate item.

- **The "8" code is for use in Section G., Physical Functioning and Structural Problems only.** The use of this code is limited to situations where the ADL activity was not performed and therefore an objective assessment of the resident's performance is not possible. Its primary use is with bed-bound residents who neither transferred from bed nor moved between locations over the entire 7 day period of observation. When the "8" code is entered for self-performance, it should also be entered for support.

CORRECTION OF ERRORS

Facilities may not "change" a previously completed MDS form as the resident's status changes during the course of the nursing home stay. Minor changes in the resident's status should be noted in the resident's record (e.g., in progress notes), in accordance with standards of clinical practice and documentation. Such monitoring and documentation is a part of the facility's responsibility to provide necessary care and services. Completion of a new MDS to reflect changes in the resident's status is not required unless the resident has had a significant change in status **(See Section 2.4 for information on Significant Change in Status Assessments)**.

The following procedures apply to the correction of errors in either paper or automated MDS 2.0 systems:

- Within a paper environment, facilities should "close" the MDS within regulatory time frames (i.e., within 14 days after admission, etc.). This is done by having the RN Coordinator sign and date the MDS at R2a and b. **Amendments may be made to any items during the next 7 day period, provided that the same Assessment Reference Date is used (A3a).** To make revisions, enter the correct response, draw a line through the previous response without obliterating it, and initial and date the corrected entry. This procedure is similar to how an entry in the medical record is corrected.

- **The concept of "factual errors," which allowed for "correction" of the paper form in certain instances at any time, has been eliminated.** Facilities operating in computerized States should seek guidance on State specific policies related to "key changes" and transmission of data for payment purposes.

The following procedures apply when a facility's MDS data are computerized[10]:

1. The clinical assessment process must be completed within the standard time frames (i.e., within 14 days after admission, etc.).

2. After completing the clinical assessment process, the facility has the next 7 days to encode the MDS in a computerized file, ensure that all MDS items pass HCFA/State edits[11] and to

---

[10]A number of States have already established automated systems and State specific requirements. These States are encouraged to modify their existing systems to conform to the above HCFA policies. However, until national specifications are established, facilities should contact their State regarding State specific requirements. HCFA is currently in the process of developing additional policies for computerization at both the facility and State level. These policies are expected to go into effect sometime in 1996.

[11]HCFA edits should be incorporated in all software products and are available to vendors and facilities through a World Wide Web site accessed through the Internet. Its address is: http://linear.chsra.wisc.edu/mds_info.htm. Vendors and facilities should also contact their State for any specific requirements.

"lock" the computer record. "Locking" the record means that no changes can be made to the MDS (i.e., either paper or electronic versions).

- Encoding process: The facility is responsible for verifying that all responses in the computer file match the responses on the paper form. Any discrepancies must be corrected in the computer file during this 7 day period.

- Editing process: The facility is responsible for running encoded MDS data against HCFA and State specific edits (which all software vendors are responsible for building into MDS Version 2.0 computer systems). For each MDS item, the response must be within the required range and also be consistent with other item responses. During this 7 day period, the facility may "correct" item responses in order to meet edits. An assessment is considered complete only if 100% of the required edits are passed. For "corrected" items, the facility must use the same "period of observation" as that used for the original item completion (i.e., the same Assessment Reference Date - A3a). Any corrections must be accurately reflected in both the electronic and paper copies of the MDS (i.e., the paper version of the MDS must be corrected).

- "Locking" process: After passing the edits, a record is then "locked." Individual MDS records must pass 100% of the edits for the record to be "locked."[12] At this point, the record cannot be changed by the facility.

After the MDS is "locked," the facility may come to realize that items in the "locked" assessment (paper or electronic versions) are in error. The facility may come to such knowledge on its own or it may have been notified by the State that the assessment record failed edits or failed other reviews at the State level. In any event, the record is "locked" and cannot be changed. The facility then has the following options:

1. A new comprehensive "significant change in status" assessment would be performed (i.e, the full MDS and RAPs) if both of the following conditions are met:

   (1) The assessment in error is the most recent assessment; and

   (2) A significant change has actually occurred (i.e., there has been a significant change in the resident's clinical status between the time of the original assessment and the time of the new assessment).

   In this case, there has been a change in the resident's status that meets the Significant Change guidelines and a new comprehensive assessment is therefore required. However, the original assessment was also in error. This new assessment requires a new observation period, a new Assessment Reference Date (A3a), and "significant change in status

[12] "Locked" records will be transferred to the State within a time frame to be determined by HCFA/State policy, pending publication of HCFA's final rule on computerization.

assessment" is coded as the reason for assessment (AA8a = 3). The "Previous Record Date"[13] in the Control Section of the new MDS record must contain the Assessment Reference Date from the original assessment that was in error.

2. If a "significant change in status" has not occurred clinically but the erroneous data in the prior MDS is major enough to warrant correction, then the facility may optionally choose to perform a new comprehensive "significant correction of prior assessment" if both of the following conditions are satisfied:

   (1) The assessment in error is the most recent assessment; and

   (2) The resident did not experience an actual "significant change in status" between the time of the original assessment and the new comprehensive assessment. However, the resident's clinical condition is different from that depicted in the assessment in error and it would otherwise appear that there had been a significant change in status.

   If the facility chooses to perform a "significant correction" assessment, then a new MDS and RAPs are required,[14] with the new MDS performed using a new observation period (i.e., a new Assessment Reference Date (A3a)), "significant correction of prior assessment" is coded as the reason for assessment (AA8a = 4), and the "Previous Record Date" in the Control Section of the new MDS record must contain the Assessment Reference Date from the original assessment that was in error.

2.8 RAPs and Care Plan Completion

RAPs

After completing the MDS portion of the RAI assessment, the assessor(s) then proceed to further identify and evaluate the resident's strengths, problems, and needs through use of the **Resident Assessment Protocol Guidelines (RAPs)** described in detail in Chapter 4 of this manual and through further investigation of any resident-specific issues not addressed in the RAI.

Completed along with the MDS, the RAPs provide the foundation upon which the care plan is formulated. There are 18 problem-oriented RAPs, each of which include MDS-based "trigger" conditions that signal the need for additional assessment and review. Triggers and their definitions for each RAP appear in **Appendix C**. Also in Appendix C are the RAP Guidelines

---

[13]The "Control Section" is part of the standardized record layout made available to facilities and vendors for development and programming of MDS data systems. It provides information that will be used when the MDS data is transferred from the facility to the State. It is not a part of the clinical MDS form.

[14]New RAPs are required because the prior inaccurate description of the resident could have misguided staff in the triggering and problem identification activities.

for additional assessment and review to determine if a care plan is appropriate to address the triggered condition.

The triggers and their definitions should provide facility staff with information to better understand the underlying cause of a problem. Often staff may be aware that a problem, warranting care planning, exists before reviewing the RAP Guidelines for a triggered condition. The Guidelines should help staff to identify the factors that have caused the resident's problem and provide direction as to what additional information is needed about the resident's problem. **After reviewing triggered RAPs, the RAP Summary form is used to document decisions about care planning and to specify where key information from the assessment for triggered RAP conditions is noted in the record.**

LINKAGE OF MDS AND RAPS TO FORMULATION OF THE CARE PLAN

For an admission (initial) assessment, the resident enters the facility on day 1 with a set of physician-based treatment orders. Facility staff typically review these orders. Questions may be raised, modifications discussed, and change orders issued. Ultimately, of course, it is the attending physician who is responsible for the orders at admission, around which significant segments of the care plan is constructed.

On day 1, facility staff also begin to assess the resident and to identify problems. Both activities provide the core of the MDS and RAP process, as staff look at issues of safety, nourishment, medications, ADL needs, continence, psychosocial status and so forth. Facility staff determine whether there are problems that require immediate intervention (e.g., providing supplemental nourishment to reverse weight loss or attending to a resident's sense of loss at entering the nursing home). For each problem, facility staff will focus on causal factors and implement an initial plan of care based on their understanding of factors affecting the resident.

The MDS and RAPs provide the clinician with additional information to assist in this preliminary care planning process. The MDS ensures that staff have timely access to a wide range of assessment data. The RAPs provide criteria that trigger review of possible problem conditions to ensure that staff identify problems in a consistent and systematic manner. Use of the RAP Guidelines helps ensure that the full range of relevant causal factors is considered.

If the admission MDS is not completed until the last date possible (i.e., at the end of calendar day 14 of the residency period), interventions will already have been implemented to address priority problems. Many of the appropriate RAP problems will have been identified, causes will have been considered, and a preliminary care plan initiated. The final written care plan, however, is not required until 7 days after the RAI assessment is completed.

For triggered problems that have already resulted in a care plan intervention, the final RAP review will ensure that all causal factors have been considered. For RAP conditions for which facility staff have not yet initiated a care program, the RAP review will focus on whether these conditions are, in fact, problems that require facility intervention. For any triggered problem, staff will apply the RAP Guidelines to evaluate the resident's status and determine whether a situation exists that warrants care planning. If it does, the RAP Guidelines will next be used to help identify the factors that should be considered for developing the care plan.

For an Annual reassessment or a Significant Change in Status assessment, the process is basically the same as that described for newly admitted residents. In these cases, however, the care plan will already be in place, and staff are unlikely to be actively instituting a new approach to care as they simultaneously complete the MDS and RAPs. Here, review of the RAPs when the MDS is complete will raise questions about the need to modify or continue services. The condition that originally triggered the RAP may no longer be present because it was resolved, or consideration of alternative causal factors may be necessary because the initial approach to a problem did not work, or was not fully implemented.

CARE PLAN COMPLETION

Facilities have 7 days after the completion of the RAI assessment to develop or revise the resident's care plan. The RN coordinator should sign and date the RAP Summary form **after all triggered RAPs have been reviewed to certify completion of the comprehensive assessment (VB1 and 2). Facilities should use this date to determine the date by which the care plan must be completed.**

The 7 day requirement for completion or modification of the care plan applies to the Admission, Significant Change in Status, or Annual RAI Assessment. A new care plan does not need to be developed after each significant change of status or annual reassessment. Rather, the facility may revise an existing care plan using the results of the latest comprehensive assessment. Facilities should also evaluate the appropriateness of the care plan after each quarterly assessment and modify the care plan if necessary. **(See Chapter 5 for more information on Care Planning.)**

Chapter 3: Item-by-Item Guide to MDS Version 2.0

3.1 Mandated Assessments, and Associated Forms

The following rules apply to HCFA's RAI, Version 2.0, as used by all nursing homes certified to participate in Medicare or Medicaid. Copies of all required forms are in Appendix B.

The content of the Minimum Data Set (MDS) Version 2.0 Nursing Home Resident Assessment is recorded on the following mandated forms: [See Appendix B for copies of all forms.]

1. The *Basic Assessment Tracking Form*. This form includes Section AA (Identification Information) Items 1-9. This form must be submitted with every *Full Assessment, Quarterly Assessment*, and State required assessment. This form provides "key" information necessary to identify and track residents in automated systems.

2. MDS Version 2.0 *Full Assessment Form*. This form contains MDS Sections A (Identification and Background Information) through Section R (Assessment Information). The full assessment is to be completed at admission, annually, and at the time of significant change in resident status. The *Full Assessment* is required more frequently by States participating in the Nursing Home Case-Mix and Quality Demonstration (NHCMQ) as well as by some other States. Contact your State RAI representative if you have any questions about when assessments are required. Additional items (if any) required by your State may appear in Section S. NHCMQ State-required material appears in Sections T and U.

    - *Background (Face Sheet) Information at Admission*. This form contains MDS Section AB (Demographic Information), Section AC (Customary Routine), and Section AD (Face Sheet Signatures). This form is to be completed at the time of the resident's initial admission to the nursing home.

3. MDS Version 2.0 *Quarterly Assessment Form*. This form contains a mandated subset of MDS items from Section A (Identification and Background Information) through Section R (Assessment Information). This form is to be completed no less frequently than once every three months between annual full assessments. Some States have mandated an expanded *Quarterly Assessment Form*, such as the optional version for RUG III found in Appendix B.

4. *RAP Summary Form*. Considered Section V of the MDS, this form is used to document triggered RAPs, the location of documentation describing the resident's clinical status and factors that impact the care planning decision, and whether a care plan has been developed for

the triggered RAP. A *Rap Summary Form* must be completed each time an RAI is required (i.e., under the Federal schedule, each time a full MDS is completed).[1]

With MDS Version 2.0, two new forms have been developed for future use in each nursing home's computerized information system to track each resident's "whereabouts" in the health care system. Once HCFA's MDS computerization requirement is in place, facilities shall use these forms. Each of these tracking forms contain Section AA (Identification Information) Items 1 through 7, and a subset of codes from Item 8, Reason for Assessment. In a computerized information system, MDS Items AA1 through 7 need to be completed only once (at admission) and saved in the system files. However, this identification information must be verified prior to "closing" the assessment record for each subsequent assessment. For each discharge from or reentry to the nursing home, it is anticipated that nursing home staff (e.g., clerk) will record the move in Item AA8, Reason for Assessment. The computer will then generate the appropriate information to accompany the type of assessment being completed. The following two forms are included in this resident tracking system:

1. The *Discharge Tracking Form*. This form includes Section AA (Identification Information) Items 1-9, but only the 3 discharge codes from Item 8, Reason for Assessment. It also contains Items AB1-2, A6, and R3-4. In a computerized system, this form must be completed whenever a resident is discharged from the facility for reasons other than a temporary visit home. This is the only form that must always be completed at the time of any discharge from the nursing home. The following is the only condition when other forms shall accompany the *Discharge Tracking Form*:

    - If the resident was discharged for any reason within 14 days of admission and you were able to complete a *Full Assessment Form* before the resident was discharged, the resident's MDS computerized file would contain a *Basic Assessment Form*, a *Background (Face Sheet) Information at Admission Form*, a *Full Assessment Form*, and a *Discharge Tracking Form*. In this scenario, enter a code of "1" Admission Assessment (required by day 14) for Item 8 (Reason for Assessment) on both the *Basic Assessment Form* and the *Full Assessment Form*; enter a code of either "6" Discharged-return not anticipated, or "7" Discharged (return anticipated) as appropriate, for Item 8 on the *Discharge Tracking Form*.

2. The *Reentry Tracking Form*. This form includes Section AA (Identification Information) Items 1-9, but only one code (ie., code designating Reentry) from Item 8, Reason for Assessment . It also contains items A4a and b, and 6. In a computerized system, this form is completed whenever a resident reenters the nursing home following temporary admission to a hospital or other health care setting. This is the only form that must always be completed at the time of reentry to the nursing home. The following is the only condition when other forms shall accompany a *Reentry Tracking Form*:

---

[1]Some States require completion of the full MDS each quarter or more frequently for payment purposes. The RAP Summary Form does not need to be completed on these occasions.

- If the resident reenters the nursing home following a temporary admission to a hospital or other health care setting AND also meets significant change criteria, a *Full Assessment* must be completed. In this case, the resident's file should contain a *Reentry Tracking Form*, a *Basic Assessment Tracking Form*, and a *Full Assessment* (significant change). In this scenario, enter a code of "9" Reentry for Item 8 (Reason for Assessment) on the Reentry Tracking Form; enter a code of "3" Significant Change Assessment for Item 8 (Reason for Assessment) on both the *Basic Assessment Tracking Form* and the *Full Assessment* form. Completion of a *Full Assessment* may also be required by the State.

3.2 Overview to the Item-by-Item Guide to MDS Version 2.0

This Chapter is to be used in conjunction with Version 2.0 of the MDS, which can be found in Chapter 1 beginning on page 1-6 and in Appendix B. Also includes in this chapter are the instructions for the supplemental items in MDS Sections S and T used in the NHCMQ demonstration States.

The changes in Version 2.0 of HCFA's MDS were made in response to comments and suggestions regarding the first version of the MDS. They were received from the nursing home industry, health professionals, advocacy groups, surveyors, etc. A few items were dropped, others modified, and still others added. This chapter includes significant new material, many more examples, and refined definitions, as compared to HCFA's original RAI Training Manual that was published in December 1990.

This chapter provides information to facilitate an accurate and uniform resident assessment. Item-by-item instructions focus on:

- The intent of items included on the MDS.
- Supplemental definitions and instructions for completing MDS items.
- Reminders of which MDS items require observation of the resident for other than the standard 7-day observation period.
- Sources of information to be consulted in completing specific MDS items.

3.3 How Can This Chapter be Used?

Use this chapter alongside the MDS Version 2.0 form, keeping the form in front of you at all times. The MDS form itself contains a wealth of information. Learn to rely on it for many of the definitions and procedural instructions necessary for good assessment. The amplifying information in this chapter should facilitate successful use of the MDS form. The items from the

MDS forms are presented in a sequential basis in this chapter. Where items are presented on a form other than the full MDS assessment form, this fact is noted in the text.

The chart that follows summarizes the recommended approach to assist you in becoming familiar with MDS Version 2.0. The initial time investment in this multi-step review process will have a major payback.

If you are familiar with the MDS and are reviewing this Chapter for new items that appear in Version 2.0 of the MDS, review the MDS form beginning on page 1-6 of Chapter 1 for new items.

New materials of the following types are presented in this Chapter: Item definitions, examples, and process recommendations regarding how to complete the assessment. Thus, you will find much useful new information regarding many of the items that were in the original MDS.

Recommended Approach for Becoming Familiar with the MDS

(A) First, review the MDS form itself.

- Notice how sections are organized and where information is to be recorded.
- Work through one section at a time.
- Examine item definitions and response categories.
- Review procedural instructions, time frames, and general coding conventions.
- ***Are the definitions and instructions clear? Do they differ from current practice at your facility? What areas require further clarification?***
- Complete the MDS assessment for a resident at your facility. Draw only on your knowledge of this individual. Enter the appropriate codes on the MDS form. Where your review could benefit from additional information, make note of that fact. ***Where might you secure additional information?***

(Continued on next page)

Recommended Approach for Becoming Familiar with the MDS (Continued)

(B) Complete the initial pass through this chapter.

- Go on to this step only after first reviewing the MDS form and trying to complete all items for a resident who is well known to you.
- As you read this chapter, clarify questions that arose as you used the MDS for the first time to assess a resident. Note sections of this manual that help to clarify coding and procedural questions you may have had.
- ***Once again, read the instructions that apply to a single section of the MDS. Make sure you understand this information before going on to another section. Review the test case you completed. Would you still code it the same? It will take time to go through all this material. Do it slowly. Do not rush. Work through the Manual one section at a time.***
- *Are you surprised by any MDS definitions, instructions, or case examples? For example, do you understand how to code ADLs? Or Mood?*
- *Do any definitions or instructions differ from what you thought you learned when you reviewed the MDS form?*
- *Would you now complete your initial case differently?*
- *Are there definitions or instructions that differ from current practice patterns in your facility?*
- Make notations next to any section(s) of this Manual you have questions about. Be prepared to discuss these issues during any formal training program you attend, or contact your State MDS resource person (see Appendix A).
- Read and complete the test cases at the end of this chapter.

(Continued on next page)

Recommended Approach for Becoming Familiar with the MDS (Continued)

In a second pass through this chapter, focus on issues that were more difficult or problematic in the first pass.

- Make notes on the MDS form of issues that warrant attention.
- Further familiarize yourself with definitions and procedures that differ from current practice patterns or seem to raise questions.
- Reread each of the case examples presented throughout this chapter.

(D) **The third pass through this chapter may occur during the formal MDS training program at your facility** and will provide you with another opportunity to review the material in this chapter. If you have questions, raise them during the training session.

(E) **Future use of information in this chapter:**

- Keep this chapter at hand during the assessment process.
- Where necessary, review the intent of each item in question.
- This Manual is a source of information. Use it to increase the accuracy of your assessments.

3.4 What is the Standard Format Used in this Chapter?

To facilitate completion of Version 2.0 of the MDS assessment and to ensure consistent interpretation of items, this chapter presents the following types of information for many **(but not all)** items:

Intent: Reason(s) for including the item (or set of items) in the MDS, including discussions of how the information will be used by clinical staff to identify resident problems and develop the plan of care.

Definition: Explanation of key terms.

Process: Sources of information and methods for determining the correct response for an item. Sources include:

- Discussion with facility staff — licensed and nonlicensed staff members
- Resident interview and observation
- Clinical records, facility records, transmittal records (at admission) — physician orders, laboratory data, medication records, treatment sheets, flow sheets (e.g., vital signs, weights, intake and output), care plans, and any similar documents in the facility record system
- Discussion with the resident's family
- Attending physician.

Coding: Proper method of recording each response, with explanations of individual response categories.

3.5 Item-by-Item Instructions for the MDS Form

This section of item-by-item instructions follows the sequence of items on the HCFA MDS, Version 2.0. Notice that an MDS section designation appears at the top of the pages that follow; this will facilitate your use of this chapter as a reference tool in the future.

IDENTIFICATION INFORMATION
SECTION AA

This section provides the key information to uniquely identify each resident, the home in which he or she resides, and the reasons for assessment. A copy of this form must accompany each Full or Quarterly Assessment submitted for computer entry in a State or Federal archiving system.

AA. IDENTIFICATION INFORMATION

1. Resident Name

Definition: Legal name in record.

Coding: Use printed letters. Enter in the following order — a.) first name, b.) middle initial, c.) last name, d.) Jr./Sr. If the resident goes by his or her middle name, enter the full middle name. If the resident has no middle initial, leave item (b) blank.

2. Gender

Coding: Enter "1" for Male or "2" for Female.

3. Birth date

Coding: Fill in the boxes with the appropriate number. Do not leave any boxes blank. If the month or day contains only a single digit, fill the first box in with a "0". For example: January 2, 1918 should be entered as:

Month		Day		Year			
0	1	0	2	1	9	1	8

4. Race/Ethnicity

Process: Enter the race or ethnic category the resident uses to identify him- or herself. Consult the resident, as necessary. For example, if parents are of two different races, consult with resident to determine how he or she wishes to be classified.

Coding: Choose only one answer.

5. Social Security and Medicare Numbers

Intent: To record resident identifier numbers.

Process: Review the resident's record. If these numbers are missing, consult with your facility's business office.

Coding: Begin writing one number per box starting with the left most box. Recheck the number to be sure you have written the digits correctly.

Social Security Number — If no Social Security number is available for the resident (e.g., if the resident is a recent immigrant or a child), enter the standard "no information" code, "NA" or a circled dash ⊖.

Medicare number (or comparable railroad insurance number) — Approximately 98% of persons age 65 or older have a Medicare number. Enter the resident's Medicare number. This number occasionally changes with marital status. If a question arises, check with your facility's business office or social worker.

In rare instances, the resident will have neither a Medicare number nor a Social Security number. When this occurs, another type of basic identification number (e.g., railroad retirement insurance number) may be substituted. In such cases, place a "C" in the left most Medicare Number box, and continue entering the number itself, one digit per box, beginning with the second box.

6. Facility Provider Numbers

Intent: To record the facility identifier numbers.

Definition: The identification numbers assigned to the nursing home by the Medicare and Medicaid programs. Some facilities will have only a Federal (Medicare) identification number; others will have Federal (Medicare) and State (Medicaid) identification numbers. Medicaid only facilities have a Federal as well as a State number. The Medicaid Federal number has a "letter" in the third box.

Process: You can obtain the facility's Medicare and Medicaid numbers from the facility's business office. Once you have these numbers, they apply to all residents of that facility.

Coding: Begin writing in the left-hand box. Enter one digit per box. Recheck the number to be sure you have entered the digits correctly. There must be at least one type of facility number entered, but there may be more than one.

7. Medicaid Number (if applicable)

Coding: Record this number if the resident is a Medicaid recipient. Begin writing one number per box in the left hand box. Recheck the number to make sure you have entered the digits correctly. *Enter a "+" in the left most box if the number is pending. If not applicable because the resident is not a Medicaid recipient, enter "N" in the left most box.*

8. Reasons for Assessment [This item also appears and must be completed on the MDS Full Assessment Form, Section A, Item 8.]

a. Primary Reason for Assessment

Intent: To document the reason for completing the assessment using the various categories of assessment types mandated by Federal regulation. Most of the types of assessments listed below will require completion of the MDS, review of triggered RAPs, and development or review of a comprehensive care plan within seven days of completing the MDS and RAPs. [Note — assessment type 5, the Quarterly review assessment, requires you to complete only a limited number of MDS items — see Appendix B for the Quarterly Assessment Form.] Please note that it is possible to select a code from both 8a (Primary reason for assessment) and 8b (Special codes).

Minimum Discharge Assessment Requirement. With the release of Version 2.0 of the MDS, a minimal list of MDS items must be completed for all discharges and facility reentries in States that are automated. These items are referenced on their own forms and item 8 (Reason for Assessment) also appears on these forms. It is listed as Item 8a in Section AA of the *Discharge Tracking* and *Reentry Tracking Form* and Item AA8a on the *Identification Information Form.*

Definition:

1. **Admission assessment.** A comprehensive assessment using the MDS and RAPs required by day 14 of the resident's stay. [Note — this code is used if resident is being readmitted subsequent to a discharge where return was not anticipated.]

2. **Annual assessment** — A comprehensive reassessment required within 12 months of the most recent full assessment. If significant change is noted, code "3" (significant change in status assessment). DO NOT code as an Annual assessment.

3. **Significant change in status assessment** — A comprehensive reassessment prompted by a "major change" that is not self-limited, that impacts on more than one area of the resident's clinical status, and that requires interdisciplinary review or revision of the care plan to ensure that appropriate care is given. When there is a significant change, the assessment must be completed by the end of the 14th calendar day following the determination that a significant change has occurred. **See procedure described later in this chapter under item A8 for assessing whether a significant change (either improvement or decline) has occurred.**

4. **Significant correction of prior assessment** —A comprehensive assessment completed at the facility's prerogative, because the previous assessment was inaccurate or completed incorrectly. This differs from a significant change in status assessment, in which there has been an actual change in the resident's health status.

5. **Quarterly Review Assessment** —The subset of MDS items specified on HCFA's *Quarterly Assessment Form*, which must be completed no less frequently than once every 3 months (i.e., between required full assessments). This assessment ensures that the care plan is correct and up to date. It also should identify instances where significant changes in resident status have occurred. If a significant change is noted, use Code "3" (Significant change in status assessment). DO NOT CODE as a Quarterly review assessment.

6. **Discharged — return not anticipated** — [This is not a code used on this form;it is used on the *Discharge Tracking Form* only.] Use this code when a resident is permanently discharged from a nursing home. This provides a means of "closing" the record of any resident at the point of discharge from the facility (without an anticipated return). **Note — until HCFA's ADP requirement is effective, this code is used only in nursing homes that are required to submit data to the State.**

7. **Discharged — return anticipated** — [This is not a code used on this form, it is used on the *Discharge Tracking Form* only.] Use this code when a resident is temporally discharged to a hospital (or other therapeutic setting). **Note — until HCFA's ADP requirement is effective, this code is used only in facilities that are required to submit data to the State.**

8. **Discharged prior to completing initial assessment** — [This is not a code used on this form, it is used on the *Discharge Tracking Form* only.] Use this code when a resident is discharged during the first 14 days of residency AND the MDS assessment remains incomplete. A subset of information is entered for all residents regardless of length of stay. *Even a very short stay resident (e.g., a person who stayed for even one day) must be tracked by the MDS system.* At the same time, remember that you have 14 days to complete the full MDS admission assessment, and by using this code you are identifying residents who have been discharged, transferred or died prior to day 14, thereby prohibiting your completion of a full assessment. **Note — until HCFA's ADP requirement is effective, this code is used only in facilities that are required to submit data to the State.**

9. **Reentry** — [This is not a code used on this form;it is used on the *Reentry Form* only.] Use this code when a resident of your facility is readmitted from a temporary discharge to a hospital or other therapeutic setting (other than for a therapeutic leave). **Note — until HCFA's ADP requirement is effective, this code is used only in facilities that are required to submit data to the State.**

0. **NONE OF ABOVE** — Use this code when your state requires you to complete one of the additional assessment types referenced in Item AA8b (below). It indicates that the assessment has been completed to comply with State-specific requirements (e.g., Case-Mix payment). Select the code under item b (below) that indicates the primary reason for assessment.

b. **Special codes for use with supplemental assessment types in Case-Mix Demonstration States or other States where required.** It is possible to select a code from both 8a and 8b (e.g., Item 8a coded "3" (Significant Change in Status assessment), and Item 8b coded "3" (60-day assessment).

1. **5 day assessment** — Required for payment reason prior to the Federally mandated admission assessment required by day 14 (Code 1, for item a).

2. **30 day assessment**

3. **60 day assessment** — In following this cycle of assessments, the initial Quarterly review assessment would be due at 90 days.

4. **Quarterly assessment using full MDS form** — Assessment completed within a 3-month interval from the last assessment, using a full (not quarterly) MDS assessment form as required by the State or NHCMQ demonstration. For Case-Mix Demonstration States, the initial Quarterly

Assessment would be due at 90 days after admission, in addition to completion of the 60-day assessment.

5. **Readmission/return assessment** — A full reassessment (i.e., MDS and RAPs) required only for residents in NHCMQ demonstration facilities (or as required by the State) who are hospitalized for more than 72 hours, or who are discharged and later readmitted to the facility from the hospital.

6. **Other state required assessment** — An example is a Utilization Review assessment. States may issue additional instructions.

Example

Mr. X resides in a nursing home in Kansas, a Case-Mix Demonstration State. He was admitted to the nursing home from an acute care hospital on 1/20/95. At the time of the admission assessment, he still exhibited some signs of delirium that had begun post-operatively in the hospital. Functionally he required extensive assistance with all ADLs. It is now time for his 60-day assessment. Cognitively, Mr. X's confusion has cleared to the point that the decisions he makes are now consistent and reasonable. His ADL performance has improved in all areas; he is either independent or receives some supervision.

Coding: Enter the number corresponding to the primary reason for assessment. For item a (Primary reason for assessment), for codes 1-9, leave first box blank, placing correct digit in the second box.

9. Signatures of Persons Completing These Items

Coding: Staff who completed parts of Section AA. Identification Information must enter their signatures, titles, and date they completed the section.

BACKGROUND (FACE SHEET) INFORMATION AT ADMISSION SECTIONS AB, AC, AD

AB. DEMOGRAPHIC INFORMATION

1. Date of Entry

Intent: Normally, the MDS Face Sheet (Sections AB and AC) is completed once, when an individual first enters the facility. However, the face sheet is also required if the person is reentering your facility after a discharge where return had not previously been expected. Do not complete the face sheet following temporary discharges to hospitals or after therapeutic leaves/home visits. ***Given this definition, enter the date the person first became a resident/patient in your facility.***

Admission and "bed-hold" policies vary among nursing homes across the country. Likewise, the way in which facilities "open" and "close" resident's medical records also varies. Some facilities choose to "close" a record when a resident is transferred for an overnight stay at an acute care hospital, and "open" a new record when the resident returns to the nursing facility. Other nursing homes maintain the resident's clinical record as open (current) even when the resident is transferred for a temporary hospital stay. **For MDS purposes, the date of entry is the date the resident entered the facility for care, regardless of how the facility chooses to "open" or "close" its medical records during the course of the stay.**

Definition: **Date the stay began** — The date the resident was most recently admitted to your facility. For example: if the resident was officially discharged in the past without the expectation of return (e.g., discharged home or to another nursing facility), enter the most recent admission date. However, if your facility begins a new record on each return from a temporary hospital stay or temporary leave, you will complete the face sheet only at the original assessment. Do not complete the face sheet at the time of return from a temporary leave, even if you are required to complete the remainder of the form (e.g., a significant change assessment is required).

Process: Review the clinical record. If dates are unclear or unavailable, ask the admissions office or medical record department at your facility.

Coding: *Use all boxes.* For a one-digit month or day, place a zero in the first box. For example: February 3, 1994, should be entered as:

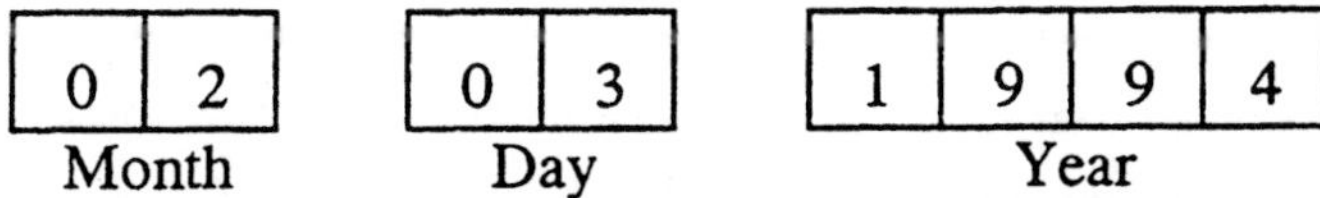

Example

Mrs. F, a diabetic, had been living with her daughter when she fractured her left hip during a fall off a footstool. She spent a few days in the local hospital after surgery, followed by an admission to a nursing facility on 5/26/94 for rehabilitation. Three weeks later (6/16/94), Mrs. F was transferred back to the hospital for an infected incision site over her left hip and general state of decline. Mrs. F returned to the nursing home eight days later. In this instance, code the following date on the original face sheet.

0	5		2	6		1	9	9	4

Rationale: The face sheet sections of the MDS — AB and AC are completed only when the resident first becomes a resident of the facility. In this case there is no need to complete a new face sheet upon return readmission from a temporary hospital stay where the resident is expected to return to the nursing home.

2. Admitted From (At Entry)

Intent: To facilitate care planning by documenting the place from which the resident was admitted to the nursing home on the date given in item AB1. For example, if the admission was from an acute care hospital, an immediate review of current medications might be warranted since the resident could be at a higher risk for delirium or may be recovering from delirium associated with acute illness, medications or anesthesia. Or, if admission was from home, the resident could be grieving due to losses associated with giving up one's home and independence. Whatever the individual circumstances, the resident's prior location can also suggest a list of contact persons who might be available for issue clarification. For example, if the resident was admitted from a private home with home health services, telephone contact with a Visiting Nurse can yield insight into the resident's situation that is not provided in the written records.

Definition: **Private home or apartment** — Any house, condominium, or apartment in the community whether owned by the resident or another person. Also included in this category are retirement communities, and independent housing for the elderly.

Home health services — Includes skilled nursing, therapy (e.g., physical, occupational, speech), nutritional, medical, psychiatric and home health aide services delivered in the home. Does not include the following services unless provided in conjunction with the services previously named: homemaker/personal care services, home delivered meals, telephone reassurance, transportation, respite services or adult day care.

Assisted Living — A non-institutional community residential setting that includes services of the following types: home health services, homemaker/personal care services, or meal services.

Other — Includes hospices and chronic disease hospitals.

Process: Review admission records. Consult the resident and the resident's family.

Coding: Choose only one answer.

Example

Mr. F, who had been living in his own home with his wife, was admitted to an acute care hospital with a CVA. From the hospital, Mr. F was transferred to this nursing home for rehabilitation. **Because Mr. F was admitted to your facility from the acute care hospital, "5" is the appropriate code.**

3. Lived Alone (Prior to Entry)

Intent: To document the resident's living arrangements prior to admission.

Definition: **In other facility** — Any institutional/supportive setting, such as a nursing home, group home, sheltered care, board and care home.

Process: Review admission records. Consult the resident and the resident's family.

Coding: If living in another facility (i.e., nursing facility, group home, board and care, assisted living) prior to admission to the nursing home, enter "2".

If the resident was not living in another facility prior to admission to the nursing home, enter "0" or "1", as appropriate.

Examples

- Mrs. H lived on her own and her daughters took turns sleeping in her home so she would never be alone at night. **Code "0" for No (did not live alone).** If, however, her daughters stayed with her only 3-4 nights per week, **Code "1" for Yes (lived alone).**
- Mr. J lived in his own second-floor apartment of a two-family home and received constant attention from his family, who lived on the first floor. **Code "0" for No (did not live alone).**
- Mr. D lived with his wife in housing for the elderly prior to admission. **Code "0" for No (did not live alone).**
- Mrs. X was the primary caregiver for her two young grandchildren, who lived with her after their parent's divorce. **Code "0" for No (did not live alone).**
- Mrs. K was admitted directly from an acute care hospital. She had been living alone in her own apartment prior to hospital stay. **Code "1" for Yes (lived alone).**
- Mr. M, who has been blind since birth, was admitted to the nursing home with his seeing eye dog, Rex. Mr. M. and Rex lived together for the past 10 years in housing for the elderly. **Code "1" for Yes (lived alone).**
- Mr. G lived in a board and care home. **Code "2" (In other facility).**

4. Zip Code of Prior Primary Residence

Definition: **Prior primary residence.** The community address where the resident last resided prior to nursing home admission. A primary residence includes a primary home or apartment, board and care home, assisted living, or group home. If the resident was admitted to your facility from another nursing home or institutional setting, the prior primary residence is the address of the resident's home prior to entering the other nursing home, etc.

Process: Review resident's admission records and transmittal records as necessary. Ask resident and family members as appropriate. Check with your facility's admissions office.

Coding: Enter one digit per box beginning with the left most box. For example, Beverly Hills, CA 90210 should be entered as:

9	0	2	1	0

Examples

- Mr. T was admitted to the nursing home from the local hospital. Prior to hospital admission he lived with his wife in a trailer park in Jensen Beach, Florida. **Enter the zip code for Jensen Beach.**
- Mrs. F was admitted to the nursing home's Alzheimer's Special Care Unit after spending 3 years living with her daughter's family in Newton, MA. Prior to moving in with her daughter, Mrs. F lived in Boston, MA for 50 years with her husband until he died. **Enter the Newton, MA zip code. Rationale:** Her daughter's home was Mrs. F's primary residence prior to nursing home admission.
- Ms. Q was admitted from a state psychiatric hospital in Illinois where she had spent the previous 16 years of her life. Prior to that, Ms. Q lived with her parents in Kansas City, Kansas. **Enter the Kansas City zip code.**

5. Residential History 5 Years Prior to Entry

Intent: To document the resident's previous experience living in institutional or group settings.

Definition: **Prior stay at this nursing home** — Resident's prior stay was terminated by discharge (without an expected return) to the community, another long-term care facility, or (in some cases) a hospitalization.

Stay in other nursing home — Prior stay in one or more nursing homes other than current facility.

Other residential facility — Examples include board and care home, group home, and assisted living.

MH/psychiatric setting — Examples include mental health facility, psychiatric hospital, psychiatric ward of a general hospital, or psychiatric group home.

MR/DD setting — Examples include mental retardation or developmental disabilities facility (including MR/DD institutions), intermediate care facilities for the mentally retarded (ICF/MRs), and group homes.

Process: Review the admission record. Consult the resident or family. Consult the resident's physician.

Coding: Check all institutional or group settings in which the resident lived for the five years prior to the current date of entry (as entered in AB1.). Exclude limited stays for treatment or rehabilitation when the resident had a primary residence to return to (i.e., the place the resident called "home" at that time). If the resident has not lived in any of these settings in the past five years, check *NONE OF ABOVE.*

6. Lifetime Occupation

Intent: To identify the resident's role or past role in life and to establish familiarity in how staff should address the resident. For example, a physician might appreciate being referred to as "Doctor". Knowing a person's lifetime occupation is also helpful for care-planning purposes. For example, a carpenter might enjoy pursuing hobby shop activities.

Coding: Enter the job title or profession that describes the resident's main occupation(s) before retiring or entering the facility. Begin printing in the left-most box.

The lifetime occupation of a person whose primary work was in the home should be recorded as "Homemaker." *When two occupations are identified, place a slash (/) between each occupation.* A person who had two careers (e.g., carpenter and night watchman) should be recorded as "Carpenter/Night Watchman". *For a resident who is a child or an MR/DD adult resident who has never been employed, record as "NONE."*

7. Education (Highest Level Completed)

Intent: To record the highest level of education the resident attained. Knowing this information is useful for assessment (e.g., interpreting cognitive patterns or language skills), care planning (e.g., deciding how to focus a planned activity program), and planning for resident education in self-care skills.

Definition: The highest level of education attained.

Technical or Trade School: Include schooling in which the resident received a non-degree certificate in any technical occupation or trade (e.g., carpentry, plumbing, acupuncture, baking, secretarial, practical/vocational nursing, computer programming, etc.).

Some College: Includes completion of some college courses, junior (community) college, or associate's degree.

Bachelor's degree: Includes any undergraduate bachelor's level college degree.

Graduate Degree: Master's degree or higher (M.S., Ph.D., M.D., J.D., etc.).

Process: Ask the resident and significant other(s). Review the resident's record.

Coding: Code for the best response. For MR/DD residents who have received special education services, code "2" (8th grade/less).

8. Language

Definition: **a. Primary language** — The language the resident primarily speaks or understands.

Process: Interview the resident and family. Observe and listen. Review the clinical record.

Coding: Enter "0" for English, "1" for Spanish, "2" for French, "3" for Other. If the resident's primary language is not listed, code "3" for Other and print the resident's primary language in item **8b** beginning with the left most box.

Example

Mrs. F emigrated with her family from East Africa several years ago. She is able to speak and understand very little English. She depends on her family to translate information in Swahili.

a. Primary Language — "3" Other

b. If other, specify

S	W	A	H	I	L	I		

9. Mental Health History

Intent: To document a primary or secondary diagnosis of psychiatric illness or developmental disability.

Definition: Resident has one of the following:

- A schizophrenic, mood, paranoid, panic or other severe anxiety disorder; somatoform disorder, personality disorder; other psychotic disorder; or another mental disorder that may lead to chronic disability; but

- Not a primary diagnosis of dementia, including Alzheimer's disease or a related disorder, or a non-primary diagnosis of dementia unless the primary diagnosis is a major mental disorder;

AND

- The disorder results in functional limitations in major life activities that would be appropriate within the past 3 to 6 months for the individual's developmental stage;

AND

- The treatment history indicates that the individual has experienced either: (a) psychiatric treatment more intensive than outpatient care more than once in the past 2 years (e.g., partial hospitalization or inpatient hospitalization); or (b) within the last 2 years due to the mental disorder, experienced an episode of significant disruption to the normal living situation, for which formal supportive services were required to maintain functioning at home, or in a residential treatment environment, or which resulted in intervention by housing or law enforcement officials.

Process: Review the resident's record only. For a "Yes" response to be entered, there must be written documentation (i.e., verbal reports from the resident or resident's family are not sufficient).

Coding: Enter "1" for Yes or "0" for No.

10. Conditions Related to MR/DD Status (Mental Retardation/ Developmental Disabilities)

Intent: To document conditions associated with mental retardation or developmental disabilities.

Definition: **For item 10e, "Other organic condition related to MR/DD"** — Examples of diagnostic conditions include congenital rubella, prenatal infection, congenital syphilis, maternal intoxication, mechanical injury at birth, prenatal hypoxia, neuronal lipid storage diseases, phenylketonuria (PKU), neurofibromatosis, microcephalus, macrencephaly, meningomyelocele, congenital hydrocephalus, etc.

Process: Review the resident's record only. For any item (10b through 10f) to be checked, the condition must be documented in the clinical record.

Coding: Check all conditions related to MR/DD status that were present before age 22. When age of onset is not specified, assume that the condition meets this criterion AND is likely to continue indefinitely.

- If an MR/DD condition is not present, check item 10a ("Not Applicable — No MR/DD") and skip to item AB-11.
- If an MR/DD condition is present, check each condition that applies.
- If an MR/DD condition is present but the resident does not have any of the specific conditions listed, check item 10f ("MR/DD with No Organic Condition").

11. Date Background Information Complete

Intent: For tracking purposes, this item should reflect the date that the *Background (Face Sheet) Information At Admission* form is completed or amended.

Coding: Enter the date the *Background (Face Sheet) Information At Admission* form is originally completed. In some circumstances (e.g., if a knowledgeable family member is not available during the 14-day assessment period), it is difficult to fill in all the background information requested on this form. However, the information is often obtained at a later date. As new or clarifying information becomes available, the facility may record additional information on the form or enter data into the computerized record. This item (AB 11) should then reflect the date that new information is recorded or existing information is revised.

Examples

Mr. B was admitted to your facility on 12/3/94 in a comatose state and therefore, unable to communicate in his own behalf. By reviewing transmittal records that accompanied him from the acute care hospital, you find that you are only able to partially complete Section AB (Demographic Information), and you are unable to complete Section AC (Customary Routine) because the records are scanty in these areas. You decide to complete what you can by the 14th day of Mr. B's residency (the date the MDS assessment is to be completed) and enter the date 12/17/94 for item AB 11. On 12/24/94 Mr. B's only relative, a daughter, visits and you are able to obtain more information from her. Enter the new information (e.g., demographic or customary routines) on the form and then enter the date 12/24/94 for item AB 11.

AC. CUSTOMARY ROUTINE

1. Customary Routine (In the year prior to DATE OF ENTRY to this nursing home, or year last in community if now being admitted from another nursing home)

Intent: These items provide information on the resident's usual community lifestyle and daily routine in the year prior to DATE OF ENTRY (AB1) to your nursing home. If the resident is being admitted from another nursing home, review the resident's routine during the last year the resident lived in the community. The items should initiate a flow of information about cognitive patterns, activity preferences, nutritional preferences and problems, ADL scheduling and performance, psychosocial well-being, mood, continence issues, etc. The resident's responses to these items also provide the interviewer with "clues" to understanding other areas of the resident's function. These clues can be further explored in other sections of the MDS that focus on particular functional domains. Taken in their entirety, the data gathered will be extremely useful in designing an individualized plan of care.

Process: Engage the resident in conversation. A comprehensive review can be facilitated by a questioning process such as described in Guidelines for Interviewing Resident that follow. Also see in Appendix D.

If the resident cannot respond (e.g., is severely demented or aphasic), ask a family member or other representative of the resident (e.g., legal guardian). For some residents you may be unable to obtain this information (e.g., a demented resident who first entered the facility many years ago and has no family to provide accurate information)

Guidelines for Interviewing Resident

Staff should regard this step in the assessment process as a good time to get to know the resident as an individual and an opportunity to set a positive tone for the future relationship. It is also a useful starting point for building trust prior to asking difficult questions about urinary incontinence, advance directives, etc.

The interview should be done in a quiet, private area where you are not likely to be interrupted. Use a conversational style to put the resident at ease. Explain at the outset why you are asking these questions ("Staff want to know more about you so you can have a comfortable stay with us." "These are things that many older people find important." "I'm going to ask a little bit about how you usually spend your day.")

Begin with a general question — e.g., "Tell me, how did you spend a typical day before coming here (or before going to the first nursing facility)?" or "What were some of the things you liked to do?" Listen for specific information about sleep patterns, eating patterns, preferences for timing of baths or showers, and social and leisure activities involvements. As the resident becomes engaged in the discussion, probe for information on each item of the Customary Routine section (i.e., cycle of daily events, eating patterns, ADL patterns, involvement patterns). Realize, however, that a resident who has been in an institutional setting for many years prior to coming to your facility may no longer be able to give an accurate description of pre-institutional routines. Some residents will persist in describing their experience in the long-term care setting, and will need to be reminded by the interviewer to focus on their usual routines prior to admission. Ask the resident, "Is this what you did before you came to live here?"

If the resident has difficulty responding to prompts regarding particular items, backtrack by re-explaining that you are asking these questions to help you understand how the resident's usual day was spent and how certain things were done. It may be necessary to ask a number of open-ended questions in order to obtain the necessary information. Prompts should be highly individualized.

Walk the resident through a typical day. Focus on usual habits, involvement with others, and activities. Phrase questions in the past tense. Periodically reiterate to the resident that you are interested in the resident's routine before nursing home admission, and that you want to know what he or she actually did, not what he or she might like to do.

(continued on next page)

Guidelines for Interviewing Resident (continued)

For example:

> After you retired from your job, did you get up at a regular time in the morning?
> When did you usually get up in the morning?
> What was the first thing you did after you arose?
> What time did you usually have breakfast?
> What kind of food did you like for breakfast?
> What happened after breakfast? (Probe for naps or regular post-breakfast activity such as reading the paper, taking a walk, doing chores, washing dishes.)
> When did you have lunch? Was it usually a big meal or just a snack?
> What did you do after lunch? Did you take a short rest? Did you often go out or have friends in to visit?
> Did you ever have a drink before dinner? Every day? Weekly?
> What time did you usually bathe? Did you usually take a shower or a tub bath?
> How often did you bathe? Did you prefer AM or PM?
> Did you snack in the evening?
> What time did you usually go to bed? Did you usually wake up during the night?

Definition: **Goes out 1+ days a week** — Went outside for any reason (e.g., socialization, fresh air, clinic visit).

Use of tobacco products at least daily — Smoked any type of tobacco (e.g., cigarettes, cigars, pipe) at least once daily. This item also includes sniffing or chewing tobacco.

Distinct food preferences — This item is checked to indicate the presence of specific food preferences, with details recorded elsewhere in the clinical record (e.g., was a vegetarian; observed kosher dietary laws; avoided red meat for health reasons; hates hot dogs; allergic to wheat and avoids bread). *Do not check this item for simple likes and dislikes.*

Use of alcoholic beverage(s) at least weekly — Drank at least one alcoholic drink per week.

Wakens to toilet all or most nights — Awoke to use the toilet at least once during the night all or most of the time.

Has irregular bowel movement pattern — Refers to an unpredictable or variable pattern of bowel elimination, regardless of whether the resident prefers a different pattern.

Bathing in PM — Took shower or bath in the evening.

Daily contact with relatives/close friends — Includes visits and telephone calls. Does not include exchange of letters only.

Usually attends church, temple, synagogue (etc.) — Refers to interaction regardless of type (e.g., regular churchgoer, watched TV evangelist, involved in church or temple committees or groups).

Daily animal companion/presence — Refers to involvement with animals (e.g. house pet, seeing-eye dog, fed birds daily in yard or park).

Unknown — If the resident cannot provide any information, no family members are available, and the admission record does not contain relevant information, check the last box in the category ("UNKNOWN"), leave all other boxes in Section AB blank.

Coding: Coding is limited to selected routines in the year prior to the resident's first admission to a nursing facility. *Code the resident's actual routine rather than his or her goals or preferences* (e.g., if the resident would have liked daily contact with relatives but did not have it, do not check "Daily contact with relatives/close friends").

Under each major category (Cycle of Daily Events, Eating Patterns, ADL Patterns, and Involvement Patterns) a *NONE OF ABOVE* choice is available. For example, if the resident did not engage in any of the items listed under Cycle of Daily Events, indicate this by checking *NONE OF ABOVE* for Cycle of Daily Events.

If an individual item in a particular category is not known (e.g."Finds strength in faith," under Involvement Patterns), enter "NA" or a circled dash ⊖.

If information is unavailable for all the items in the entire Customary Routine section, check the final box "UNKNOWN" — Resident/family unable to provide information". If UNKNOWN is checked, no other boxes in the Customary Routine section should be checked.

AD. FACE SHEET SIGNATURES

a. Signature of RN Assessment Coordinator

Coding: The RN Assessment Coordinator who worked on the *Background (Face Sheet) Information at Admission* sections of the MDS must enter his or her signature on the day this part of the MDS form is complete. Also, to the right of the name enter the date the form was signed.

b-g. Signature of Others Who Completed Part of Background Assessment Sections AB and AC

Coding: Other staff who completed parts of the Background sections of the MDS must enter their signatures, the sections they completed, and the date they completed their assigned sections.

MINIMUM DATA SET FOR NURSING HOME RESIDENT ASSESSMENT AND CARE SCREENING (MDS)

FUNCTIONAL ASSESSMENT

Sections A – R

SECTION A. IDENTIFICATION AND BACKGROUND INFORMATION

1. Resident Name

Definition: Legal name in record.

Coding: Print the resident's name in the following order — a.) first name, b.) middle initial, c.) last name, d.) Jr./Sr. If the resident goes by his or her middle name, enter the full middle name. If the resident has no middle initial, leave item (b) blank.

2. Room Number

Intent: Another identifying number for tracking purposes.

Definition: The number of resident's room in the facility.

Coding: Start in the left most box, use as many boxes as needed.

Example

Mr. F lives in Room N305 at your facility. The N stands for New Building in your

N	3	0	5	

two building complex. The three hundred series of rooms are on the third floor.

3. Assessment Reference Date

Intent: To establish a common temporal reference point for all staff participating in the resident's assessment. Although staff members may work on completing a resident's MDS on different days, establishment of the assessment reference date ensures the commonality of the assessment period (i.e., "starting the clock" so that all assessment items refer to the resident's objective performance and health status during the same period of time).

Definition: **a. Last day of MDS observation period.** This date refers to a specific end-point in the MDS assessment process. Almost all MDS items refer to the resident's status over a designated time period, most frequently the seven day period ending on this date. The date sets the designated endpoint of the common observation period, and all MDS items refer back in time from this point. Some cover the 14 days ending on this day, some 30 days ending on this date, and so forth.

Coding: The first coding task is to enter the observation reference date (i.e., the end point date of the observation period). For an admission assessment, this date can be any day up to the 14th day following admission (the last possible date for completing the admission assessment). For a followup assessment, select a common reference date within the period the assessment must be completed. This date is the endpoint to which all MDS items must refer.

For an admission assessment, staff may begin to gather some information on the day of admission. An observation end date will be set, often a date prior to day 14.

RAPs must be completed within regulatory required time frames for completion of the RAI.

Examples of Assessment Reference Date for an Admission Assessment

Mrs. M was admitted to your facility on 8/20/94. Your facility's policy states that all MDS assessments for new admissions shall be completed by the 7th day of residency. Therefore, staff decided to conduct their observations, tests, interviews with resident, family and other staff, and chart reviews during the first 7 days of the resident's stay. During this time they record pertinent findings in the resident's record and, where appropriate, on the MDS form. They record the endpoint of the MDS observation period as follows, giving staff another 7 days in which to complete the RAPs:

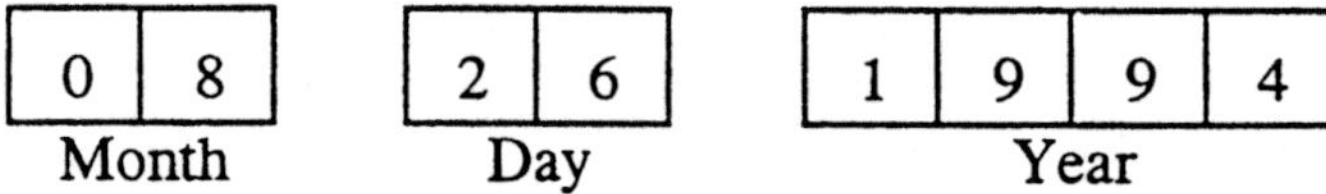

Mr. S was admitted to your facility on 8/20/94. Your facility's policy states that all MDS assessments for new admissions shall be completed by the 14th day of residency. The interdisciplinary team on the new resident's unit decides to take the full 14 days to complete the assessment. Of course they conduct observations, tests, necessary interviews, and chart reviews necessary for care planning. During this time they record pertinent findings in the resident's record. They record the endpoint of the MDS observation period as follows, with the stipulation that the RAPs must also be completed on that date:

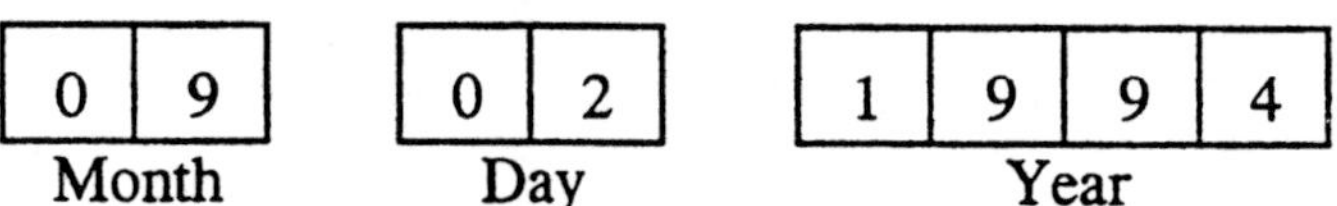

Rationale: As 9/2/94 is the 14th day of residency, the period of review for the MDS items will be the 7 days prior to that date, plus the period that ends on that date (or the period from 8/27 through 9/2/94).

For an annual assessment, staff are likely to have extensive data on hand. In such cases, a designated observation period of seven days is usually established. The date on which the observation period ends is the Assessment Reference Date. All staff who participate in the assessment must, however, agree that their description of the resident reflects the resident's status in this seven day period.

For the month and day of the assessment, enter two digits each, using zero, ("0") as a filler. Use four digits for the year.

Example of Assessment Reference Date for an Annual Assessment

Mr. X has been living at your facility for the past 2 years. The date of his last full MDS assessment was approximately 1 year ago (9/27/93). It is time to think about scheduling another full assessment. The MDS RN coordinator posts a notice to the interdisciplinary team stating Mr. X's next full assessment date is 9/20/94. This means that the team should be evaluating Mr. X during the 7 day period that ends on this date for most MDS items (i.e., from 9/14/94 to 9/20/94). Record the endpoint of the MDS observation period as:

0	9		2	0		1	9	9	4
Month			Day			Year			

Remember, an annual assessment must be completed within 12 months of the most recent MDS assessment.

B. Original (0) or corrected copy of form (enter number of corrections): Reserved for use in assessment data correction and transmission to State/HCFA. Further instructions will be issued when HCFA's proposed automated data processing (ADP) requirement goes into effect.

4. Date of reentry

Intent: To track the date of the resident's readmission to the facility following a temporary discharge to a hospital.

Definition: The date the resident was most recently readmitted to your facility after being temporarily discharged for hospital stay in last 90 days (or since last assessment or admission if less than 90 days).

Process: Review the clinical record. If dates are unclear or unavailable, ask the admissions office or medical record department.

Coding: If the resident has not been hospitalized in last 90 days, leave blank. Otherwise, use all boxes. For a one-digit month or day, place a zero in the first box. For example: February 3, 1994, should be entered as:

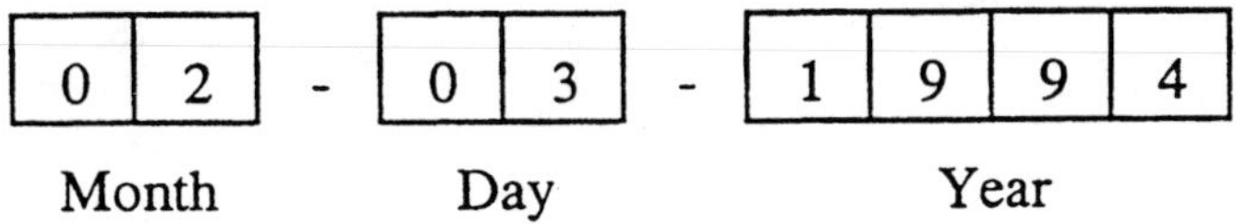

5. Marital Status

Coding: Choose the answer that describes the current marital status of the resident.

6. Medical Record Number

Definition: This number is the unique identifier assigned by the facility for the resident. Get it from the facility's admissions office, business office, or medical records department.

7. Current Payment Source(s) for Nursing Home Stay

Intent: To determine payment source(s) that cover the daily per diem or ancillary services for the resident's stay in the nursing facility over the last 30 days.

Definition: **Per diem** — Room, board, nursing care, activities, and services included in the routine daily charge.

Ancillary — Services such as medications, equipment for treatments, or supplies billed outside of the daily routine per diem charge.

Self (or family) pays — full — Includes full private pay by resident or family.

Self (or family) pays — co-pay — The resident is responsible for a co-payment.

Private insurance — The resident's private insurance company is covering daily charges.

Other — Examples include Commission for the Blind, Alzheimer's Association.

Process: Check with the billing office to review current payment sources. Do not rely exclusively on information recorded in the resident's clinical record, as the resident's clinical condition may trigger different sources of payment over time. Usually business offices track such information.

Coding: For each payment source, check the corresponding answer box.

Example of Current Payment Sources

Mr. F. was recently admitted to your facility from an acute care hospital. Medicare (Part A) has partially covered his per diem and ancillary services, and private insurance has covered the remainder of his charges. Mr. F. does not belong to a managed care program.

Check "b", Medicare per diem, "c", Medicare ancillary, and "i", Private insurance.

8. Reasons for Assessment

a. Primary Reason for Assessment

Intent: To document the key reason for completing the assessment, using the various categories of assessment types mandated by Federal regulation. Most of the types of assessments listed below will require completion of the MDS, review of triggered RAPs, and development or review of a comprehensive care plan within seven days of completing the RAI. [Note — assessment type 5 requires you to complete only a limited number of MDS items.] Please note that it is possible to select a code from both 8a (Primary reason for assessment) and 8b (Special codes).

Minimum Discharge Assessment Requirement. With the release of Version 2.0 of the MDS, a minimal list of MDS items must be completed for all discharges and facility reentries. These items are referenced on their own forms and item 8 also appears on these forms — it is listed as Item 8 in Section AA of the *Discharge Tracking and Reentry Tracking Forms*; it is also Item AA8 on the *Basic Assessment Tracking Form.*

Definition:

1. **Admission assessment.** A comprehensive assessment using the MDS and RAPs required by day 14 of the resident's stay. Note, this code is used if the resident is being readmitted subsequent to a discharge where return was not anticipated.

2. **Annual assessment** — A comprehensive reassessment required within 12 months of the most recent full assessment. If significant change is noted, code "3" (significant change in status assessment). DO NOT code as an Annual assessment.

3. **Significant change in status assessment** — A comprehensive reassessment prompted by a "major change" that is not self-limited, that impacts on more than one area of the resident's health status, and that requires interdisciplinary review or revision of the care plan to ensure that

appropriate care is given. When there is a significant change, the assessment must be completed by the end of the 14th calendar day following the determination that a significant change has occurred. **See procedure described below for assessing whether a significant change (either improvement or decline) has occurred.**

4. **Significant correction of prior assessment** —A comprehensive assessment completed at the facility's prerogative, because the previous assessment was inaccurate or completed incorrectly. This differs from a significant change in status assessment, in which case there has been an actual change in the resident's health status.

5. **Quarterly Assessment** —The subset of MDS items specified on HCFA's Quarterly Assessment Form, which must be completed no less frequently than once every 3 months (i.e., between required full assessments). This assessment ensures that the care plan is correct and up to date. It also should identify instances where significant changes have occurred. If significant change is noted, Code "3" (Significant change in status assessment). DO NOT CODE as Quarterly review assessment.

Minimum Discharge Information — Until HCFA's ADP requirement is effective, this code is used only by facilities that are already required to submit data to the State. A subset of MDS items must be completed for all residents who are discharged or are out of the facility over night. Differentiate whether return is anticipated, not anticipated, or whether the resident has been discharged prior to completing an initial assessment. These items are referenced below.

6. **Discharged — return not anticipated** — [This is not a code used on this form; it is used on the *Discharge Tracking Form* only.] Use this code whenever a resident is permanently discharged from a nursing facility. This is a means of "closing" the record of any resident at the point of discharge from the facility (without an anticipated return). **Note — until HCFA's ADP requirement is effective, this code is used only in facilities that are required to submit data to the State.**

7. **Discharged — return anticipated** — [This is not a code used on this form; it is used on the *Discharge Tracking Form* only.] Use this code when a resident is temporarily discharged to a hospital (or other therapeutic setting). Also use this code when a respite patient returns home, with an anticipated return to this facility at a later date. **Note — until HCFA's ADP requirement is effective, this code is used only in facilities that are required to submit data to the State.**

8. **Discharged prior to completing initial assessment** — [This is not a code used on this form; it is used on the *Discharge Tracking Form* only.] Use this code when the resident is discharged during the first 14 days of residency AND the MDS assessment remains incomplete. A subset of information is entered for all residents regardless of length of stay. *Even a very short stay resident (e.g., a person who stayed for even one day) must be tracked by the MDS system.* At the same time, remember that you have 14 days to complete the full MDS admission assessment, and by using this code you are identifying residents who have been discharged, transferred or died prior to day 14, thereby prohibiting your completion of a full assessment. **Note — until HCFA's ADP requirement is effective, this code is used only in facilities that are required to submit data to the State.**

Minimum Reentry Information — Until HCFA's ADP requirement is effective, this code is used only by facilities that are already required to submit data to the State. A subset of MDS items must be completed for residents "reentering" the facility after a temporary absence (other than a therapeutic leave) in order to reenter the resident into the State database.

9. **Reentry**— [This is not a code used on this form; it is used on the *Reentry Tracking Form* only.] Use this code when a resident of your facility is readmitted from a temporary discharge to a hospital or other therapeutic setting (other than for a therapeutic leave). **Note — until HCFA's ADP requirement is effective, this code is used only in facilities that are required to submit data to the State.**

0. **NONE OF ABOVE** — Use this code when your state requires you to complete one of the additional assessment types referenced in Item AA8 (below). It indicates that the assessment has been completed to comply with State-specific requirements (e.g., case-mix payment). Select the code under item b (below) that indicates the primary reason for assessment.

b. **Special codes for use with supplemental assessment types in Case-Mix Demonstration States or other States where required.** It is possible to select a code from both 8a and 8b (e.g., Item 8a coded "3" (Significant Change in Status assessment), and Item 8b coded "3" (60-day assessment).

1. **5 day assessment** — Required for payment reasons prior to the Federally mandated admission assessment required by day 14 (Code 1, for item a).

2. **30 day assessment**

3. **60 day assessment** -- In following this cycle of assessments, the initial Quarterly review assessment would be due at 90 days.

4. **Quarterly assessment using full MDS form** — Assessment completed within a 3-month interval from the last assessment, using a full (not quarterly) MDS assessment form as required by the State or NHCMQ demonstration.

5. **Readmission/return assessment** — A full reassessment (i.e., MDS and RAPs) required only for residents in NHCMQ demonstration facilities (or as required by the State) who are hospitalized for more than 72 hours, or who are discharged and later readmitted to the facility from the hospital.

6. **Other state required assessment** — An example is a Utilization Review assessment. States may issue additional instructions.

Coding: Enter the number corresponding to the primary reason for assessment. For item a (Primary reason for assessment), for codes 1-9, leave first box blank, placing correct digit in the second box.

Additional Comments on Significant Change Assessment

Facilities have an ongoing responsibility to assess the resident's status and intervene to assist the resident to attain or maintain the highest practicable level of physical, mental, and psychosocial well-being. Staff have the responsibility of deciding whether a change they have noted (either an improvement or decline) is significant.

A "significant change" is defined as a major change in the resident's status that:

- Is not self-limiting;
- Impacts on more than one area of the resident's health status; and
- Requires interdisciplinary review and/or revision of the care plan.

The following indicate conditions under which a significant change reassessment is required. The terms referenced are based on items (and definitions) found in Version 2.0 of the MDS. Other situations can apply; this list is not exhaustive, and other situations may also meet significant change definition. [Note -- in an end stage disease status, a full reassessment is optional, depending on a clinical determination of whether or not the resident would benefit from the reassessment.]

A significant change may occur at any point during the resident's stay, although facilities may most commonly identify that a significant change has occurred while constructing the resident's scheduled quarterly review. Over a six-month period, depending on the resident population, one in five residents typically declines in two or more of these areas. The goal of the significant change reassessment is to ensure that residents are being appropriately monitored and necessary changes in care instituted. Also see discussion in Chapter 2.

SIGNIFICANT CHANGE CRITERIA*

A significant change assessment is required if a decline (or improvement) change is consistently noted in two or more areas of decline, or two or more areas of improvement.

DECLINE

- Any **decline in ADL physical functioning** where a resident is **newly** coded as 3, 4, or 8 (Extensive assistance; Total dependency; Activity did not occur).
- Increase in number of areas where Behavioral symptoms are coded as not easily altered (increase in number of code 1's for E4B).
- **Resident's** decision making **changes** from 0 **or** 1 to 2 **or** 3.
- **Resident's** incontinence **pattern changes** from 0 **or** 1 to 2, 3, **or** 4, or placement of an indwelling catheter.
- Emergence of sad or anxious mood as a problem that is not easily altered.
- Emergence of an unplanned weight loss problem (5% change in 30 days or 10% **change** in 180 days)
- Begin to use a trunk restraint or a chair that prevents rising **for a resident when it was not used before**.
- Emergence of a condition/disease **in which** resident is judged to be unstable.
- Emergence of a pressure ulcer at Stage II or higher, when no ulcers were previously present at that stage or higher.
- Overall deterioration **of resident's condition; resident** receives more support, (e.g., in performing ADLs, or in decision making).

IMPROVEMENT

- Any **improvement in ADL physical functioning** where a resident is **newly** coded as 0, 1, or 2 when previously scored as a 3, 4, or 8.
- Decrease in number of areas where Behavioral symptoms of sad or anxious mood are coded as not easily altered.
- **Resident's** decision making **changes** from 2 or 3 to 0 **or** 1.
- **Resident's** incontinence **pattern changes** from 2, 3, **or** 4 to 0 **or** 1.
- Overall improvement **of resident's condition; resident** receives fewer supports.

* This is not an exhaustive list.

9. Responsibility/Legal Guardian

Intent: To record who has responsibility for participating in decisions about the resident's health care, treatment, financial affairs, and legal affairs. Depending on the resident's condition, multiple options may apply. For example, a resident with moderate dementia may be competent to make decisions in certain areas, although in other areas a family member will assume decision-making responsibility. Or a resident may have executed a limited power of attorney to someone responsible only for legal affairs. Legal oversight such as guardianship, durable power of attorney, and living wills are generally governed by State law. The descriptions provided here are for general information only. Refer to the law in your State and to the facility's legal counsel, as appropriate, for additional clarification.

Definition: **Legal guardian** — Someone who has been appointed after a court hearing and is authorized to make decisions for the resident, including giving and withholding consent for medical treatment. Once appointed, the decision-making authority of the guardian may be revoked only by another court hearing.

Other legal oversight — Use this category for any other program in your State whereby someone other than the resident participates in or makes decisions about the resident's health care and treatment.

Durable power of attorney/health care — Documentation that someone other than the resident is legally responsible for health care decisions if the resident becomes unable to make decisions. This document may also provide guidelines for the agent or proxy decision-maker, and may include instructions concerning the resident's wishes for care. Unlike a guardianship, durable power of attorney/health care proxy terms can be revoked by the resident at any time.

Durable power of attorney/financial — Documentation that someone other than the resident is legally responsible for financial decisions if the resident becomes unable to make decisions.

Family member responsible — Includes immediate family or significant other(s) as designated by the resident. Responsibility for decision-making may be shared by both resident and family.

Patient responsible for self — Resident retains responsibility for decisions. In the absence of guardianship or legal documents indicating that decision-making has been delegated to others, always assume that the resident is the responsible party.

Process: Legal oversight such as guardianship, durable power of attorney, and living wills are generally governed by state law. The descriptions provided here are for general information only. Refer to the law in your State and to the facility's legal counsel, as appropriate, for additional clarification.

Consult the resident and the resident's family. Review records. Where the legal oversight or guardianship is court ordered, a copy of the legal document must be included in the resident's record in order for the item to be checked on the MDS form.

Coding: Check all that apply.

10. Advanced Directives

Intent: To record the legal existence of directives regarding treatment options for the resident, whether made by the resident or a legal proxy. Documentation must be available in the record for a directive to be considered current and binding. The absence of pre-existing directives for the resident should prompt discussion by clinical staff with the resident and family regarding the resident's wishes. Any discrepancies between the resident's current stated wishes and what is said in legal documents in the resident's file should be resolved immediately.

Definition: **Living will** — A document specifying the resident's preferences regarding measures used to prolong life when there is a terminal prognosis.

Do not resuscitate — In the event of respiratory or cardiac failure, the resident, family or legal guardian has directed that no cardiopulmonary resuscitation (CPR) or other life-saving methods will be used to attempt to restore the resident's respiratory or circulatory function.

Do not hospitalize — A document specifying that the resident is not to be hospitalized even after developing a medical condition that usually requires hospitalization.

Organ donation — Instructions indicating that the resident wishes to make organs available for transplantation, research, or medical education upon death.

Autopsy request — Document indicating that the resident, family or legal guardian has requested that an autopsy be performed upon death. The family or responsible party must still be contacted upon the resident's death and re-asked if they want an autopsy to be performed.

Feeding restrictions — The resident or responsible party (family or legal guardian) does not wish the resident to be fed by artificial means (e.g., tube, intravenous nutrition) if unable to be nourished by oral means.

Medication restrictions — The resident or responsible party (family or legal guardian) does not wish the resident to receive life-sustaining medications (e.g., antibiotics, chemotherapy). These restrictions may not be appropriate, however, when such medications could be used to ensure the resident's comfort. In these cases, the directive should be reviewed with the responsible party.

Other treatment restrictions — The resident or responsible party (family or legal guardian) does not wish the resident to receive certain medical treatments. Examples include, but are not limited to, blood transfusion, tracheotomy, respiratory intubation, and restraints. Such restrictions may not be appropriate to treatments given for palliative reasons (e.g., reducing pain or distressing physical symptoms such as nausea or vomiting). In these cases, the directive should be reviewed with the responsible party.

Process: You will need to familiarize yourself with the legal status of each type of directive in your State. In some states only a health care proxy is formally recognized; other jurisdictions allow for the formulation of living wills and the appointment of individuals with durable power of attorney for health care decisions. Facilities should develop a policy regarding documents drawn in other states, respecting them as important expressions of the resident's wishes until their legal status is determined.

Review the resident's record for documentation of the resident's advance directives. Documentation must be available in the record for a directive to be considered current and binding.

Some residents at the time of admission may be unable to participate in decision-making. Staff should make a reasonable attempt to determine whether the new resident has ever created an advance directive (e.g., ask family members, check with the primary physician). Lacking any directive, treatment decisions will likely be made in concert with the resident's closest family members or, in their absence or in case of conflict, through legal guardianship proceedings.

Coding: The following comments provide further guidance on how to code these directives. You will also need to consider State law, legal interpretations, and facility policy.

- The resident (or proxy) should always be involved in the discussion to ensure informed decision-making. If the resident's preference is known and the attending physician is aware of the preference, but the preference is not recorded in the record, check the MDS item only after the preference has been documented.

- If the resident's preference is in areas that require supporting orders by the attending physician (e.g., do not resuscitate, do not hospitalize, feeding restrictions, other treatment restrictions), check the MDS item only if the document has been recorded or after the physician provides the necessary order. Where a physician's current order is recorded but resident's or proxy's preference is not indicated, discuss with the resident's physician and check the MDS item only after documentation confirming that the resident's or proxy's wishes have been entered into the record.

- If your facility has a standard protocol for withholding particular treatments from all residents (e.g., no facility staff member may resuscitate or perform CPR on any resident; facility does not use feeding tubes), check the MDS item only if the advanced directive is the individual preference of the resident (or legal proxy), regardless of the facility's policy or protocol.

Coding: Check all that apply. If none of the directives are verified by documentation in the medical records, check *NONE OF ABOVE*.

SECTION B. COGNITIVE PATTERNS

Intent: To determine the resident's ability to remember, think coherently, and organize daily self-care activities. These items are crucial factors in many care-planning decisions. Your focus is on resident performance, including a demonstrated ability to remember recent and long-past events and to perform key decision making skills.

Questions about cognitive function and memory can be sensitive issues for some residents who may become defensive or agitated or very emotional. These are not uncommon reactions to performance anxiety and feelings of being exposed, embarrassed, or frustrated if the resident knows he or she cannot answer the questions cogently.

Be sure to interview the resident in a private, quiet area without distractions — i.e., not in the presence of other residents or family, unless the resident is too agitated to be left alone. Using a nonjudgmental approach to questioning will help create a needed sense of trust between staff and resident. After eliciting the resident's responses to the questions, return to the resident's family or others, as appropriate, to clarify or validate information regarding the resident's cognitive function over the last seven days. For residents with limited communication skills or who are best understood by family or specific care givers, you will need to carefully consider their insights in this area.

- Engage the resident in general conversation to help establish rapport.

- Actively listen and observe for clues to help you structure your assessment. Remember — repetitiveness, inattention, rambling speech, defensiveness, or agitation may be challenging to deal with during an interview, but they provide important information about cognitive function.

- Be open, supportive, and reassuring during your conversation with the resident (e.g., "Do you sometimes have trouble remembering things? Tell me what happens. We will try to help you").

  If the resident becomes really agitated, sympathetically respond to his or her feelings of agitation and STOP discussing cognitive function. The information-gathering process does not need to be completed in one sitting but may be ongoing during the entire assessment period. Say to the agitated resident, for example, "Let's talk about something else now," or "We don't need to talk about that now. We can do it later". Observe the resident's cognitive performance over the next few hours and days and come back to ask more questions when he or she is feeling more comfortable.

1. Comatose

Intent: To record whether the resident's clinical record includes a documented neurological diagnosis of coma or persistent vegetative state.

Coding: Enter the appropriate number in the box.

If the resident has been diagnosed as comatose or in a persistent vegetative state, code "1". ***Skip to Section G.*** If the resident is not comatose or is semi-comatose, code "0" and proceed to the next item (B2).

2. Memory

Intent: To determine the resident's functional capacity to remember both recent and long-past events (i.e., short-term and long-term memory).

Process: a. **Short-Term Memory:** Ask the resident to describe a recent event that both of you had the opportunity to remember. Or, you could use a more structured short-term memory test. For residents with limited communication skills, ask staff and family about the resident's memory status. Remember, if there is no positive indication of memory ability, (e.g., remembering multiple items over time or following through on a direction given five minutes earlier) the correct response is "1", Memory Problem.

Examples

Ask the resident to describe the breakfast meal or an activity just completed.

Ask the resident to remember three items (e.g., book, watch, table) for a few minutes. After you have stated all three items, ask the resident to repeat them (to verify that you were heard and understood). Then proceed to talk about something else — do not be silent, do not leave the room. In five minutes, ask the resident to repeat the name of each item. If the resident is unable to recall all three items, code "1." For persons with verbal communication deficits, non-verbal responses are acceptable (e.g., when asked how many children they have, they can tap out a response of the appropriate number).

b. Long-Term Memory: Engage in conversation that is meaningful to the resident. Ask questions for which you can validate the answers (from your review of record, general knowledge, the resident's family). For residents with limited communication skills, ask staff and family about the resident's memory status. Remember, if there is no positive indication of memory ability, the correct response is "1", Memory Problem.

Example

Ask the resident, "Where did you live just before you came here?" If "at home" is the reply, ask "What was your address?" If "another nursing home" is the reply, ask "What was the name of the place?" Then ask: "Are you married?" "What is your spouse's name?" "Do you have any children?" "How many?" "When is your birthday?" "In what year were you born?"

Coding: Enter the numbers that correspond to the observed responses.

3. Memory/Recall Ability

Intent: To determine the resident's memory/recall performance within the environmental setting. A resident may have intact social graces and respond to staff and others with a look of recognition, yet have no idea who they are. This item will enable staff to probe beyond first, perhaps mistaken, impressions.

Definition: **Current season** — Able to identify the current season (e.g., correctly refers to weather for the time of year, legal holidays, religious celebrations, etc.).

Location of own room — Able to locate and recognize own room. It is not necessary for the resident to know the room number, but he or she should be able to find the way to the room.

Staff names/faces — Able to distinguish staff members from family members, strangers, visitors, and other residents. It is not necessary for the resident to know the staff member's name, but he or she should recognize that the person is a staff member and not the resident's son or daughter, etc.

That he/she is in a nursing home — Able to determine that he or she is currently living in a nursing home. To check this item, it is not necessary that the resident be able to state the name of the facility, but he/she should be able to refer to the facility by a term such as a "home for older people", a "hospital for the elderly", "a place where older people live", etc.

Process: Test memory/recall. Use information obtained from clinical records or staff. Ask the resident about each item. For example, "What is the current season? "What is the name of this place?" "What is this kind of place?" If the resident is not in his or her room, ask "Will you show me to your room?" Observe the resident's ability to find the way.

Coding: For each item that the resident can recall, check the corresponding answer box. If the resident can recall none, check *NONE OF ABOVE*.

4. Cognitive Skills for Daily Decision-Making

Intent: To record the resident's actual performance in making everyday decisions about tasks or activities of daily living.

Examples

Choosing items of clothing; knowing when to go to scheduled meals; using environmental cues to organize and plan (e.g., clocks, calendars, posted listings of upcoming events); in the absence of environmental cues, seeking information appropriately (i.e., not repetitively) from others in order to plan the day; using awareness of one's own strengths and limitations in regulating the day's events (e.g., asks for help when necessary); making the correct decision concerning how to get to the lunchroom; acknowledging need to use a walker, and using it faithfully.

Process: Review the clinical record. Consult family and nurse assistants. Observe the resident. *The inquiry should focus on whether the resident is actively making these decisions, and not whether staff believe the resident might be capable of doing so. Remember the intent of this item is to record what the resident is doing (performance).* Where a staff member takes decision-making responsibility away from the resident regarding tasks of everyday living, or the resident does not participate in decision-making, whatever his or her level of capability may be, the resident should be considered to have impaired performance in decision-making.

This item is especially important for further assessment and care planning in that it can alert staff to a mismatch between a resident's abilities and his or her current level of performance, or that staff may be inadvertently fostering the resident's dependence.

Coding: Enter one number that corresponds to the most correct response.

0. **Independent** — The resident's decisions in organizing daily routine and making decisions were consistent, reasonable, and organized reflecting lifestyle, culture, values.

1. **Modified Independence** — The resident organized daily routine and made safe decisions in familiar situations, but experienced some difficulty in decision-making when faced with new tasks or situations.

2. **Moderately Impaired** — The resident's decisions were poor; the resident required reminders, cues, and supervision in planning, organizing, and correcting daily routines.

3. **Severely Impaired** — The resident's decision-making was severely impaired; the resident never (or rarely) made decisions.

5. Indicators of Delirium — Periodic Disordered Thinking/Awareness

Intent: To record behavioral signs that may indicate that delirium is present. Frequently, delirium is caused by a treatable illness such as infection or reaction to medications.

The characteristics of delirium are often manifested behaviorally and therefore can be observed. For example, disordered thinking may be manifested by rambling, irrelevant, or incoherent speech. Other behaviors are described in the definitions below.

A recent change (deterioration) in cognitive function is indicative of delirium (acute confusional state), which may be reversible if detected and treated in a timely fashion. Signs of delirium can be easier to detect in a person with intact cognitive function at baseline. However, when a resident has a pre-existing cognitive impairment or pre-existing behaviors such as restlessness, calling out, etc., detecting signs of delirium is more difficult. Despite this difficulty, it is possible to detect signs of delirium in these residents by being attuned to recent changes in their usual functioning. For example, a resident who is usually noisy or belligerent may suddenly become quiet, lethargic, and inattentive. Or, conversely, one who is normally quiet and content may suddenly become restless and noisy. Or, one who is usually able to find his or her way around the unit may begin to get "lost".

Definitions:

a. **Easily distracted** (e.g., difficulty paying attention; gets sidetracked)

b. **Periods of altered perception or awareness of surroundings** (e.g., moves lips or talks to someone not present; believes he/she is somewhere else; confuses night and day)

c. **Episodes of disorganized speech** (e.g., speech is incoherent, nonsensical, irrelevant, or rambling from subject to subject; loses train of thought)

d. **Periods of restlessness** (e.g., fidgeting or picking at skin, clothing, napkins, etc.; frequent position changes; repetitive physical movements or calling out)

e. **Periods of lethargy** (e.g., sluggishness, staring into space; difficult to arouse; little body movement)

f. **Mental function varies over the course of the day** (e.g., sometimes better, sometimes worse; behaviors sometimes present, sometimes not)

Coding:

Code for resident's behavior in the last seven days regardless of what you believe the cause to be — focusing on when the manifested behavior first occurred.

0. Behavior not present
1. Behavior present, not of recent onset
2. Behavior present over last 7 days appears different from resident's usual functioning (e.g., new onset or worsening)

Case Example 1

Mrs. K is a 92 year old widow of 30 years who has severe functional dependency secondary to heart disease. Her primary nurse assistant has reported during the last two days Mrs. K has "not been herself." She has been napping more frequently and for longer periods during the day. She is difficult to arouse and has mumbling speech upon awakening. She also has difficulty paying attention to what she is doing. For example, at meals instead of eating as she usually does, she picks at her food as if she doesn't know what to do with a fork. Then stops and closes her eyes after a few minutes. Alternatively, Mrs. K has been waking up at night believing it to be daytime. She has been calling out to staff demanding to be taken to see her husband (although he is deceased). On 3 occasions Mrs. K was observed attempting to climb out of bed over the foot of the bed.

Indicators	Coding
a. Easily distracted	2 (present, new)
b. Periods of altered perception or awareness of surroundings	2 (present, new)
c. Episodes of disorganized speech	2 (present, new)
d. Periods of restlessness	2 (present, new)
e. Periods of lethargy	2 (present, new)
f. Mental function varies over the course of the day	2 (present, new)

Case Example 2

Mr. D has a history of Alzheimer's disease. His skills for decision making have been poor for a long time. He often has difficulty paying attention to tasks and activities and usually wanders away from them. He rarely speaks to others, and when he does it is garbled and the contents are nonsensical. He is often observed mumbling and moving his lips as if he's talking to someone. Although Mr. D is often restless and fidgety this behavior is not new for him and it rarely interferes with a good night's sleep.

Indicators	Coding
a. Easily distracted	1 (present, not new)
b. Periods of altered perception or awareness of surroundings	1 (present, not new)
c. Episodes of disorganized speech	1 (present, not new)
d. Periods of restlessness	1 (present, not new)
e. Periods of lethargy	0 (behavior not present)
f. Mental function varies over the course of the day	1 (present, not new)

6. Change in Cognitive Status

Intent: To document changes in the resident's cognitive status, skills, or abilities as compared to his or her status of 90 days ago (or since last assessment if less than 90 days ago). These can include, but are not limited to, changes in level of consciousness, cognitive skills for daily decision-making, short-term or long-term memory, thinking or awareness, or recall. Such changes may be permanent or temporary; their causes may be known (e.g., a new pain or psychotropic medication) or unknown. If the resident is a new admission to the facility, this item includes changes during the period prior to admission.

Coding: Record the number corresponding to the most correct response. Enter "0" for No change, "1" for Improved, or "2" for Deteriorated.

Examples of Change in Cognitive Status

Mrs. G experienced delirium (acute confusion) secondary to pneumonia approximately 30 days ago. With appropriate antibiotic therapy, hydration, and a quiet supportive milieu, she recovered. Although Mrs. G's cognitive skills did not increase beyond the level that existed prior to her pneumonia, and she remains unable to make daily decisions, she has steadily improved to her pre-pneumonia status. **Code "0" for No Change.**

Ms. P is intellectually intact. About two and one-half months ago she was informed by her daughter that her neighbor and lifelong friend had died while on a trip to Europe. Ms. P took the news very hard; she was stunned and seemed to be confused and bewildered for days. With support of family and staff, confusion passed. Although she continued to grieve, her cognitive status returned to what it was prior to her receiving the bad news. **Code "0" for No change.**

Mr. D was admitted to the nursing home three months ago upon discharge from the hospital with signs of post-operative delirium. Since that time he no longer requires frequent reminders and re-orientation throughout each day. His decision-making skills have improved. **Code "1" for Improved.**

Mr. F has Alzheimer's disease. He did well until two months ago, when his primary nurse assistant reported that he can no longer find his way back to his room, which he was able to do three months ago. He often gets lost now while trying to find his way to the unit activity/dining room. **Code "2" for Deteriorated.**

(continued on next page)

Examples of Change in Cognitive Status (continued)

Mrs. F was admitted to the facility six weeks ago. Upon admission she had modified independence in daily decision-making skills, intact short and long term memory, and good recall abilities. Since that time, Mrs. F has had a stroke, which has left her with deficits in these areas. Within this Significant Change assessment period, her decisions have become poor. She is not aware of her new physical limitations and has taken unreasonable safety risks in transferring and locomotion. She receives supervision at all times. **Code "2" for Deteriorated.**

MDS Cognitive Performance Scale©

Many facilities have asked for a system to combine MDS cognitive items into an overall Cognitive Performance Scale. Such a scale has been produced — The MDS Cognitive Performance Scale (CPS)© **[see Appendix F]**. Five MDS items are used in assigning residents to one of seven CPS categories. The CPS categories are highly related to residents' average scores on the Folstein Mini-Mental Status Examination (MMSE), which has a score range of zero (worst) to thirty (best). According to Folstein, an MMSE score of 23 or lower usually suggests cognitive impairment but it may be lower for persons with an eighth grade education or less.

SECTION C. COMMUNICATION/HEARING PATTERNS

Intent: To document the resident's ability to hear (with assistive hearing devices, if they are used), understand, and communicate with others.

There are many possible causes for the communication problems experienced by elderly nursing home residents. Some can be attributed to the aging process; others are associated with progressive physical and neurological disorders. Usually the communication problem is caused by more than one factor. For example, a resident might have aphasia as well as long standing hearing loss; or he or she might have dementia and word finding difficulties and a hearing loss. The resident's physical, emotional, and social situation may also complicate communication problems. Additionally, a noisy or isolating environment can inhibit opportunities for effective communication.

Deficits in one's ability to understand (receptive communication deficits) can involve declines in hearing, comprehension (spoken or written), or recognition of facial expressions. Deficits in ability to make one's self understood (expressive communication deficits) can include reduced voice volume and difficulty in producing sounds, or difficulty in finding the right word, making sentences, writing, and gesturing.

1. Hearing

Intent: To evaluate the resident's ability to hear (with environmental adjustments, if necessary) during the past seven-day period.

Process: Evaluate hearing ability after the resident has a hearing appliance in place, if the resident uses an appliance. Review the clinical record. Interview and observe the resident, and ask about the hearing function. Consult the resident's family, direct care staff, and speech or hearing specialists. Test the accuracy of your findings by observing the resident during your verbal interactions.

Be alert to what you have to do to communicate with the resident. For example, if you have to speak more clearly, use a louder tone, speak more slowly, or use more gestures, or if the resident needs to see your face to know what you are saying, or if you have to take the resident to a more quiet area to conduct the interview — all of these are cues that there is a hearing problem, and should be so indicated in the coding.

Also, observe the resident interacting with others and in group activities. Ask the activities personnel how the resident hears during group leisure activities.

Coding: Enter one number that corresponds to the most correct response.

0. **Hears adequately** — The resident hears all normal conversational speech, including when using the telephone, watching television, and engaged in group activities.

1. **Minimal difficulty** — The resident hears speech at conversational levels but has difficulty hearing when not in quiet listening conditions or when not in one-on-one situations.

2. **Hears in special situations only** — Although hearing-deficient, the resident compensates when the speaker adjusts tonal quality and speaks distinctly; or the resident can hear only when the speaker's face is clearly visible.

3. **Highly impaired/absence of useful hearing** — The resident hears only some sounds and frequently fails to respond even when the speaker adjusts tonal quality, speaks distinctly, or is positioned face to face. There is no comprehension of conversational speech, even when the speaker makes maximum adjustments.

2. Communication Devices/Techniques

Definition: **Hearing aid, present and used** — A hearing aid or other assistive listening device is available to the resident and is used regularly.

Hearing aid, present and not used regularly — A hearing aid or other assistive listening device is available to the resident and is not regularly used (e.g., resident has a hearing aid that is broken or is used only occasionally).

Other receptive communication technique used (e.g., lip reading) — A mechanism or process is used by the resident to enhance interaction with others (e.g., reading lips, touching to compensate for hearing deficit, writing by staff member, use of communication board).

Process: Consult with the resident and direct care staff. Observe the resident closely during your interaction.

Coding: Check all that apply. If the resident does not have a hearing aid or does not regularly use compensatory communication techniques, check *NONE OF ABOVE*.

3. Modes of Expression

Intent: To record the types of communication techniques (verbal and non-verbal) used by the resident to make his or her needs and wishes known.

Definition: **Writing messages to express or clarify needs** — Resident writes notes to communicate with others.

Signs/gestures/sounds — This category includes nonverbal expressions used by the resident to communicate with others.

- Actions may include pointing to words, objects, people; facial expressions; using physical gestures such as nodding head twice for "yes" and once for "no" or squeezing another's hand in the same manner.

- Sounds may include grunting, banging, ringing a bell, etc.

Communication board — An electronic, computerized or other home-made device used by the resident to convey verbal information, wishes, or commands to others.

Other — Examples include flash cards or various electronic assistive devices.

Process: Consult with the primary nurse assistant and other direct-care staff from all shifts, if possible. Consult with the resident's family. Interact with the resident and observe for any reliance on non-verbal expression (physical gestures, such as pointing to objects), either in one-on-one communication or in group situations.

Coding: Check the boxes for each method used by the resident to communicate his or her needs. If the resident does not use any of the listed items, check *NONE OF ABOVE.*

4. Making Self Understood

Intent: To document the resident's ability to express or communicate requests, needs, opinions, urgent problems, and social conversation, whether in speech, writing, sign language, or a combination of these.

Process: Interact with the resident. Observe and listen to the resident's efforts to communicate with you. Observe his or her interactions with others in different settings (e.g., one-on-one, groups) and different circumstances (e.g., when calm, when agitated). Consult with the primary nurse assistant (over all shifts) if available, the resident's family, and speech-language pathologist.

Coding: Enter the number corresponding to the most correct response.

0. **Understood** — The resident expresses ideas clearly.

1. **Usually Understood** — The resident has difficulty finding the right words or finishing thoughts, resulting in delayed responses; or the resident requires some prompting to make self understood.

2. **Sometimes Understood** — The resident has limited ability, but is able to express concrete requests regarding at least basic needs (e.g., food, drink, sleep, toilet).

3. **Rarely or Never Understood** — At best, understanding is limited to staff interpretation of highly individual, resident-specific sounds or body language (e.g., indicated presence of pain or need to toilet).

5. Speech Clarity

Intent: To document the quality of the resident's speech, not the content or appropriateness — just words spoken.

Definition: **Speech** — the expression of articulate words.

Process: Listen to the resident. Confer with primary assigned caregivers.

Coding: Enter the number corresponding to the most correct response.

0. **Clear speech** — utters distinct, intelligible words.
1. **Unclear speech** — utters slurred or mumbled words.
2. **No speech** — absence of spoken words.

6. Ability to Understand Others

Intent: To describe the resident's ability to comprehend verbal information whether communicated to the resident orally, by writing, or in sign language or braille. This item measures not only the resident's ability to hear messages but also to process and understand language.

Process: Interact with the resident. Consult with primary direct care staff (e.g., nurse assistants) over all shifts if possible, the resident's family, and speech-language pathologist.

Coding: Enter the number corresponding to the most appropriate response.

0. **Understands** — The resident clearly comprehends the speaker's message(s) and demonstrates comprehension by words or actions/behaviors.
1. **Usually Understands** — The resident may miss some part or intent of the message but comprehends most of it. The resident may have periodic difficulties integrating information but generally demonstrates comprehension by responding in words or actions.

2. **Sometimes Understands** — The resident demonstrates frequent difficulties integrating information, and responds adequately only to simple and direct questions or directions. When staff rephrase or simplify the message(s) and/or use gestures, the resident's comprehension is enhanced.

3. **Rarely/Never Understands** — The resident demonstrates very limited ability to understand communication. Or, staff have difficulty determining whether the resident comprehends messages, based on verbal and nonverbal responses. Or, the resident can hear sounds but does not understand messages.

7. Change in Communication/Hearing

Intent: To document any change in the resident's ability to express, understand, or hear information compared to his or her status of 90 days ago (or since last assessment if less than 90 days ago). If the resident is a new admission to the facility, this item includes changes during the period prior to admission.

Process: In addition to consulting primary care staff (over all shifts if possible), consulting the family of new admissions, and reviewing prior Quarterly reviews when available, ask the resident if he or she has noticed any changes in the ability to hear, talk, or understand others. Sometimes, residents do not complain of changes being experienced because they attribute them to "old age". Therefore, it is important that they be asked directly. Some types of deterioration are easily corrected (e.g., by new hearing aid batteries or removal of ear wax).

Coding: Enter the number corresponding to the most correct response. Enter "0" for No change, "1" for Improved, or "2" for Deteriorated.

Examples of Change in Communication/Hearing

Mrs. L has had expressive aphasia for two years. Although she periodically says a word or phrase that is understood by others, this is not new for her. During the last 90 days her communication status has essentially remained unchanged. **Code "0" for No change.**

Mrs. R's hearing is severely impaired. Five months ago the occupational therapist developed flash cards for staff to use when communicating with her. This was a tremendous boost for both Mrs. R and staff. Her ability to understand others continues to improve. **Code "1" for Improved.**

Mr. S has complained for the last two weeks of ringing in his ears, saying "Please do something, it's driving me crazy! **Code "2" for Deteriorated.**

Upon admission two months ago Mrs. T had difficulty hearing unless the speaker adjusted his or her tone of voice and spoke more distinctly. She has worn hearing aids in the past but lost them during a hospital admission. Since admission to the nursing home, Mrs. T was tested and fitted with hew hearing aids. She hears much better with the aids though she is still trying to adjust to wearing them. **Code "1" for Improved.**

SECTION D. VISION PATTERNS

Intent: To record the resident's visual abilities and limitations over the past seven days, assuming adequate lighting and assistance of visual appliances, if used.

1. Vision

Intent: To evaluate the resident's ability to see close objects in adequate lighting, using the resident's customary visual appliances for close vision (e.g., glasses, magnifying glass).

Definition: **"Adequate" lighting** — What is sufficient or comfortable for a person with normal vision.

Process:

- Ask direct care staff over all shifts if possible, if the resident has manifested any change in usual vision patterns over the past seven days — e.g., is the resident still able to read newsprint, menus, greeting cards, etc.?

- Then ask the resident about his or her visual abilities.

- Test the accuracy of your findings by asking the resident to look at regular-size print in a book or newspaper with whatever visual appliance he or she customarily uses for close vision (e.g., glasses, magnifying glass). Then ask the resident to read aloud, starting with larger headlines and ending with the finest, smallest print.

- Be sensitive to the fact that some residents are not literate or are unable to read English. In such cases, ask the resident to read aloud individual letters of different size print or numbers, such as dates or page numbers, or to name items in small pictures.

- If the resident is unable to communicate or follow your directions for testing vision, observe the resident's eye movements to see if his or her eyes seem to follow movement and objects. Though these are gross measurements of visual acuity, they may assist you in assessing whether the resident has any visual ability.

Coding: Enter the number corresponding to the most correct response.

0. **Adequate** — The resident sees fine detail, including regular print in newspapers/books.

1. **Impaired** — The resident sees large print, but not regular print in newspapers/books.

2. **Moderately Impaired** — The resident has limited vision, is not able to see newspaper headlines, but can identify objects in his or her environment.

3. **Highly Impaired** — The resident's ability to identify objects in his or her environment is in question, but the resident's eye movements appear to be following objects (especially people walking by).

Note: Many residents with severe cognitive impairment are unable to participate in vision screening because they are unable to follow directions or are unable to tell you what they see. However, many such residents appear to "track" or follow moving objects in their environment with their eyes. For residents who appear to do this, use code "3", Highly Impaired. With our current limited technology, this is the best assessment you can do under the circumstances.

4. **Severely Impaired** — The resident has no vision; sees only light colors or shapes; or eyes do not appear to be following objects (especially people walking by).

2. Visual Limitations/Difficulties

Intent: To document whether the resident experiences visual limitations or difficulties related to diseases common in aged persons (e.g., cataracts, glaucoma, macular degeneration, diabetic retinopathy, neurologic diseases). It is important to identify whether these conditions are present. Some eye problems may be treatable and reversible; others, though not reversible, may be managed by interventions aimed at maintaining or improving the resident's residual visual abilities.

Process: **Side vision problems** — Observe the resident during his or her daily routine (e.g., eating meals, traveling down a hallway). Also, ask the resident about any vision problems (e.g., spilling food, bumping into objects and people). Ask the primary nurse assistant and other direct-care staff on each shift if possible, whether the resident appears to have difficulties related to decreased peripheral vision (e.g., leaves food on one side of tray, has difficulty traveling, bumps into people and objects, misjudges placement of chair when seating self).

Experiences any of the following — Ask the resident directly if he or she is seeing halos or rings around lights, flashes of light, or "curtains" over the eyes. Ask staff members if the resident complains about any of these problems.

Coding: Check all that apply. If none apply, check *NONE OF ABOVE*.

3. Visual Appliances

Intent: To determine if the resident uses visual appliances regularly.

Definition: Glasses; contact lenses; magnifying glass — Includes any type of corrective device used at any time during the last seven days.

Coding: Enter "1" if the resident used glasses, contact lenses, or a magnifying glass during the past seven days. Enter "0" if none apply.

SECTION E.
MOOD AND BEHAVIOR PATTERNS

Mood distress is a serious condition and is associated with significant morbidity. Associated factors include poor adjustment to the nursing home, functional impairment, resistance to daily care, inability to participate in activities, isolation, increased risk of medical illness, cognitive impairment, and an increased sensitivity to physical pain. It is particularly important to identify signs and symptoms of mood distress among elderly nursing home residents because they are very treatable.

In many facilities, staff have not received specific training in how to evaluate residents who have distressed mood or behavioral symptoms. Therefore, many problems are underdiagnosed and undertreated. In facilities where such training has not occurred, an in-service program under the direction of a professional mental health specialist is recommended. At a minimum, staff in such facilities have found the various mental health RAPs (e.g., Mood, Behavior) to be helpful and these should be carefully reviewed.

1. Indicators of Depression, Anxiety, Sad Mood

Intent: To record the frequency of indicators observed in the last 30 days, irrespective of the assumed cause of the indicator (behavior).

Definition: Feelings of psychic distress may be expressed directly by the resident who is depressed, anxious, or sad. However, statements such as "I'm so depressed" are rare in the older nursing home population. Rather, distress is more commonly expressed in the following ways:

VERBAL EXPRESSIONS OF DISTRESS

a. **Resident made negative statements** — e.g., "Nothing matters; Would rather be dead; What's the use; Regrets having lived so long; Let me die."

b. **Repetitive questions** — e.g., "Where do I go; What do I do?"

c. **Repetitive verbalizations** — e.g., Calling out for help, ("God help me").

d. **Persistent anger with self or others** — e.g., easily annoyed, anger at placement in nursing home; anger at care received.

e. **Self deprecation** — e.g., "I am nothing; I am of no use to anyone".

f. **Expressions of what appear to be unrealistic fears** — e.g., fear of being abandoned, left alone, being with others.

g. **Recurrent statements that something terrible is about to happen** — e.g., believes he or she is about to die, have a heart attack.

h. **Repetitive health complaints** — e.g., persistently seeks medical attention, obsessive concern with body functions.

I. **Repetitive anxious complaints/concerns (non-health related)** — e.g., persistently seeks attention/reassurance regarding schedules, meals, laundry, clothing, relationship issues.

DISTRESS MAY ALSO BE EXPRESSED NON-VERBALLY AND IDENTIFIED THROUGH OBSERVATION OF THE RESIDENT IN THE FOLLOWING AREAS DURING USUAL DAILY ROUTINES:

SLEEP CYCLE ISSUES — Distress can also be manifested through disturbed sleep patterns.

j. **Unpleasant mood in morning**

k. **Insomnia/change in usual sleep pattern** — e.g., difficulty falling asleep, fewer or more hours of sleep than usual, waking up too early and unable to fall back to sleep

SAD, APATHETIC, ANXIOUS APPEARANCE

l. **Sad, pained, worried facial expressions** — e.g., furrowed brows

m. **Crying, tearfulness**

n. **Repetitive physical movements** — e.g., pacing, hand wringing, restlessness, fidgeting, picking

LOSS OF INTEREST. These items refer to a change in resident's usual pattern of behavior.

o. **Withdrawal from activities of interest** — e.g., no interest in long standing activities or being with family/friends

p. **Reduced social interaction** — e.g., less talkative, more isolated

Process: Initiate a conversation with the resident. Some residents are more verbal about their feelings than others and will either tell someone about their distress, or tell someone only when directly asked how they feel. Other residents may be unable to articulate their feelings (i.e., cannot find the words to describe how they feel, or lack insight or cognitive capacity). Observe residents carefully for any indicator. Consult with direct-care staff over all shifts, if possible, and family who have direct knowledge of the resident's behavior. Relevant information may also be found in the clinical record.

Coding: For each indicator apply one of the following codes based on interactions with and observations of the resident in the last 30 days. Remember, code regardless of what you believe the cause to be.

0. Indicator not exhibited in last 30 days
1. Indicator of this type exhibited up to five days a week (*i.e., exhibited at least once during the last 30 days but less than 6 days a week*).
2. Indicator of this type exhibited daily or almost daily (6, 7 days a week)

Example

Mr. F is a new admission who becomes upset and angry when his daughter visits (3 times a week). He complains to her and staff caregivers that 'she put me in this terrible dump.' He chastizes her 'for not taking him into her home', and berates her 'for being an ungrateful daughter.' After she leaves, he becomes remorseful, sad looking, tearful, and says "What's the use. I'm no good. I wish I died when my wife did." **Coding "1" for a. (Resident made negative statements), d. (Persistent anger with self or others), e. (Self deprecation), m. (Crying, tearfulness); remaining Mood items would be coded "0".**

2. Mood Persistence

Intent: To identify if one or more indicators of depressed, sad or anxious mood were not easily altered by attempts to "cheer up", console, or reassure the resident over the last seven days.

Process: Observe the resident and discuss the situation with direct caregivers over all shifts, if possible, and family members or friends who visit frequently or have frequent telephone contact with the resident.

Coding: Enter "0" if the resident did not exhibit any mood indicators over last 7 days, "1" if indicators were present and easily altered by staff interactions with the resident or "2" if any indicator was present but not easily altered (e.g., behavior persisted despite staff efforts to console resident).

3. Change in Mood

Intent: To document changes in the resident's mood as compared to his or her status of 90 days ago (or since last assessment if less than 90 days ago). If the resident is a new admission to the facility, this item includes changes during the period prior to admission.

Definition: **Change in Mood** — Refers to status of any of the symptoms (new onset, improvement, worsening) described in item E1 (verbal expressions of distress, sleep cycle issues, sad apathetic, anxious appearance, loss of interest or other signs) and item E2 (mood persistence). Such changes include:

- increased or decreased **numbers** of expressions or signs of distress
- increased or decreased **frequency** of distress occurrence
- increased or decreased **intensity** of expressions or signs of distress

Process: Review the clinical records including the last Quarterly Assessment findings and transmittal records of newly admitted residents. Interview and observe the resident. Consult with staff from all shifts, if possible, to clarify your observations.

Coding: Code "0" if No Change, "1" if Improved, or "2" if Deteriorated as compared to status of 90 days ago.

Examples of Changes in Mood

Mrs. Y has bipolar disease. Historically, she has responded well to lithium and her mood state has been stable for almost a year. About two months ago, she became extremely sad and withdrawn, expressed the wish that she were dead, and stopped eating. She was transferred to a psychiatric hospital for evaluation and treatment. Since her return to the nursing home three weeks ago, her mood and appetite have improved while on a new lithium dose and an additional antidepressant drug. She is back to her "old self" of 90 days ago. **Code "0" for No change.**

During the admission assessment period of 90 days ago, Mr. M was tearful and expressed great sadness and anger over entering the nursing home. He had difficulties falling asleep at night, was restless off and on during the night, and awakened too early in the morning, upset that he couldn't fall back to sleep. Since that time, Mr. M has been involved in a twice weekly support group, and has been enjoying socializing in activities with new friends. He is currently sleeping through the night and feels well in the morning. Although he still expresses sadness and anger over his need for nursing home care, it is less frequent and intense. **Code "1" for Improved.**

Mrs. D has a long history of depression. Two months ago she had an adverse reaction to a psychoactive drug. She expressed fears that she was going out of her mind and was observed to be quite agitated. Her attention span diminished and she stopped attending group activities because she was too restless. After the medication was discontinued, intensity of feelings and behaviors diminished and she has less frequent episodes of agitation. Mrs. D is better than she was, but she still has feelings of sadness. Mrs. D is now better than her worst status two months ago, but she has not fully recovered to her status of 90 days ago. **Code "2" for Deteriorated.**

During the admission assessment 6 weeks ago, Mrs. Z was very agitated. She had multiple daily complaints of vague aches and pains. She repetitively asked the nurses to "Call the doctor, I'm sick". After no physical problems could be identified, Mrs. Z was evaluated by a psychiatrist who diagnosed a clinical depression and prescribed an antidepressant drug. Its effect on Mrs. Z has been dramatic. During this Significant Change assessment, Mrs. Z had many fewer complaints about her health and was more involved in unit activities. **Code "1" for Improved.**

4. Behavioral Symptoms

Intent: To identify a.) the frequency and b.) alterability of behavioral symptoms in the last seven days that cause distress to the resident, or are distressing or disruptive to facility residents or staff members. Such behaviors include those that are potentially harmful to the resident himself or herself or disruptive in the environment, even if staff and other residents appear to have adjusted to them (e.g.,

"Mrs. R's calling out isn't much different than others on the unit. There are many noisy residents;" or "Mrs. L doesn't mean to hit me. She does it because she's confused.")

Acknowledging and documenting the resident's behavioral symptom patterns on the MDS provides a basis for further evaluation, care planning, and delivery of consistent, appropriate care towards ameliorating the behavioral symptoms. Documentation in the clinical record of the resident's current status may not be accurate or valid, and it is not intended to be the one and only source of information. (See Process below). However, once the frequency and alterability of behavioral symptoms is accurately determined, subsequent documentation should more accurately reflect the resident's status and response to interventions.

Definition: **Wandering** — Locomotion with no discernible, rational purpose. A wandering resident may be oblivious to his or her physical or safety needs. Wandering behavior should be differentiated from purposeful movement (e.g., a hungry person moving about the unit in search of food). Wandering may be manifested by walking or by wheelchair.

Do not include pacing as wandering behavior. Pacing back and forth is not considered wandering, and if it occurs, it should be documented in Item E1n, "Repetitive physical movements".

Verbally Abusive Behavioral Symptoms — Other residents or staff were threatened, screamed at, or cursed at.

Physically Abusive Behavioral Symptoms — Other residents or staff were hit, shoved, scratched, or sexually abused.

Socially Inappropriate/Disruptive Behavioral Symptoms — Includes disruptive sounds, excessive noise, screams, self-abusive acts, or sexual behavior or disrobing in public, smearing or throwing food or feces, hoarding, rummaging through others' belongings.

Resists care — Resists taking medications/injections, ADL assistance or help with eating. This category does not include instances where the resident has made an informed choice not to follow a course of care (e.g., resident has exercised his or her right to refuse treatment, and reacts negatively as staff try to reinstitute treatment).

Signs of resistance may be verbal and/or physical (e.g., verbally refusing care, pushing caregiver away, scratching caregiver). These behaviors are not necessarily positive or negative, but are intended to provide information about the resident's responses to nursing interventions and to prompt further investigation of causes for care planning purposes (e.g., fear of pain, fear of falling, poor comprehension, anger, poor relationships, eagerness for greater participation in care decisions, past experience with medication errors and unacceptable care, desire to modify care being provided).

Process: Take an objective view of the resident's behavioral symptoms. The coding for this item focuses on the resident's actions, not intent. It is often difficult to determine the meaning behind a particular behavioral symptom. Therefore, it is important to start the assessment by recording any behavioral symptoms. The fact that staff have become used to the behavior and minimize the resident's presumed intent ("He doesn't really mean to hurt anyone. He's just frightened.") is not pertinent to this coding. Does the resident manifest the behavioral symptom or not? Is the resident combative during personal care and strike out at staff or not?

Observe the resident. Observe how the resident responds to staff members' attempts to deliver care to him or her. Consult with staff who provide direct care on all three shifts. A symptomatic behavior can be present and the RN Assessment Coordinator might not see it because it occurs during intimate care on another shift. Therefore, it is especially important that input from all nurse assistants having contact with the resident be solicited.

Also, be alert to the possibility that staff might not think to report a behavioral symptom if it is part of the unit norm (e.g., staff are working with severely cognitively and functionally impaired residents and are used to residents' wandering, noisiness, etc.). Focus staff attention on what has been the individual resident's actual behavior over the last seven days. Finally, although it may not be complete, review the clinical record for documentation.

Coding: **(A) Behavioral symptom frequency in last 7 days.**

Record the frequency of behavioral symptoms manifested by the resident across all three shifts.

Code "0" if the described behavioral symptom was not exhibited in last seven days.

For each type of behavior described on the MDS form, Code "0" if the resident did not exhibit that type of symptom in the last seven days. This code applies to residents who have never exhibited the behavioral symptom or those who have previously exhibited the symptom but now no longer exhibit it, including those whose behavioral symptoms are fully managed by psychotropic drugs, restraints, or a behavior-management program. For example: A "wandering" resident who did not wander in the last seven days because he was restricted to a geri-chair would be coded "0" — Behavioral symptom not exhibited in last seven days. The questionable clinical practice of restricting wandering by placing a person in a geri-chair to restrict movement would then be evaluated using the Physical Restraints RAP.

Code "1" if the described behavioral symptom occurred 1 to 3 days, in last 7 days.

Code "2" if the described behavioral symptom occurred 4 to 6 days, but less than daily.

Code "3" if the described behavioral symptom occurred daily or more frequently (i.e., multiple times each day).

(B) Behavioral symptom alterability in last 7 days.

Code "0" if either the behavioral symptom was not present or the behavioral symptom was easily altered with current interventions.

Code "1" if the described behavioral symptom occurred with a degree of intensity that is not responsive to staff attempts to reduce the behavioral symptom through limit setting, diversion, adapting unit routines to the resident's needs, environmental modification, activities programming, comfort measures, appropriate drug treatment, etc. For example: A cognitively impaired resident who hits staff during morning care and swears at staff with each physical contact on multiple occasions per day, and the behavior is not easily altered, would be coded "1".

Examples for Wandering	(A) Frequency	(B) Alterability
Ms. T has dementia and is severely impaired in making decisions about daily life on her unit. She is dependent on others to guide her through each day. When she is not involved in some type of activity (leisure, dining, ADLs, etc.) she wanders about the unit. Despite the repetitive, daily nature of her wandering, this behavior is easily channeled into other activities when staff redirect Ms. T by inviting her to activities. Ms. T is easily engaged and is content to stay and participate in whatever is going on.	3	0
Mr. W has dementia and is severely impaired in making daily decisions. He wanders all around the residential unit throughout each day. He is extremely hard of hearing and refuses to wear his hearing aid. He is easily frightened by others and cannot stay still for activities programs. Numerous attempts to redirect his wandering have been met with Mr. W hitting and pushing staff. Over time, staff have found him to be most content while he is wandering within a structured setting.	3	1

5. Change in Behavioral Symptoms

Intent: To document whether the behavioral symptoms or resistance to care exhibited by the resident remained stable, increased or decreased in frequency of occurrence or alterability as compared to his or her status of 90 days ago (or since last assessment if less than 90 days ago). Consider changes in any area, including (but not limited to) wandering, symptoms of verbal or physical abuse or aggressiveness, socially inappropriate behavior, or resistance to care. If the resident is a new admission to the facility, this item includes changes during the period prior to admission.

Definition: **Change in behavioral symptoms** — refers to the status (new onset, improvement, worsening) of any of the symptoms described in item E4 (Behavioral Symptoms). Such changes include:

- increased or decreased **numbers** of behavioral symptoms
- increased or decreased **frequency** of behavioral symptoms occurrence
- increased or decreased **intensity** of behavioral symptoms
- increased or decreased **alterability** of behavioral symptoms.

Process: Review nursing notes and resident's records, including the last Quarterly Assessment findings and transmittal records of newly admitted residents. Observe the resident. Consult with direct care staff across all shifts, if possible, and family to clarify your observations.

Coding: **Code "0"** if no change has occurred in behavioral symptoms. This code should also be used for the resident who has no behavioral symptoms currently or 90 days ago.

Code "1" (Improved) if the behavioral symptoms became fewer, less frequent, less intense, and were not complicated by the onset of additional behavioral symptoms as compared to 90 days ago.

Code "2" (Deteriorated) if the behavioral symptoms became more frequent or more intense or were complicated by the onset of additional behavioral symptoms as compared to 90 days ago.

Examples of Change in Behavioral Symptoms

Despite staff efforts to provide support and structure over the last 90 days, Mrs. H continues to hoard food in her room every day. Staff understand the needs of this formerly homeless woman, but because they have found ants and cockroaches in her room, they feel a need to reevaluate their approach to care. **Code "0" for No change since last assessment.**

During the seven day assessment period, Mrs. D had a difficult time with bowel regularity. She had a history of constipation that became worse during an episode of pneumonia and poor fluid intake that resulted in dehydration. During this time Mrs. D was more confused and subdued. She was found on several occasions during the assessment period disimpacting herself and smearing feces (Socially Inappropriate/Disruptive Behavior). Upon examination Mrs. D was found to have a fecal impaction. She received treatment and was placed on a bowel regimen. The program was successful in eliminating the socially inappropriate behavioral symptoms that was induced by discomfort. However, once Mrs. D started to feel better and was more alert, she resumed her former daily wandering (of 4 months ago), pushing others and rummaging through their dresser drawers. **Code "0" for No change since last assessment.**

Mrs. F has always been a quiet passive woman who has never exhibited any behavioral symptoms since her admission to the nursing home. During this Significant Change assessment following Mrs. F's stroke, no problematic behavioral symptoms were noted. **Code "0" for No change since last assessment.**

(continued on next page)

Examples of Change in Behavioral Symptoms (continued)

Mr. C wanders in and out of other residents' rooms and rummages through their belongings at least once a day and sometimes more often. Despite this behavior, during the last few weeks, he has been easier to work with now that he is more familiar with staff. Although wandering and rummaging continue, he no longer screams, curses, and shoves residents and staff who try to stop this behavior as he did 90 days ago. **Code "1" for Improved.**

Ninety days ago Mrs. R banged her cane loudly and repetitively on the dining/activity room table about once a week. In the past week, staff have noticed that this socially inappropriate behavioral symptom (disruptive sounds) now occurs multiple times daily. **Code "2" for Deteriorated.**

SECTION F. PSYCHOSOCIAL WELL-BEING

Intent: To determine the resident's emotional adjustment to the nursing facility, including his or her general attitude, adaptation to surroundings, and change in relationship patterns.

1. Sense of Initiative/Involvement

Intent: To assess the degree to which the resident is involved in the life of the nursing home and takes initiative in participating in various social and recreational programs, including solitary pursuits.

Definitions: **At ease interacting with others** — Consider how the resident behaves during the time you are together, as well as reports of how the resident behaves with other residents, staff, and visitors. A resident who tries to shield himself or herself from being with others, spends most time alone, or becomes agitated when visited, is not "at ease interacting with others."

At ease doing planned or structured activities — Consider how the resident responds to organized social or recreational activities. A resident who feels comfortable with the structure or not restricted by it is "at ease doing planned or structured activities." A resident who is unable to sit still in organized group activities and either acts disruptive or makes attempts to leave, or refuses to attend any such activities, is not "at ease doing planned or structured activities."

At ease doing self-initiated activities — These include leisure activities (e.g., reading, watching TV, talking with friends), and work activities (e.g., folding personal laundry, organizing belongings). A resident who spends most of his or her time alone and unoccupied, or who is always looking for someone to find something for him or her to do, is not "at ease doing self-initiated activities."

Establishes own goals — Consider statements the resident makes, such as "I hope I am able to walk again," or "I would like to get up early and visit the beauty parlor." Goals can be as traditional as wanting to learn how to walk again following a hip replacement, or wanting to live to say goodbye to a loved one. However, some goals may not actually be verbalized by the resident, but inferred in that the resident is observed to have an individual way of living at the facility (e.g., organizing own activities or setting own pace).

Pursues involvement in life of facility — In general, consider whether the resident partakes of facility events, socializes with peers, and discusses activities as if he or she is part of things. A resident who conveys a sense of belonging to the community represented by the nursing home or the particular nursing unit is "involved in the life of the facility."

Accepts invitations into most group activities — A resident who is willing to try group activities even if later deciding the activity is not suitable and leaving, or who does not regularly refuse to attend group programs, "accepts invitations into most group activities."

Process: Selected responses should be confirmed by objective observation of the resident's behavior (either verbal or nonverbal) in a variety of settings (e.g., in own room, in unit dining room, in activities room) and situations (e.g., alone, in one-on-one situations, in groups) over the past seven days. The primary source of information is the resident. Talk with the resident and ask about his or her perception (how he or she feels), how he or she likes to do things, and how he or she responds to specific situations. Then talk with staff members who have regular contact with the resident (e.g., nurse assistants, activities personnel, social work staff, or therapists if the person receives active rehabilitation). Remember, it is possible for discrepancies to exist between how the resident sees himself or herself and how he or she actually behaves. Use your best clinical judgment as a basis for planning care.

Coding: Check all that apply. None of the choices are to be construed as negative or positive. Each is simply a statement to be checked if it applies and not checked if it does not apply. If you do not check any items in Section F1, check *NONE*

OF ABOVE. For individualized care-planning purposes, remember that information conveyed by unchecked items is no less important than information conveyed by checked items.

2. Unsettled Relationships

Intent: To indicate the quality and nature of the resident's interpersonal contacts (i.e., how the resident interacts with staff members, family, and other residents).

Definition: **Covert/open conflict with or repeated criticism of staff** — The resident chronically complains about some staff members to other staff members, verbally criticizes staff members in therapeutic group situations causing disruption within the group, or constantly disagrees with routines of daily life on the unit. Checking this item does not require any assumption about why the problem exists or how it might be remedied.

Unhappy with roommate — This category also includes "bathroom mate" for residents who share a private bathroom. Unhappiness may be manifested by frequent requests for roommate changes, or grumbling about "bathroom mate" spending too long in the bathroom, or complaints about roommate rummaging in one's belongings, or complaints about physical, mental, or behavioral status of roommate. Other examples of roommate compatibility issues include early bedtime vs. staying up and watching TV, neat vs. sloppy maintenance of personal area, roommate spending too much time on the telephone, or snoring, or odors from incontinence or poor hygiene.

Unhappy with residents other than roommate — May be manifested by chronic complaints about the behaviors of others, poor quality of interaction with other residents, or lack of peers for socialization. This definition refers to conflict or disagreement outside of the range of normal criticisms or requests (i.e., repetitive, ongoing complaints beyond a reasonable level).

Openly expresses conflict/anger with family/friends — Includes expressions of feelings of abandonment, ungratefulness on part of family, lack of understanding by close friends, or hostility regarding relationships with family or friends.

Absence of personal contact with family/friends — Absence of visitors or telephone calls from others in the last seven days.

Recent loss of close family member/friend — Includes relocation of family member/friend to a more distant location, even temporarily (e.g., for the winter months), incapacitation or death of a significant other, or a significant relationship that recently ceased (e.g., a favorite nurse assistant transferred to work on another unit).

Does not adjust easily to change in routines — Signs of anger, prolonged confusion, or agitation when changes in usual routines occur (e.g., staff turnover or reassignment; new treatment or medication routines; changes in activity or meal programs; new roommate).

Example

For the past 6 months Mrs. A has been receiving 2 white pills, 1 blue pill, 1 yellow pill and 2 puffs of medication from an orange hand-held aerosol inhaler. The drug company that makes the inhaler recently changed its packaging. When Mrs. G is given the new blue inhaler to use and is told that it is the same drug with a different color holder, she becomes very agitated and upset. It takes a lot of patience and reassurance by the nurse before Mrs. G uses the new inhaler. This happened for several days during the past week.

Process: Ask the resident for his or her point of view. Is he or she generally content in relationships with staff and family, or are there feelings of unhappiness? If the resident is unhappy, what specifically is he or she unhappy about?

It is also important to talk with family members who visit or have frequent telephone contact with the resident. How have relationships with the resident been in the last seven days?

During routine nursing care activities, observe how the resident interacts with staff members and other residents. Do you see signs of conflict? Talk with direct-care staff (e.g., nurse assistants, dietary aides who assist in the dining room, social work staff, or activities aides) and ask for their observations of behavior that indicate either conflicted or harmonious interpersonal relationships. Consider the possibility that some staff members describing these relationships may be biased. As the evaluator, you are seeking to gain an overall picture, a consensus view.

Coding: Check all that apply over the last seven days. If none apply, check *NONE OF ABOVE.*

3. Past Roles

Intent: To document the resident's recognition or acceptance of feelings regarding previous roles or status now that he or she is living in a nursing home.

Definition: ***Strong identification with past roles and life status*** — *This may be indicated*, for example, when the resident enjoys telling stories about his or her past, or takes pride in past accomplishments or family life, or continues to be connected with prior lifestyle (e.g., celebrating family events, carrying on life-long traditions).

Expresses sadness/anger/empty feeling over lost roles/status — Resident expresses feelings such as "I'm not the man I used to be" or "I wish I had been a better mother to my children" or "It's no use, I'm not capable of doing things I like to do anymore." Resident cries when reminiscing about past failures, accomplishments, memories.

Resident perceives that daily routine (customary routine, activities) is very different from prior pattern in the community — In general, the resident's pattern of routines is perceived by the resident not to be comparable with his or her previous lifestyle.

Examples

In the nursing home, resident takes a shower 2 mornings a week vs. taking a daily tub bath before going to bed as she did at home.

The resident now retires at 7 pm whereas at home he stayed up to watch the 11 pm news.

In the community Mrs. L enjoyed multiple daily telephone conversations with her 5 daughters. In the nursing home there is only one public telephone that seems to be in constant use by residents and staff. Mrs. L now speaks with each daughter only once a week.

Process: Initiate a conversation with the resident about life prior to nursing home admission. It is often helpful to use environmental cues to prompt discussions (e.g., family photos, grandchildren's letters or art work). This information may emerge from discussions around other MDS topics (e.g., Customary Routine, Activity Pursuits, ADLs). Direct care staff and family visitors may also have useful insights.

Coding: Check item if it applies over the last seven days. If none apply, Check *NONE OF ABOVE*.

SECTION G. PHYSICAL FUNCTIONING AND STRUCTURAL PROBLEMS

Most nursing home residents are at risk of physical decline. Most residents also have multiple chronic illnesses and are subject to a variety of other factors that can severely impact self-sufficiency. For example, cognitive deficits can limit ability or willingness to initiate or participate in self-care or constrict understanding of the tasks required to complete ADLs. A wide range of physical and neurological illnesses can adversely affect physical factors important to self-care such as stamina, muscle tone, balance, and bone strength. Side effects of medications and other treatments can also contribute to needless loss of self-sufficiency.

Due to these many, possibly adverse influences, a resident's potential for maximum functionality is often greatly underestimated by family, staff, and the resident himself or herself. Thus, all residents are candidates for nursing-based rehabilitative care that focuses on maintaining and expanding self-involvement in ADLs. Individualized plans of care can be successfully developed only when the resident's self-performance has been accurately assessed and the amount and type of support being provided to the resident by others has been evaluated.

1. (A) Activities of Daily Living (ADL) Self-Performance

Intent: To record the resident's self-care performance in activities of daily living (i.e., what the resident actually did for himself or herself and/or how much verbal or physical help was required by staff members) during the **last seven days**.

Definition: **ADL SELF-PERFORMANCE** — Measures what the resident actually did (not what he or she might be capable of doing) within each ADL category over the last seven days according to a performance-based scale.

Bed Mobility — How the resident moves to and from a lying position, turns side to side, and positions body while in bed.

Transfer — How the resident moves between surfaces — i.e., to/from bed, chair, wheelchair, standing position. Exclude from this definition movement to/from bath or toilet, which is covered under Toilet Use and Bathing.

Walk in room — How resident walks between locations in his/her room.

Walk in corridor — How resident walks in corridor on unit.

Locomotion on unit — How the resident moves between locations in his or her room and adjacent corridor on the same floor. If the resident is in a wheelchair, locomotion is defined as self-sufficiency once in the chair.

Locomotion off unit — How the resident moves to and returns from off unit locations (e.g., areas set aside for dining, activities, or treatments). If the facility has only one floor, locomotion off the unit is defined as how the resident moves to and from distant areas on the floor. If in wheelchair, self-sufficiency once in chair.

Dressing— How the resident puts on, fastens, and takes off all items of street clothing, including donning/removing a prosthesis.

Eating — How the resident eats and drinks, regardless of skill. Includes intake of nourishment by other means (e.g., tube feeding, total parenteral nutrition).

Toilet Use — How the resident uses the toilet room, commode, bedpan, or urinal, transfers on/off toilet, cleanses, changes pad, manages ostomy or catheter, and adjusts clothes.

Personal Hygiene — How the resident maintains personal hygiene, including combing hair, brushing teeth, showering, applying makeup, and washing/drying face, hands, and perineum. Exclude from this definition personal hygiene in baths and showers, which is covered under Bathing.

Bathing— How the resident takes a full-body bath/shower, sponge bath, and transfers in/out of tub/shower. Exclude washing of back and hair.

Process: In order to be able to promote the highest level of functioning among residents, clinical staff must first identify what the resident actually does for himself or herself, noting when assistance is received and clarifying the types of assistance provided (verbal cueing, physical support, etc.)

A resident's ADL self-performance may vary from day to day, shift to shift, or within shifts. There are many possible reasons for these variations, including mood, medical condition, relationship issues (e.g., willing to perform for a nurse assistant he or she likes), and medications. The responsibility of the person completing the assessment, therefore, is to capture the total picture of the resident's ADL self-performance over the seven day period, 24 hours a day — i.e., not only how the evaluating clinician sees the resident, but how the resident performs on other shifts as well.

In order to accomplish this, it is necessary to gather information from multiple sources — i.e., interviews/discussion with the resident and direct care staff on all three shifts, including weekends and review of documentation used to communicate with staff across shifts. Ask questions pertaining to all aspects of the ADL activity definitions. For example, when discussing Bed Mobility with a nurse assistant, be sure to inquire specifically how the resident moves to and from a lying position, how the resident turns from side to side, and how the resident positions himself or herself while in bed. A resident can be independent in one aspect of Bed Mobility yet require extensive assistance in another aspect. Since accurate coding is important as a basis for making decisions on the type and amount of care to be provided, be sure to consider each activity definition fully.

The wording used in each coding option is intended to reflect real-world situations in nursing homes, where slight variations are common. Where variations occur, the coding ensures that the resident is not assigned to an excessively independent or dependent category. For example, by definition, codes 0, 1, 2, and 3 (Independent, Supervision, Limited Assistance, and Extensive Assistance) permit one or two exceptions for the provision of heavier care. This is clinically useful and increases the likelihood that staff will code ADL Self-Performance items consistently and accurately.

Because this section involves a two-part evaluation (Item G1A. ADL Self-Performance and Item G1B, ADL Support), each using its own scale, it is recommended that you complete the Self-Performance evaluation for all ADL Self-Performance activities before beginning the ADL Support evaluation.

To evaluate a resident's ADL Self-Performance, begin by reviewing the documentation in the clinical record. Talk with clinical staff from each shift to ascertain what the resident does for himself or herself in each ADL activity as well as the type and level of staff assistance being provided. As previously noted, be alert to differences in resident performance from shift to shift, and apply the ADL codes that capture these differences. For example, a resident may be independent in Toilet Use during daylight hours but receive non-weight bearing physical assistance every evening. In this case, the resident would be coded as “2” (Limited Assistance) in Toilet Use.

The following chart provides general guidelines for recording accurate ADL Self-Performance and ADL Support assessments.

Guidelines for Assessing ADL Self-Performance and ADL Support

- The scales in Items G1A and G1B are used to record the resident's actual level of involvement in self-care and the type and amount of support actually received during the last seven days.

- Do not record your assessment of the resident's capacity for involvement in self-care — i.e., what you believe the resident might be able to do for himself or herself based on demonstrated skills or physical attributes. An assessment of potential capability is covered in Item G8 ("ADL Functional Rehabilitation Potential").

- Do not record the type and level of assistance that the resident "should" be receiving according to the written plan of care. The type and level of assistance actually provided may be quite different from what is indicated in the plan. Record what is actually happening.

- Engage direct care staff from all shifts who have cared for the resident over the last seven days in discussions regarding the resident's ADL functional performance. Remind staff that the focus is on the last seven days only. To clarify your own understanding and observations about each ADL activity (bed mobility, locomotion, transfer, etc.), ask probing questions, beginning with the general and proceeding to the more specific.

Here is a typical conversation between the RN Assessment Coordinator and a nurse assistant regarding a resident's Bed Mobility assessment:

R.N. "Describe to me how Mrs. L positions herself in bed. By that I mean, once she is in bed, how does she move from sitting up to lying down, lying down to sitting up, turning side to side, and positioning herself?"

N.A. "She can lay down and sit up by herself, but I help her turn on her side."

R.N. "She lays down and sits up without any verbal instructions or physical help?"

N.A. "No, I have to remind her to use her trapeze every time. But once I tell her how to do things, she can do it herself."

R.N. "How do you help her turn side to side?"

N.A. "She can help turn herself by grabbing onto her siderail. I tell her what to do. But she needs me to lift her bottom and guide her legs into a good position."

R.N. "Do you lift her by yourself or does someone help you?"

N.A. "I do it by myself."

R.N. "How many days during the last week did you give this type of help?

N.A. "Every day."

Provided that ADL function in Bed Mobility was similar on all shifts, Mrs. L would receive an ADL Self-Performance Code of "3" (Extensive Assistance) and an ADL Support Provided Code of "2" (one person physical assist).

Now review the first two exchanges in the conversation between the RN Assessment Coordinator and nurse assistant. If the RN did not probe further, he or she would not have received enough information to make an accurate assessment of either the resident's skills or the nurse assistant's actual workload, or whether the current plan of care was being implemented.

Coding: For each ADL category, code the appropriate response for the resident's actual performance during the past seven days. Enter the code in column (A), labeled "SELF-PERF." Consider the resident's performance during all shifts, as functionality may vary. In the pages that follow two types of supplemental instructional material are presented to assist you in learning how to use this code: a schematic flow chart for scoring ADL Self Performance and a series of case examples for each ADL.

In your evaluations, you will also need to consider the type of assistance known as "set-up help" (e.g., comb, brush, toothbrush, toothpaste have been laid out at the bathroom sink by the nurse assistant). Set-up help is recorded under ADL Support Provided (Item G1B). But in evaluating the resident's ADL Self-Performance, include set-up help within the context of the "0" (Independent) code. For example: If a resident grooms independently once grooming items are set up for him, code "0" (Independent) in Personal Hygiene.

0. **Independent** — No help or staff oversight -OR- Staff help/oversight provided only one or two times during the last seven days.

1. **Supervision** — Oversight, encouragement, or cueing provided three or more times during last seven days -OR- Supervision (3 or more times) plus physical assistance provided only one or two times during last seven days.

2. **Limited Assistance** — Resident highly involved in activity, received physical help in guided maneuvering of limbs or other nonweight-bearing assistance on three or more occasions -OR- limited assistance (3 or more times) plus more help provided only one or two times during last seven days.

3. **Extensive Assistance** — While the resident performed part of activity over last seven days, help of following type(s) was provided three or more times:

   — Weight-bearing support provided three or more times
   — Full staff performance of activity (3 or more times) during part (but not all) of last seven days

4. **Total Dependence** — Full staff performance of the activity during entire seven-day period. Complete non-participation by the resident in all aspects of the ADL definition.

   For example: For a resident to be coded as totally dependent in Eating, he or she would be fed all food and liquids at all meals and snacks (including tube feeding delivered totally by staff), and never initiate any subtask of eating (e.g., picking up finger foods, giving self tube feeding or assisting with procedure) at any meal.

8. **Activity did not occur during the entire 7-day period** — Over the last seven days, the ADL activity was not performed by the resident or staff. In other words, the particular activity did not occur at all.

   For example: The definition of Dressing specifies the wearing of street clothes. During the seven day period, if the resident did not wear street clothing, a code of "8" would apply (i.e., the activity did not occur during the entire seven day period). Likewise, a resident who was restricted to bed for the entire seven day period and was never transferred from bed would receive a code of "8" for Transfer.

   However, do not confuse a resident who is totally dependent in an ADL activity (code 4 — Total Dependence) with the activity itself not occurring. For example: Even a resident who receives tube feedings and no food or fluids by mouth is engaged in eating (receiving nourishment), and must be evaluated under the Eating category for his or her level of assistance in the process. A resident who is highly involved in giving himself a tube feeding is not totally dependent and should not be coded as "4".

   Each of these ADL Self-Performance codes is exclusive; there is no overlap between categories. Changing from one self-performance category to another demands an increase or decrease in the number of times that help is provided. Thus, to move from Independent to Supervision to Limited Assistance, non weight-bearing supervision or physical assistance must increase from one or two times up to three or more times during the last seven days.

There will be times when no one type or level of assistance is provided to the resident 3 or more times during a 7-day period. However, the sum total of support of various types will be provided 3 or more times. In this case, code for the least dependent self-performance category where the resident received that level or more dependent support 3 or more times during the 7-day period.

Examples

The resident received supervision for walking in the corridor on two occasions and non weight-bearing assistance on two occasions. **Code "1" for Supervision in Walking in Corridor. Rationale:** Supervision is the least dependent category.

The resident received supervision in dressing on one occasion, non weight-bearing assistance (IE, putting a hat on resident's head) on two occasions, and weight-bearing assistance (IE, lifting resident's arm into a sleeve) on one occasion during the last 7 days. **Code "2" for Limited Assistance in Dressing. Rationale:** There were 3 episodes of physical assistance in the last 7 days: 2 non-weight-bearing episodes, and 1 weight-bearing episode. Limited Assistance is the correct code because it reflects the least dependent support category that encompasses 3 or more activities that were at least at that level of support.

SCORING ADL SELF PERFORMANCE

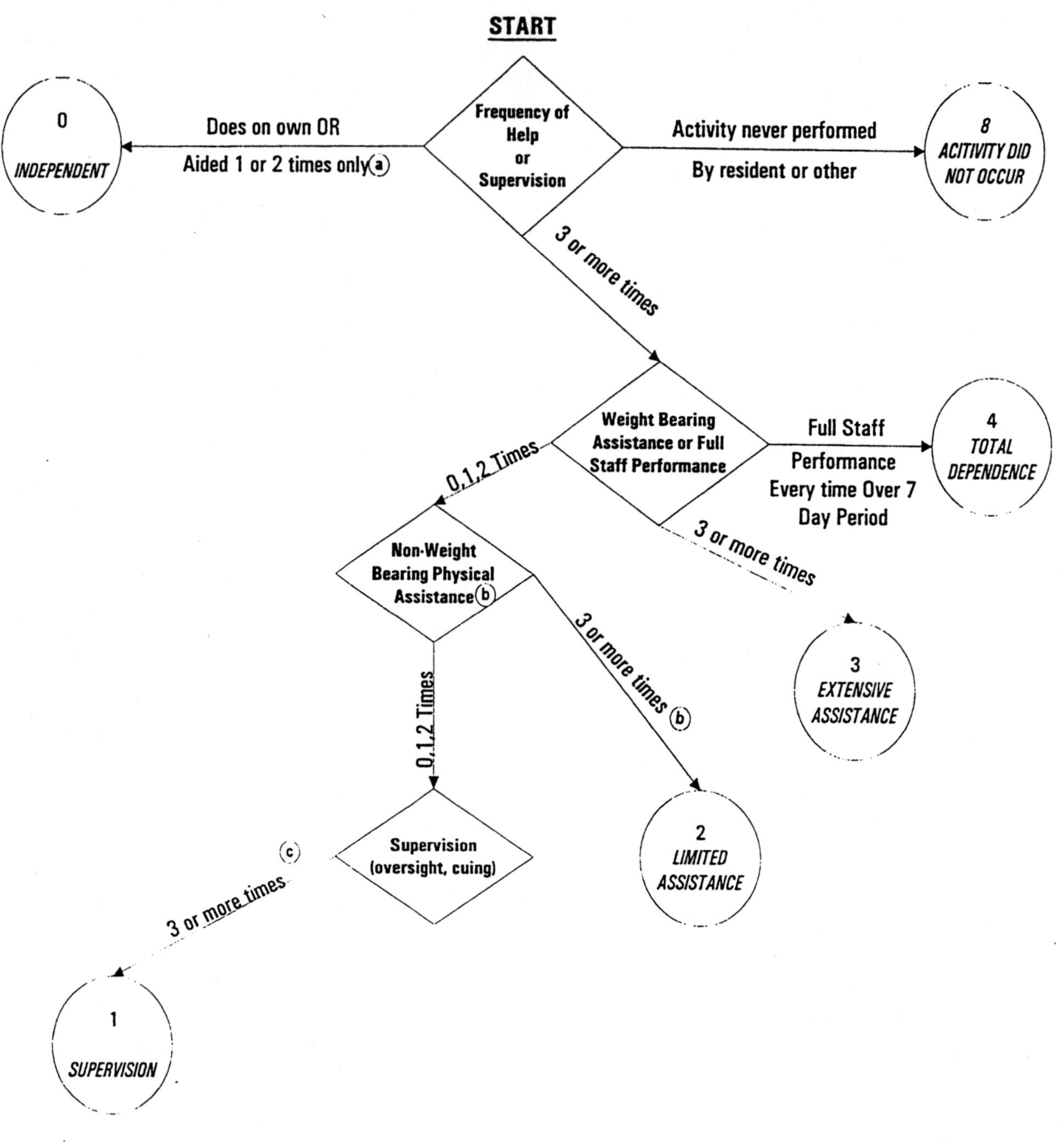

---

a. Can include one or two events where received supervision, non-weight bearing help, or weight bearing help.

b. Can include one or two episodes of weight bearing help--e.g., two events with non-weight bearing plus two of weight bearing would be coded as a "2".

c. Can include one or two episodes where physical help received--e.g., two episodes of supervision, one of weight bearing, and one of non-weight bearing would be coded as a "1".

1. (B) ADL Support Provided

Intent: To record the type and highest level of support the resident received in each ADL activity over the last seven days.

Definition: **ADL Support Provided** — Measures the highest level of support provided by staff over the last seven days, even if that level of support only occurred once. This is a different scale, and is entirely separate from the ADL Self-Performance assessment.

Set-up help — The type of help characterized by providing the resident with articles, devices or preparation necessary for greater resident self-performance in an activity. This can include giving or holding out an item that the resident takes from the caregiver.

Examples of Setup Help

- **For bed mobility** — handing the resident the bar on a trapeze.
- **For transfer** — giving the resident a transfer board or locking the wheels on a wheelchair for safe transfer.
- **For locomotion:**

  Walking — handing the resident a walker or cane.

  Wheeling— unlocking the brakes on the wheelchair or adjusting foot pedals to facilitate foot motion while wheeling.
- **For dressing** — retrieving clothes from closet and laying out on the resident's bed; handing the resident a shirt.
- **For eating** — cutting meat and opening containers at meals; giving one food category at a time.
- **For toilet use** — handing the resident a bedpan or placing articles necessary for changing ostomy appliance within reach.
- **For personal hygiene** — providing a wash basin and grooming articles.
- **For bathing** — placing bathing articles at tub side within the resident's reach; handing the resident a towel upon completion of bath.

Process: For each ADL category, code the maximum amount of support the resident received over the last seven days irrespective of frequency, and enter in the "SUPPORT" column. Be sure your evaluation considers all nursing shifts, 24 hours per day, including weekends. Code independently of the resident's Self-Performance evaluation. For example, a resident could have been Independent in ADL Self-Performance in Transfer but received a one-person physical assist one or two times during the seven-day period. Therefore, the ADL Self-Performance Coding for Transfer would be "0" (Independent), and the ADL Support coding "2" (One person physical assist).

Coding: Note: The highest code of physical assistance in this category (other than the "8" code) is a code of "3" not "4" as in Self-Performance.

0. **No setup or physical help from staff**

1. **Setup help only** — The resident is provided with materials or devices necessary to perform the activity of daily living independently.

2. **One person physical assist**

3. **Two+ persons physical assist**

8. **ADL activity itself did not occur during the entire 7-days** — When an "8" code is entered for an ADL Support Provided category, enter an "8" code for ADL Self-Performance in the same category.

For example, if a resident never left the unit during the assessment period, code "8" for locomotion off unit. The activity did not occur, there was no help provided.

The examples that follow clarify coding for both Self-Performance and Support. The answers appear to the right of the resident descriptions. Cover the answers, read and score the example, and then compare your answers with those provided.

Examples: ADL Self-Performance and Support	Self-Perf.	Support
Bed Mobility		
Resident was physically able to reposition self in bed but had a tendency to favor and remain on his left side. He received frequent reminders and monitoring to reposition self while in bed.	1	0
Resident received supervision and verbal cueing for using a trapeze for all bed mobility. On two occasions when arms were fatigued, he received heavier physical assistance of two persons.	1	3
Resident usually repositioned himself in bed. However, because he sleeps with the head of the bed raised 30 degrees, he occasionally slides down towards the foot of the bed. On 3 occasions the night nurse assistant helped him to reposition by providing weight-bearing support as he bent his knees and pushed up off the footboard.	3	2
To turn over, the resident always began by reaching for a side rail for support. He received physical assistance of one person to guide his legs into position and complete the turn by guiding him with a turn sheet (using weight-bearing assistance).	3	2
Resident independently turned on his left side whenever he wanted. Because of left-sided weakness he received physical weight bearing help of 1-2 persons to turn to his right side or sit up in bed.	3	3
Because of severe, painful joint deformities, resident was totally dependent on two persons for all bed mobility. Although unable to contribute physically to positioning process, she was able to cue staff for the position she wanted to assume and at what point she felt comfortable.	4	3

Examples: ADL Self-Performance and Support	Self-Perf.	Support
Transfer		
Despite bilateral above-the-knee amputations, resident almost always moved independently from bed to wheelchair (and back to bed) using a transfer board he retrieves independently from his bedside table. On one occasion in the past week, staff had to remind resident to retrieve the transfer board. On one other occasion, the resident was lifted by a staff member from the wheelchair back into bed.	0	2
Resident was physically independent for all transfers. However, he would not get up in the morning until the nurse assistant rearranged his bed covers and released the half side rail on his bed.	0	1
Once someone correctly positioned the wheelchair in place and locked the wheels, the resident transferred independently to and from the bed.	0	1
Resident moved independently in and out of armchairs but always received light physical guidance of one person to get in and out of bed safely.	2	2
Transferring ability varied throughout each day. Resident received no assistance at some times and heavy weight-bearing assistance of one person at other times.	3	2

Examples: ADL Self-Performance and Support	Self-Perf.	Support
Walk in room		
Resident walked in his/her room while holding on to furniture for support.	0	0
Resident walked independently during the day and received non-weight bearing physical help of 1 person for getting to the bathroom in room at night.	2	2
Resident received non-weight bearing physical assistance of one person for all walking in own room.	2	2
Resident did not walk but wheeled self independently in own room.	8	8
Walk in corridor		
A timid, fearful resident is usually physically independent in walking. During the last week she was very anxious and fearful of falling, and therefore received reassurance and encouragement from someone walking next to her while walking back to her room from meals in the unit dining room.	1	0
A resident with memory loss ambulated independently on the unit corridor albeit with a walker. Several times a day she left her walker in the bathroom, in the dining room, etc., necessitating that someone return it to her and offer her reminders to use it for safety.	1	1
Resident walked in corridor on unit by supporting self on one side with the handrail along the wall and receiving verbal cues from another person.	1	0
Resident walked twice daily 4-6 feet in the corridor outside his room. He received weight bearing assistance of 1 person for each walk.	3	2
Resident walked in room for short distances with heavy assistance of 2 persons but traveled independently in corridor on unit by wheelchair.	8	8

Examples: ADL Self-Performance and Support	Self-Perf.	Support
Locomotion on unit		
Resident ambulated slowly on unit pushing a wheelchair for support, stopping to rest every 15–20 feet. She has good safety awareness and has never fallen. Staff felt she was reliable enough to be on her own.	0	0
A resident with a history of falling and an unsteady gait always received physical guidance (non-weight-bearing) of one person for all ambulation. Two nights last week the resident was found in his bathroom after getting out of bed and walking independently.	2	2
Resident ambulated independently around the unit "ad lib," socializing with others and attending activities during the day. Loves dancing and yoga. Because she can become afraid at night, she received contact guard of one person to walk her to the bathroom at least twice every night.	2	2
During last week resident was learning to walk short distances with new leg prosthesis with heavy partial weight-bearing assistance of two persons. He refuses to ride in a wheelchair.	3	3
Locomotion off unit		
Resident independently walked with a cane to all meals in the Main Dining Room (off the unit) and social and recreational activities in the nearby hobby shop. Received no set-up or physical help during the assessment period.	0	0
Resident walked independently to the off unit dining room for all meals. For one visit to a clinic held at the opposite end of the building she was given a ride in a wheelchair by a volunteer. She was wheeled to the clinic and after her session she was wheeled back to her unit.	0	2
Resident is independent in walking about her residential unit. She does get lost and has difficulty finding her room but enjoys stopping to chat with others. Because she would get lost, she was always accompanied by a staff member for her daily walks around the facility.	1	0
Resident did not leave the residential unit during the 7-day assessment period.	8	8

Examples: ADL Self-Performance and Support	Self-Perf.	Support
Dressing		
Resident usually dressed self. After a seizure, she received total help from several staff members once during the week.	0	3
Resident is totally independent in dressing herself except for donning and removing TED stockings. Nurse assistant applied the TED stockings each AM and removed them at bedtime.	3	2
Nurse assistant provided physical weight-bearing help with dressing every morning. Later each day, as resident felt better (joints were more flexible), she required staff assistance only to undo buttons and guide her arms in/out of sleeves every pm.	3	2
A 325 lb. resident received total care by two persons in dressing. He did not participate by putting arms through sleeves, lifting legs into shoes, etc.	4	3
Eating		
Resident arose daily after 9:00 am, preferring to skip breakfast and just munch on fresh fruit later in the morning. She ate lunch and dinner independently in the facility's main dining room.	0	0
Resident on long standing tube feedings via gastrostomy tube was completely independent in self-administration including self-medication via the tube once set up by staff.	0	1
Resident with a history of dysphagia and choking, ate independently as long as a staff member sat with him during every meal (stand-by assistance if necessary).	1	0
Resident is blind and confused. He ate independently once staff oriented him to types and whereabouts of food on his tray and instructed him to eat.	1	1
Cognitively impaired resident ate independently when given one food item at a time and monitored to assure adequate intake of each item.	1	1
Resident fed self solid foods independently at all meals and snacks. Self-administered all fluids and medications via G-tube with supervision once set up appropriately.	1	1
Resident with difficulty initiating activity always ate independently after someone guided her hand with the first few bites and then offered encouragement to continue.	3	2

Examples: ADL Self-Performance and Support	Self-Perf.	Support
Eating continued		
Resident with fine motor tremors fed self finger foods (e.g., sandwiches, raw vegetables and fruit slices, crackers) but always received supervision and total physical assistance with liquids and foods requiring utensils.	3	2
Resident fed self with staff monitoring at breakfast and lunch but tired later in day. She was fed totally by nursing assistant at supper meal.	3	2
Resident who was being weaned from gastrostomy tube feedings continued to receive total care for twice daily tube feedings. Additionally, she ate small amounts of food by mouth with staff supervision.	3	2
Resident received tube feedings via a jejunostomy for all nutritional intake. Feedings were given by a nurse.	4	2
Toileting Use		
Resident used bathroom independently once up in a wheelchair; used bedpan independently at night after it was set up on bedside table.	0	1
In the toilet room resident is independent. As a safety measure, the nurse assistant stays just outside the door, checking with her periodically.	1	0
Resident uses the toilet independently but occasionally required minor physical assistance for hygiene and straightening clothes afterwards. She received such help twice during the last week.	0	2
When awake, resident was toileted every two hours with minor assistance of one person for all toileting activities (e.g., contact guard for transfers to/from toilet, drying hands, zipping/buttoning pants). She required total care of one person several times each night after incontinence episodes.	3	2
Resident received heavy assistance of two persons to transfer on/off toilet. He was able to bear weight partially, and required only standby assistance with hygiene (e.g., being handed toilet tissue or incontinence pads).	3	3
Obese, severely physically and cognitively impaired resident receives a hoyer lift for all transfers to and from her bed. It is impossible to toilet her and she is incontinent. Complete personal hygiene is provided at least every 2 hours by 2 persons.	4	3

Examples: ADL Self-Performance and Support	Self-Perf.	Support
Personal Hygiene		
New resident, in nursing home adjustment phase, liked to sleep in his clothes in case of fire. He remained in the same clothes for 2–3 days at a time. He cleaned his hands and face independently and would not let others help with any personal hygiene activities.	0	0
Once grooming articles were laid out and arranged by staff, resident regularly performed the tasks of personal hygiene by receiving verbal directions from one person throughout each task.	1	1
Resident carried out personal hygiene but was not motivated. She received daily cueing and positive feedback from nursing staff to keep self clean and neat. Once started, she could be left alone to complete tasks successfully.	1	0
Resident shaves self with an electric razor, washes his face and hands, brushes his teeth, and combs his hair. Because he is losing his sight, staff stand-by to hand grooming articles to the resident and return articles to their proper location.	1	1
Resident performed all tasks of personal hygiene except shaving. The facility barber visited him on the unit three times a week to shave his thick beard.	3	2
Resident required total daily help combing her long hair and arranging it in a bun. Otherwise she was independent in personal hygiene.	3	2

2. Bathing

Bathing is the only ADL activity for which the ADL Self-Performance codes in item G1A do not apply. A unique set of Self-Performance codes, to be used only in the Bathing assessment, are described below. The Self-Performance codes for the other ADL items would not be applicable for bathing given the normal frequency with which the bathing activity is carried out during a one-week period. Assuming that the average frequency of bathing during a seven-day period would be one or two baths, the coding for the other ADL Self- Performance items, which permits one or two exceptions of heavier care, would result in the inaccurate classification of almost all residents as "Independent" for Bathing.

The ADL Support Provided codes given in item G1B, however, continue to apply to the Bathing activity.

Intent: To record the resident's Self-Performance and Support provided in bathing, including how the resident transfers into and out of the tub or shower.

Definition: **Bathing** — How the resident takes a full body bath, shower, or sponge bath, including transfers in and out of the tub or shower. The definition does not, however, include the washing of back or hair.

Coding: **A. Bathing Self-Performance Codes** -- Record the resident's self-performance in bathing according to the codes listed below. When coding, apply the code number that reflects the maximum amount of assistance the resident received during bathing episodes.

0. **Independent** — No help provided
1. **Supervision** — Oversight help only.
2. **Physical help limited to transfer only**
3. **Physical help in part of bathing activity**
4. **Total dependence**
8. **Activity itself did not occur during entire 7 days**

B. Support -- Next, score the maximum amount of support provided in bathing activities using the ADL Support Scale (Item G1B).

Examples: ADL Self-Performance and Support	Self-Perf.	Support
Bathing		
Resident received verbal cueing and encouragement to take twice-weekly showers. Once staff walked resident to bathroom, he bathed himself with periodic oversight.	1	0
On Monday, one staff member helped transfer resident to tub and washed his legs. On Thursday, resident had physical help of one person to get into tub but washed himself completely.	3	2
Resident afraid of hoyer lift. Given full sponge or bed bath by nurse assistant twice weekly. Actively involved in this activity.	3	2
For one bath, resident received light guidance of one person to position self in bathtub. However, due to her fluctuating moods, she received total help for her other bath. ***Rationale:*** The coding directions for bathing state, "code for most dependent in self performance and support."	4	2

3. Test for Balance

Residents with impaired balance in standing and sitting are at greater risk of falling. It is important to assess an individual's balance abilities so that interventions can be implemented to prevent injuries (e.g., strength training exercises; safety awareness; restorative nursing; nursing-based rehabilitation).

Intent: To record the resident's capacity of a.) balance while standing (not walking) without an assistive device or assistance of a person, and b.) balance while sitting without using the back or arms of the chair for support.

Process **a. Balance While Standing**

Preparation:

- Obtain a watch with a second hand to time the test.
- Pick a time to test the resident when he or she is likely to be at his or her best. If the resident refuses, negotiate a better time and try again later.
- Place a chair directly behind the resident in case the resident needs to sit down.
- Stand close to the resident while testing balance in order to catch or balance the resident, if necessary.
- If the resident is heavy or tall or seems frail, ask another staff person to stand by with you in case the resident needs assistance.
- Test balance without assistive devices (but with prostheses, if used). For residents who use walkers, make sure the walker is placed directly in front of the resident within easy reach in case it is needed for rebalancing.

Conducting the tests:

- DO each of the following tests (10 seconds each) on residents who are able to stand without physical help.
- DO NOT attempt to test residents who cannot stand by themselves. Code these residents as "3", Not able to attempt test without physical help.
- For persons with visual impairment who may not be able to see your demonstrations of feet placement, provide rich verbal descriptions.

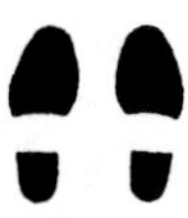

Position 1 —

"I would like you to stand with your feet together, side-by-side, like this (demonstrate as illustrated). [Note, in this and all tests, both feet should be firmly on the floor for support.]

"Do not move your feet until I say stop. Ready, OK, begin." If the resident is ABLE to maintain this position for 10 seconds, proceed to test resident in Position 2. **If the resident is NOT ABLE to maintain this position for 10 seconds, stop testing here.** Do not proceed with Position 2 for balance testing.

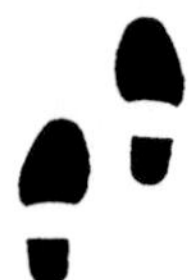

Position 2 —

"Now I would like you to stand with one foot halfway in front of the other like this" (demonstrate as illustrated).

"You may use either foot, whichever is more comfortable for you. Ready, OK, begin." If the resident is ABLE to maintain this position for 10 seconds, proceed to test resident in Position 3. **If the resident is NOT ABLE to do this, stop testing here.**

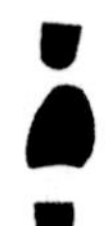

Position 3 —

"Now I would like you to stand with the heel of one foot in front of you touching the toes of the other foot like this (demonstrate as illustrated). You may use either foot, whichever is more comfortable for you. Ready, OK, begin."

Coding:

0. **Maintained position as required in test** — Resident was able to maintain all 3 standing positions for 10 seconds without moving feet out of position.

1. **Unsteady, but able to rebalance self without physical support** — Resident was unable to maintain one or more standing positions for 10 seconds each without moving feet out of position. Resident was unsteady but was able to rebalance self without physical support from others or from an assistive device in at least the first position.

2. **Partial physical support during test, or stands but does not follow directions for test** — While the resident performed part of the activity, resident was unable to maintain one or more standing positions without physical support from other(s) or from an assistive device. This category also includes residents who can stand but are unable or refuse to follow your directions to perform a test of balance.

3. **Not able to attempt test without physical help** — Resident is not able to stand without physical help from another person or an assistive device.

Examples of Balance Testing

Mrs. R usually walks with a walker. After completing the test preparation steps for safety, which include placing Mrs. R's walker directly in front of her in case she needs it during the test, you briefly explain to Mrs. R what you are going to ask her to do. You also demonstrate the actions. Once Mrs. R is standing, start to test her in Position 1 by giving her the brief directions and your demonstration of the position. You start timing her once you say, "Ready, OK, begin".

Results: During the 10-second test, Mrs. R moves her feet out of position to rebalance herself.

How to proceed: Tell Mrs. R, "That was a good try." STOP the test because the next 2 positions are harder to perform. If Mrs. R cannot maintain Position 1, it is unlikely she will be able to maintain Positions 2 or 3.

Coding: "1", Unsteady, but able to rebalance self without physical support.
Rationale: Mrs. R moved her feet out of position but did not need to hold her walker, or lean against the chair behind her, or receive assistance from you during the 10 seconds.

Mr. C has cognitive and hearing impairment and restlessness. He usually walks independently (wandering) and occasionally stands at the nurses' station to be with the unit secretary. Therefore, you know he can stand, but you do not know if he would be able to maintain his balance if her were asked to "hold" specific standing positions for 10 seconds each. After completing the test preparation, and steps for safety, you give Mr. C the brief directions and demonstration for testing position 1.

Results: During your interaction with Mr. C he becomes agitated, says "No, no" and walks away.

How to proceed: STOP the test.

Coding: "2", Partial physical support during test or stands but does not follow directions for test. ***Rationale:*** This is the best you can do under the circumstances. Although Mr. C did not need physical help to balance, you really do not know what his true balance capacity is. All you know is that he is able to stand, but you can't test his balance capacity because he refuses and is unable to follow directions.

Ms. M has multiple sclerosis and has been confined to her bed and reclining chair for the last 2 years.

How to proceed: DO NOT perform any standing balance tests. Ms. M cannot stand.

Coding: "3", Not able to attempt test without physical help.

Process: **b. Balance while sitting — position, trunk control**

Preparation

- Obtain a watch with a second hand to time the test.
- Do not conduct sitting balance in wheelchair. Find a chair with a firm, solid seat to conduct the test.
- The height of the chair seat should be low enough to allow the bottom of the resident's feet to rest on the floor for support. (Of course, this does not apply to persons with bilateral leg amputations.)
- It is safer to use a chair with arms in case the resident needs physical support during the test.
- Stand close to the resident while testing sitting balance in order to catch or balance the resident, if necessary.
- If the resident is heavy or tall or seems frail, ask another staff person to stand by with you in case the resident needs assistance.

Conducting the test:

- DO NOT attempt to test residents who are clearly unable to sit without physical help. Code these residents as "3", Not able to attempt test without physical help.
- Instruct the resident to sit in a chair with arms folded across his or her chest without using the back or arms of the chair for support. Make sure the resident's feet are both flat on the floor for support. Demonstrate the action to the resident. Observe balance for 10 seconds, then ask resident to stop.

Coding:

0. **Maintained position as required in test** — Resident was ABLE to sit for 10 seconds without touching the back or sides of the chair for support.
1. **Unsteady, but able to rebalance self without physical support.** — Resident was unable to maintain sitting balance for 10 seconds without touching the back or sides of the chair for support. Resident was unsteady but was ABLE to rebalance self.
2. **Partial physical support by others during test or sits but does not follow directions for test** — While resident performed part of activity, resident was UNABLE to maintain sitting balance without physical support **from**

other(s) or from touching the backs or sides of the chair for support. This category also includes residents who can sit but are unable or refuse to follow your directions to perform this test of sitting balance.

3. **Not able to attempt test without physical help** — Resident is not able to sit without physical help from another, or an assistive/adaptive device, or chair back/arms for support.

Examples of Sitting Balance

Ms. Z spends a lot of time sitting in a wheelchair on a gel cushion for pressure relief. She has a left-sided below-the-knee amputation. She does not have a leg prosthesis. She also has a left-sided hemiparesis from a CVA 1 year ago. You complete the test preparation activities for safety, assist Ms. Z to transfer into a chair with a firm seat, and ask her to place her right foot firmly on the floor. You instruct her to cross her arms over her chest. She cannot lift her left arm across her chest but is able to hold it across her abdomen. You instruct her to "sit up in the chair without leaning on the chair back or arms for support". You demonstrate this activity from another chair. Once the resident begins, you time for 10 seconds.

Results: Ms. Z maintained the position for the full 10 seconds without touching the chair back/arms for support.

How to proceed: Tell Ms. Z, "You did an excellent job. That's all we have to do." STOP testing. The test is complete.

Coding: "0", Maintained position as required in test.

4. Functional Limitation in Range of Motion

(A) Limitation in range of motion.

Intent: **Limitation in the range of motion** — To record the presence of (A) functional limitation in range of joint motion or (B) loss of voluntary movement.

Definition: Limitation that interferes with daily functioning (particularly with activities of daily living), or places the resident at risk of injury.

Process: **Assessing for functional limitations.** This test is a screening item used to determine the need for a more intensive evaluation. It does not need to be performed by a physical therapist. Rather, it can be administered by a member of any clinical discipline in accordance with these instructions.

- Do each of the following tests on all residents unless contraindicated (e.g., recent fracture or joint replacement).

- Perform each test on both sides of the resident's body.

- If the resident is unable to follow verbal directions demonstrate each movement (e.g., Ask the resident to do what you're doing).

- If resident is still unable to perform the activity after your demonstration, move the resident's joints through slow, active assisted range of motion to assess for limitations. In active assistive range of motion exercises, the health professional provides support and direction with the resident performing some of the activity.

- STOP if a resident experiences pain.

Neck — With resident seated in a chair, ask him or her to turn the head slowly, looking side to side. Then ask the resident to return head to center and then try to reach the right ear towards the right shoulder, then left ear towards left shoulder.

Arm — including shoulder or elbow — With resident seated in a chair instruct him or her to reach with both hands and touch palms to back of the head (mimics the action needed to comb hair). Then ask the resident to touch each shoulder with the opposite hand. Alternatively, observe the resident donning or removing a shirt over the head.

Hand— including wrist or fingers — For each hand, instruct the resident to make a fist, then open the hand (useful actions for grasping utensils, letting go).

Leg — including hip or knee — While resident is lying supine in a flat bed, instruct the resident to lift his or her leg (one at a time), bending it at the knee. [The knee will be at a right angle (90 degrees)]. Then ask the resident to slowly lower his or her leg, and extend it flat on the mattress.

Foot — including ankle or toes — While supine in bed, instruct the resident to flex (pull toes up towards head) and extend (push toes down away from head) each foot.

Other limitation or loss — Decreased mobility in spine, jaw, or other joints that are not listed.

Coding: For each body part, code the appropriate response for the resident's active (or assisted passive) range of motion function during the past seven days. Enter the code in the column labeled (A). If the resident has an amputation on one side of the body, use Code "1", Limitation on one side of the body. If there are bilateral amputations, use code "2", Limitation on both sides of the body.

0. **No limitation** — Resident has full function range of motion on the right and left side.

1. **Limitation on one side of the body (either right or left side).**

2. **Limitation on both sides of the body.**

Example of Coding for
(A) Limitation in Range of Motion

Mr. O was admitted to the nursing home for rehabilitation following right knee surgery. His right leg is in an immobilizer. With the exception of his right leg, Mr. O has full active range of motion in all other areas.

Coding (A)

Neck	0
Arm	0
Hand	0
Leg	1
Foot	0
Other	0

(B) Loss of voluntary movement.

Definition: **Loss of voluntary movement** — Impairment in purposeful (intentional) functional movement. This category refers to a range of impairments exhibited when a resident tries to perform a task and includes deficits such as incoordination, tremors, spasms, muscular rigidity, "freezing", choreiform movements (jerking) as well as lack of initiation of movement. Impairments in voluntary movement are often due to injury or disease of muscles, bones, nerves, spinal cord or the brain and can place a resident at risk for functional disability and injury.

Process: While performing the assessment of range of motion in item G4(A) above, observe the resident for impairment(s) in purposeful movement on each side of the resident's body.

Coding: For each body part, code the appropriate response for the resident's function during the past seven days. Enter the code in the column labelled (B). If the body part is missing on one side (e.g., left above knee amputation), code "1",

Partial loss of voluntary movement. If missing bilaterally, code "2", Full loss of voluntary movement.

0. **No loss of voluntary movement** — Resident moves body part to complete the required task. Movements are smooth and coordinated.

1. **Partial loss of voluntary movement** — Resident is able to initiate and complete the required task but movements are slow, spastic, uncoordinated, rigid, choreiform frozen, etc. on one or both sides.

2. **Full loss of voluntary movement** — Resident is not able to initiate the required task. There is no voluntary movement on either side.

Example of Function Limitation

Mrs. X is a diabetic who sustained a CVA 2 months ago. She can only turn her head slightly from side to side and tip her head towards each shoulder (limited neck range of motion). She can perform all arm, hand, and leg motions on the right side, with smooth coordinated movements. She is unable to move her left side (limited arm, hand, and leg motion) as she has a flaccid left hemiparesis. She is able to extend her legs flat on the bed. She has no feet. She has no other limitations.

Coding

	(A) Limitation in Range of Motion	**(B) Loss of Voluntary Movement**
a. Neck	1	0
b. Arm	1	1
c. Hand	1	1
d. Leg	1	1
e. Foot	2	2
f. Other	0	0

5. Modes of Locomotion

Intent: To record the type(s) of appliances, devices, or personal assistance the resident used for locomotion (on and off unit).

Definition: **Cane/walker/crutch** — Also check this item in those instances where the resident walks by pushing a wheelchair for support.

Wheeled self — Includes using a hand-propelled or motorized wheelchair, as long as the resident takes responsibility for self-mobility, even for part of the time.

Other person wheeled — Another person pushed the resident in a wheelchair.

Wheelchair primary mode of locomotion — Even if resident walks some of the time, he or she is primarily dependent on a wheelchair to get around. The wheelchair may be motorized, self-propelled, or pushed by another person.

Coding: Check all that apply during the last 7 days. If no appliances or assistive devices were used, check *NONE OF ABOVE*.

6. Modes of Transfer

Intent: To record the type(s) of appliances or assistive devices the resident used for transferring in and out of bed or chair, and for bed mobility.

Definition: **Bedfast all or most of the time** — Resident is in bed or in a recliner in own room for 22 hours or more per day. This definition also includes residents who are primarily bedfast but have bathroom privileges. For care planning purposes this information is useful for identifying residents who are at risk of developing physical and functional problems associated with restricted mobility, as well as cognitive, mood, and behavior impairment related to social isolation. **Code this item when it was true on at least 4 of the last 7 days.**

Bed rail(s) used for bed mobility or transfer — Refers to any type of side rail(s) attached to the bed USED by the resident as a means of support to facilitate turning and repositioning in bed, as well as for getting in and out of bed. **Do not check this item if resident did not use rails for this purpose.**

Lifted manually — The resident was completely lifted by one or more persons.

Lifted mechanically — The resident was lifted by a mechanical device (e.g., Hoyer lift). Does not include a bath lift.

Transfer Aid — Includes devices such as slide boards, trapezes, canes, walkers, braces and other assistive devices.

Coding: Check all that apply. If none of these items apply, check *NONE of ABOVE*.

7. Task Segmentation

Intent: To identify residents who are more involved and independent in personal care tasks (such as eating, bathing, grooming, dressing) because they have received help in breaking tasks down into smaller steps. Some residents become overwhelmed and anxious when there are expectations for greater independence and they are no longer able to perform the steps necessary to complete an ADL activity. Such residents are at great risk for becoming dependent on others unless activities are made easier for them to manage by task segmentation. These residents usually have some deficits in memory, thinking, or paying attention to the task consequent to problems such as dementia, head injury, CVA, or depression. Other residents receive task segmentation care because of body-control problems, poor stamina, or other physical difficulties that limit self-performance.

Definition: **Task segmentation** provides the resident with directions — such as verbal cues, physical cues, or verbal and physical cues — for performing each constituent step in an ADL activity.

Verbal cueing involves giving a verbal direction to complete the first step in a task, and once the step is accomplished, giving another verbal direction to complete the next step. Verbal encouragement, praise, and feedback for the resident's successful completion of the steps are usually given by the direct care staff person prior to providing the next verbal cue. For example, "That looks good. Now put on this skirt."

Physical cueing involves giving the resident an object as a reminder of what needs to be done — e.g., handing the resident some toilet paper as a cue to wipe self, or placing an item from a food tray in front of the resident and handing him or her a fork as a cue to eat the item.

Physical and verbal cueing involves use of objects and words to stimulate action — e.g., giving the resident one item of clothing at a time and saying "Put this shirt on," which is less confusing to a cognitively impaired resident than putting all clothing items before him or her and saying "Get dressed."

Examples	
Task Segmentation	**No Task Segmentation**
• When handed a soapy face cloth and asked, "Would you please wash your face?", the resident washes her face.	• When a wash basin, a face cloth, a towel, and various grooming supplies are placed before the resident, the resident becomes overwhelmed.
• When a nurse assistant sets a mirror in front of the resident, and hands him a brush, the resident brushes his hair.	• When a nurse assistant places the resident's clothes for the day on the bed and says, "Get dressed," the resident becomes confused and is unable to dress self.
• When the nurse assistant hands the resident a sock and says "Put this sock on this foot" and upon completion of the step hands the resident another sock and says "Put this sock on this foot," the resident dons his socks.	• When a tray containing an entire meal and several different utensils are placed before the resident on a table, the resident becomes confused and is unable to eat by herself.
• When single food items and only one utensil are presented to the resident in succession, the resident eats independently. • When a nurse assistant gives verbal directions for each step in transferring from a wheelchair (e.g., "Lock the brakes... Hold onto the arms of the chair and push yourself up... Hold onto your walker with both hands like this [demonstrates]"), the resident succeeds in transferring himself from a seated to a standing position.	• When a nurse assistant lifts a resident from a sitting to a standing position and does not involve the resident in the process of self-care in the activity, the resident becomes more physically dependent on the nurse assistant.
For all above examples, **Code "1" for Yes.**	For all above examples, **Code "0" for No.**

Process: Ask the nurse assistant to think about how the resident completes activities of daily living, or ways the nurse assistant helped the resident complete an activity of daily living over the last seven days. Specifically: Did the nurse assistant break the ADL activity into subtasks (smaller steps) so that the resident could perform them? Did this occur in the last seven days?

Coding: Code "0" if task segmentation was not done. Code "1" if ADLs were broken into a series of subtasks so that resident could perform them.

8. ADL Functional Rehabilitation Potential

Intent: To describe beliefs and characteristics related to the resident's functional status that may indicate he or she has the capacity for greater independence and involvement in self-care in at least some ADL areas. Even if highly independent in an activity, the resident may believe he or she can do better (e.g., walk longer distances, shower independently).

Process: Ask if the resident thinks he or she could be more self-sufficient given more time. Listen to and record what the resident believes, even if it appears unrealistic. Also, as a clue to whether the resident might do better all the time, ask if his or her ability to perform ADLs varies from time to time, or if ADL function or joint range of motion has declined or improved in the last three months.

Ask direct care staff (e.g., nurse assistants on all shifts) who routinely care for the resident if they think he or she is capable of greater independence, or if the resident's performance in ADLs varies from time to time. Ask if ADL function or range of motion of joints declined or improved in the last three months. You may need to prompt staff to consider such factors as:

- Has self-performance in any ADL varied over the last week (e.g., the resident usually requires two-person assistance but on one day transferred out of bed with assistance of one person)?
- Has resident's performance varied during the day (e.g., more involved and independent in the afternoon than in the morning)?
- Was the resident so slow in performing some activities that staff members intervened and performed the task or activity? Is the resident capable of increased self-performance when given more time? - OR - Is the resident capable of increased self-performance when tasks are broken into manageable steps?

- Does the resident tire noticeably during most days?
- Does the resident avoid an ADL activity even though physically or cognitively capable (e.g., refuses to walk alone for fear of falling, demands that others attend to personal care because they do it better)?
- Has the resident's performance in any ADL improved?

Coding: Check all that apply. If none of these items apply check *NONE OF ABOVE.*

Examples

Mr. N, who is cognitively impaired, receives limited physical assistance in locomotion for safety purposes. However, he believes he is capable of walking alone and often gets up and walks by himself when staff aren't looking. **Check "a" (Resident believes he/she capable of increased independence).**

The nurse assistant who totally feeds Mrs. W has noticed in the past week that Mrs. W has made several attempts to pick up finger foods. She believes Mrs. W could become more independent in eating if she received close supervision (cueing) in a small group for restorative care in eating. **Check "b" (Direct care staff believes resident is capable of increased independence).**

Mrs. Y has demonstrated the ability to get dressed, but has missed breakfast on several occasions because she was slow getting organized. Therefore, every morning her nurse assistant physically helped her to dress so that she would be ready for breakfast. **Check "c" (Resident able to perform task but is very slow).**

Mrs. F remained continent during day shifts while receiving supervision in toileting. During the evening and night shifts she was incontinent because she was not helped out of bed to the toilet room. After incontinence episodes, direct-care staff provided total help in hygiene. **Check "d" (Difference in ADL self-performance or ADL support, comparing mornings to evenings).**

Mr. K has hemiplegia secondary to a CVA. He receives extensive assistance in bed mobility transfer, dressing, toilet use, personal hygiene and eating. He is totally dependent in locomotion (wheelchair). Whenever he has tried to do more for himself he has experienced chest pain and shortness of breath. Both Mr. K and direct care staff believe that he is involved in self-care as much as he is physically able. **Check "e" (*NONE OF ABOVE*).**

9. Change in ADL Function

Intent: To document any changes occurring in the resident's overall ADL self-performance, as compared to status of 90 days ago (or since last assessment if less than 90 days ago). These include, but are not limited to, changes in the resident's level of involvement in ADL activities as well as the amount and the type of support received by staff. If the resident is a new admission to the facility, this item includes changes during the period prior to admission.

Process: Review the record for indications of a change. Consult with the resident and direct care staff. Review Section G from the last assessment and compare these findings with current findings. For new residents, consult with the primary family caregiver.

Coding: Code "0" if there has been no change. Code "1" if the resident's ADL function has improved. Code "2" if the resident's function has deteriorated. You may find that some ADLs have improved, some deteriorated, and others remain unchanged. You must weigh all of the information and make an overall clinical judgment (e.g., in general, the resident's ADL function has...).

Examples

Dr. B had been highly involved in self-care in most ADL activities. Seven weeks ago he slipped, fell, and bruised his right wrist. For several weeks he received more extensive assistance with dressing, grooming, and eating. However, in the last three weeks he is functioning at the same level of involvement in ADLs as before the fall. **Code "0" for No change.**

Ms. A participated in a structured feeding group during the past six weeks. With lots of encouragement and supervision from the group leader, she has progressed from requiring extensive assistance to feeding herself under staff supervision. Her performance in other ADLs remains unchanged. **Code "1" for Improved.**

Since fracturing her left hip three weeks ago, Mrs. Z receives more weight bearing help with transfers, locomotion, dressing, toileting, personal hygiene, and bathing. However, she has made strides in OT and PT. Her improvement in self-care has been steady although she still has a long way to go to reach her Self-Performance level of 90 days ago. **Code "2" for Deteriorated.**

(continued on next page)

Examples (continued)

Mr. L's favorite nurse (Miss McC) transferred to another unit 30 days ago. Although he says he's happy for her, he has become more passive and withdrawn. He no longer dresses himself in a suit and tie. His personal hygiene habits have deteriorated and he now must be frequently coaxed to shave and wash himself and comb his hair. Because he now wears stained clothing, staff have started to select and set out his clothes each day. Despite these losses, Mr. L is now somewhat more self-sufficient in locomotion, making twice-a-week trips to see Miss McC on her new unit. **Code "2" for Deteriorated.** The ***rationale*** for the coding decision is that although some improvement is noted in one ADL activity (locomotion) it only occurs twice weekly. In general, Mr. L has deteriorated in his self-care performance in two ADL activities (dressing and personal hygiene) that require multiple daily tasks.

During a Significant Change assessment for severe mood distress, Mrs. M was found to be more dependent on others for physical assistance in personal hygiene, dressing and toileting. She also received more coaxing and encouragement to eat. These changes represented less involvement in self-care since the last assessment two months ago. **Code "2" for Deteriorated.**

SECTION H. CONTINENCE IN LAST 14 DAYS

1. Continence Self-Control Categories

Note: This section differs from the other ADL assessment items in that the time period for review has been extended to 14 days. Research has shown that 14 days are the minimum required to obtain an accurate picture of bowel continence patterns. For the sake of consistency, both bowel continence and bladder continence are evaluated over 14 days.

Intent: To determine and record the resident's pattern of bladder and bowel continence (control) over the last 14 days.

Definition: **Bladder and Bowel Continence** — Refers to control of urinary bladder function and/or bowel movement. This item describes the resident's bowel and bladder continence pattern even with scheduled toileting plans, continence training programs, or appliances. It does not refer to the resident's ability to toilet self — e.g., a resident can receive extensive assistance in toileting and yet be continent, perhaps as a result of staff help. The resident's self-performance in toilet use is recorded in Item G1iA.

Process: Review the resident's clinical record and any urinary or bowel elimination flow sheets (if available). Validate the accuracy of written records with the resident. Make sure that your discussions are held in private. Control of bladder and bowel function are sensitive subjects, particularly for residents who are struggling to maintain control. Many people with poor control will try to hide their problems out of embarrassment or fear of retribution. Others will not report problems to staff because they mistakenly believe that incontinence is a natural part of aging and that nothing can be done to reverse the problem. Despite these common reactions to incontinence, many elders are relieved when a health care professional shows enough concern to ask about the nature of the problem in a sensitive, straightforward manner.

- Validate continence patterns with people who know the resident well (e.g., primary family caregiver of newly admitted resident; direct care staff).

- Remember to consider continence patterns over the last 14 day period, 24 hours a day, including weekends. If staff assignments change frequently, consider initiating and maintaining a bladder and bowel elimination flow sheet in order to gather more accurate information as a basis for coding decisions and, ultimately, care planning.

A five-point coding scale is used to describe continence patterns. Notice that in each category, different frequencies of incontinent episodes are specified for bladder and bowel. The reason for these differences is that there are more episodes of urination per day and week, whereas bowel movements typically occur less often.

0. **Continent** — Complete control (including control achieved by care that involves prompted voiding, habit training, reminders, etc.).

1. **Usually Continent** — Bladder, incontinent episodes occur once a week or less; Bowel incontinent episodes occur less than once a week.

2. **Occasionally Incontinent** — Bladder incontinent episodes occur two or more times a week but not daily; Bowel incontinent episodes occur once a week.

3. **Frequently Incontinent** — Bladder incontinent episodes tend to occur daily, but some control is present (e.g., on day shift); Bowel incontinent episodes occur two to three times per week.

4. **Incontinent** — Has inadequate control. Bladder incontinent episodes occur multiple times daily; Bowel incontinent is all (or almost all) of the time.

Coding: Choose one response to code level of bladder continence and one response to code level of bowel continence for the resident over the last 14 days.

Code for the resident's actual bladder and bowel continence pattern — i.e., the frequency with which the resident is wet and dry during the 14 day assessment period. Do not record the level of control that the resident might have achieved under optimal circumstances.

For bladder incontinence, the difference between a code of "3" (Frequently Incontinent) and "4" (Incontinent) is determined by the presence ("3") or absence ("4") of any bladder control.

Examples of Bladder Continence Coding

Mr. Q was taken to the toilet after every meal, before bed, and once during the night. He was never found wet and is considered continent. **Code "0" for "Continent" — Bladder.**

Mr. R had an indwelling catheter in place during the entire 14 day assessment period. He was never found wet and is considered continent. **Code "0" for "Continent" — Bladder.**

Although she is generally continent of urine, every once in a while (about once in 2 weeks) Mrs. T doesn't make it to the bathroom to urinate in time after receiving her daily diuretic pill. **Code "1" for "Usually Continent" — Bladder.**

Mrs. A has less than daily episodes of urinary incontinence, particularly late in the day when she is tired. **Code "2" for "Occasionally Incontinent" — Bladder.**

Mr. S is comatose. He wears an external (condom) catheter to protect his skin from contact with urine. This catheter has been difficult for staff to manage as it keeps slipping off. They have tried several different brands without success. During the last 14 days Mr. S has been found wet at least twice daily on the day shift. **Code "3" for "Frequently Incontinent" — Bladder.**

Mrs. U is terminally ill with end-stage Alzheimer's disease. She is very frail and has stiff, painful contractures of all extremities. She is primarily bedfast on a special water mattress, and is turned and re-positioned hourly for comfort. She is not toileted and is incontinent of urine for all episodes. **Code "4" for Incontinent" — Bladder.**

2. Bowel Elimination Pattern

Intent: To record the effectiveness of resident's bowel function.

Definition: **Bowel elimination pattern regular** — Resident has at least one movement every three days.

Constipation — Resident passes two or fewer bowel movements per week, or strains more than one out of four times when having a bowel movement.

Diarrhea — Frequent elimination of watery stools from any etiology (e.g., diet, viral or bacterial infection).

Fecal impaction — The presence of hard stool upon digital rectal exam. Fecal impaction may also be present if stool is seen on abdominal x-ray in the sigmoid colon or higher, even with a negative digital exam or documentation in the clinical record of daily bowel movement.

Process: Ask the resident. Examine, if necessary. Review the clinical record, particularly any documentation flow sheets of bowel elimination patterns. Ask direct care staff (e.g., nurse assistants from all shifts).

Coding: Check all that apply in the last 14 days. If no items apply, check *NONE OF ABOVE*.

3. Appliances and Programs

Definition: **Any scheduled toileting plan** — A plan whereby staff members at scheduled times each day either take the resident to the toilet room, or give the resident a urinal, or remind the resident to go to the toilet. Includes habit training and/or prompted voiding.

Bladder retraining program — A retraining program where the resident is taught to consciously delay urinating (voiding) or resist the urgency to void. Residents are encouraged to void on a schedule rather than according to their urge to void. This form of training is used to manage urinary incontinence due to bladder instability.

External (condom) catheter — A urinary collection appliance worn over the penis.

Indwelling catheter — A catheter that is maintained within the bladder for the purpose of continuous drainage of urine. Includes catheters inserted through the urethra or by supra-pubic incision.

Intermittent catheter — A catheter that is used periodically for draining urine from the bladder. This type of catheter is usually removed immediately after the bladder has been emptied. Includes intermittent catheterization whether performed by a licensed professional or by the resident. Catheterization may occur as a one-time event (e.g., to obtain a sterile specimen) or as part of a bladder emptying program (e.g., every shift in a resident with an underactive or acontractile bladder muscle).

Did not use toilet room/commode/urinal — Resident never used any of these items during the last 14 days, nor used a bed pan.

Pads/brief used — Any type of absorbent, disposable or reusable undergarment or item, whether worn by the resident (e.g., diaper, adult brief) or placed on the bed or chair for protection from incontinence. Does not include the routine use of pads on beds when a resident is never or rarely incontinent.

Enemas/irrigation — Any type of enema or bowel irrigation, including ostomy irrigations.

Ostomy present — Any type of ostomy of the gastrointestinal or genitourinary tract.

Process: Check the clinical record. Consult with nurse assistant and the resident. Be sure to ask about any items that are usually hidden from view because they are worn under street clothing (e.g., pads or briefs).

Coding: Check all that apply. If none of the items apply, check *NONE OF ABOVE.*

4. Change in Urinary Continence

Intent: To document changes in the resident's urinary continence status as compared to 90 days ago (or since last assessment if less than 90 days ago), including any changes in self-control categories, appliances, or programs. If the resident is a new admission to the facility, this item includes changes during the period prior to admission.

Process: Review the resident's clinical record and Bladder Continence patterns as recorded in the last assessment (if available). Validate findings with the resident and direct care staff on all shifts. For new residents, consult with the primary family caregiver.

Coding: Code "0" for No change, "1" for Improvement, or "2" for Deteriorated. A resident who was incontinent 90 days ago who is now continent by virtue of a catheter should be coded as "1", Improved. See fourth example in the box below.

Examples of Change in Urinary Continence

During an outbreak of gastroenteritis at the nursing home six weeks ago, Mrs. L, who is usually continent, became totally incontinent of bladder and bowel. This problem lasted only two weeks and she has been continent for the last month. **Code "0" for No change.**

Dr. R had prostate surgery three months ago. Prior to surgery, he was frequently incontinent. Upon returning from the hospital, his indwelling catheter was discontinued. Although he initially experienced incontinence, he now remains dry with only occasional incontinence. He sings the praises of surgery to his peers. **Code "1" for Improved.**

Mrs. B is a new admission. Both she and her daughter report that she has never been incontinent of urine. By her third day of residency, her urinary incontinence became evident, especially at night. **Code "2" for Deteriorated.**

Two weeks ago Mr. K returned from the hospital following plastic surgery for a pressure ulcer. Prior to hospital admission, Mr. K was totally incontinent of urine. He is now continent with an indwelling catheter in place. **Code "1" for Improved.** ***Rationale:*** Although one could perceive that Mr. K had "deteriorated" because he now has a catheter for bladder control, remember that the MDS definition for bladder continence states "Control of bladder function with appliances (e.g., foley) or continence programs, if employed."

SECTION I. DISEASE DIAGNOSES

Intent: To document the presence of diseases that have a relationship to the resident's current ADL status, cognitive status, mood or behavior status, medical treatments, nursing monitoring or risk of death. In general, these are conditions that drive the current care plan. Do not include conditions that have been resolved or no longer affect the resident's functioning or care plan. In many facilities, clinical staff and physicians neglect to update the list of resident's "active" diagnoses. There may also be a tendency to continue old diagnoses that are either resolved or no longer relevant to the resident's plan of care. One of the important functions of the MDS assessment is to generate an updated, accurate picture of the resident's health status.

Definition: **Nursing monitoring** — Includes clinical monitoring by a licensed nurse (e.g., serial blood pressure evaluations, medication management, etc.)

1. Diseases

Definition: **Diabetes mellitus** — Includes insulin-dependent diabetes mellitus (IDDM) and diet-controlled diabetes mellitus (NIDDM or AODM).

Cardiac dysrhythmias — Disorder of heart rate or heart rhythm.

Peripheral vascular disease — Vascular disease of the lower extremities that can be of venous and/or arterial origin.

Arthritis — Includes degenerative joint disease (DJD), osteoarthritis (OA), and rheumatoid arthritis (RA). Record more specific forms of arthritis (e.g., Sjogren's syndrome; gouty arthritis) in Item I3 (with ICD-9-CM code).

Hip fracture — Includes any hip fracture that occurred at any time that continues to have a relationship to current status, treatments, monitoring, etc. Hip fracture diagnoses also include femoral neck fractures, fractures of the trochanter, subcapital fractures.

Missing limb (e.g., amputation) — Includes loss of any part of any upper or lower extremity.

Pathological bone fracture — Fracture of any bone due to weakening of the bone, usually as a result of a cancerous process.

Aphasia — A speech or language disorder caused by disease or injury to the brain resulting in difficulty expressing thoughts (i.e., speaking, writing), or understanding spoken or written language.

Cerebral palsy — Paralysis related to developmental brain defects or birth trauma.

Cerebrovascular accident (CVA/Stroke) — A vascular insult to the brain that may be caused by intracranial bleeding, cerebral thromboses, infarcts, emboli.

Dementia other than Alzheimer's — Includes diagnoses of organic brain syndrome (OBS) or chronic brain syndrome (CBS), senility, senile dementia, multi-infarct dementia, and dementia related to neurologic diseases other than Alzheimer's (e.g., Picks, Creutzfeld-Jacob, Huntington's disease, etc.).

Hemiplegia/hemiparesis — Paralysis/partial paralysis (temporary or permanent impairment of sensation, function, motion) of both limbs on one side of the body. Usually caused by cerebral hemorrhage, thrombosis, embolism, or tumor. There must be a diagnosis of hemiplegia or hemiparesis in the resident's record.

Paraplegia — Paralysis (temporary or permanent impairment of sensation, function, motion) of the lower part of the body, including both legs. Usually caused by cerebral hemorrhage, thrombosis, embolism, tumor, or spinal cord injury. There must be a diagnosis of paraplegia in the resident's record.

Quadriplegia — Paralysis (temporary or permanent impairment of sensation, function, motion) of all four limbs. Usually caused by cerebral hemorrhage, thrombosis, embolism, tumor, or spinal cord injury. There must be a diagnosis of quadriplegia in the resident's record.

Transient ischemia attack — A sudden, temporary, inadequate supply of blood to a localized area of the brain. Often recurrent.

Traumatic brain injury — Damage to the brain as a result of physical injury to the head.

Manic depressive (bipolar disease) — Includes documentation of clinical diagnoses of either manic depression or bipolar disorder. "Bipolar disorder" is the current term for manic depressive illness.

Emphysema/COPD — Includes COPD (chronic obstructive pulmonary disease) or COLD (chronic obstructive lung disease), chronic restrictive lung diseases such as asbestosis, and chronic bronchitis.

Allergies— Any hypersensitivity caused by exposure to a particular allergen. Includes agents (natural and artificial) to which the resident is susceptible for an allergic reaction, not only those to which he or she currently reacted to in the last seven days. This item includes allergies to drugs (e.g., aspirin, antibiotics), foods (e.g., eggs, wheat, strawberries, shellfish, milk), environmental substances (e.g., dust, pollen), animals (e.g., dogs, birds, cats), and cleaning products (e.g., soap, laundry detergent), etc. Hypersensitivity reactions include but are not limited to, itchy eyes, runny nose, sneezing, contact dermatitis, etc.

Anemia — Includes anemia of any etiology.

Process: Consult transfer documentation and medical record (including current physician treatment orders and nursing care plans). If the resident was admitted from an acute care or rehabilitation hospital, the discharge forms often list diagnoses and corresponding ICD-9-CM codes that were current during the hospital stay. If these diagnoses are still active, record them on the MDS form. Also, accept statements by the resident that seem to have clinical validity. Consult with physician for confirmation and initiate necessary physician documentation.

Physician involvement in this part of the assessment process is crucial. The physician should be asked to review the items in Section I at the time of visit closest to the scheduled MDS assessment. Use this scheduled visit as an opportunity to ensure that active diagnoses are noted and "inactive" diagnoses are designated as resolved. This is also an important opportunity to share the entire MDS assessment with the physician. In many nursing facilities physicians are not brought into the MDS review and assessment process. It is the responsibility of facility staff to aggressively solicit physician input. Inaccurate or missed diagnoses can be a serious impediment to care planning. Thus, you should share this section of the MDS with the physician and ask for his or her input. Physicians completing a portion of the MDS assessment should sign in Item R2 (Signatures of Those Completing the Assessment).

Full physician review of the most recent MDS assessment or ongoing input into the assessment currently being completed can be very useful. For the physician, the MDS assessment completed by facility staff can provide insights that would have otherwise not been possible. For staff, the informed comments of the physician may suggest new avenues of inquiry, or help to confirm existing observations, or suggest the need for additional follow-up.

Check a disease item only if the disease has a relationship to current ADL status, cognitive status, behavior status, medical treatment, nursing monitoring, or risk of death. For example, it is not necessary to check "hypertension" if one episode occurred several years ago unless the hypertension is either currently being controlled with medications, diet, biofeedback, etc., or is being regularly monitored to prevent a recurrence.

Coding: Do not record any conditions that have been resolved and no longer affect the resident's functional status or care plan.

Check all that apply. If none of the conditions apply, check *NONE OF ABOVE*. ***If you have more detailed information available in the clinical record for a more definitive diagnosis than is provided in the list in Section I1, check the more general diagnosis in I1 and then enter the more detailed diagnosis (with ICD-9-CM code) under I3.***

For example: If the record reveals that the resident has "osteoarthritis" you check item I1l (Arthritis) and record "Osteoarthritis" with 1CD-9-CM Code 715.00 in Section I3.

Consult the resident's transfer documentation (in the case of new admissions or re-admissions) and current medical record including current nursing care plans. There will be times when a particular diagnosis will not be documented in the medical record. If that is the case, as indicated above, accept statements by the resident that seem to have clinical validity, consult with the physician for confirmation, and initiate necessary physician documentation.

For example: If a new resident says he or she had a severe depression and was seeing a private psychiatrist in the community, this information may have been missed if the information was not carried forward in records accompanying the resident from an acute care hospital to the nursing home.

The following chart of ICD-9-CM codes for diseases listed in Item I1 is intended to clarify the level of specificity represented when the disease item is checked. This is also the list to use in computer applications of the MDS.

ICD-9-CM Codes for Diseases Listed in Section I1

ICD-9-CM Code	Disease Condition
ENDOCRINE/METABOLIC/NUTRITIONAL	
250.00	Diabetes mellitus
242.9[0 or1]	Hyperthyroidism
244.9	Hypothyroidism
HEART/CIRCULATION	
414.00 through 414.03	Arteriosclerotic heart disease (ASHD)
427.9	Cardiac dysrhythmia
428.0	Congestive heart failure
453.8	Deep vein thrombosis
401.9	Hypertension (unspecified)
458.9	Hypotension (unspecified)
443.9	Peripheral vascular disease (unspecified)
429.2	Other cardiovascular disease
MUSCULOSKELETAL	
716.90	Arthritis (unspecified site)
820.9	Hip fracture (unspecified site or NOS [not otherwise specified])
736.89	Missing limb (e.g., amputation)
733.00	Osteoporosis (unspecified)
733.10	Pathological bone fracture (unspecified sites)

(Continued on next page)

ICD-9-CM Codes for Diseases Listed in Section I1
(Continued)

ICD-9-CM Code	Disease Condition
NEUROLOGICAL	
331.0	Alzheimer's disease
784.3	Aphasia
343.90	Cerebral palsy (unspecified)
436	Cerebrovascular accident (stroke) (NOS acute)
290.0	Dementia other than Alzheimer's (Senile Dementia, NOS)
342.90 through 342.92	Hemiplegia/Hemiparesis
340	Multiple sclerosis (NOS)
344.1	Paraplegia
332.0	Parkinson's disease
344.00 through 344.09	Quadriplegia
780.3	Seizure disorder
435.9	Transient ischemic attack (TIA) (unspecified)
854.00	Traumatic brain injury (unspecified)
PSYCHIATRIC/MOOD	
300.00	Anxiety disorder (unspecified)
311	Depression
296.8	Manic depression (bipolar disease)
295.90	Schizophrenia (unspecified)
PULMONARY	
493.90	Asthma (unspecified)
492.8	Emphysema
496	COPD
SENSORY	
366.9	Cataracts (unspecified)
362.01, 362.02 and 250.50 through 250.53	Diabetic retinopathy
365.9	Glaucoma (unspecified)
362.50	Macular degeneration (unspecified)
OTHER	
995.3	Allergies (unspecified)
285.9	Anemia
199.1	Cancer (unspecified as to site or stage)
586	Renal failure (unspecified)

ICD-9-CM: The International Classification of Diseases – 9th Revision – Clinical Modification. Ann Arbor, Michigan: Edward Brothers, Inc., October, 1989.

2. Infections

Definition: **Antibiotic resistant infection** (e.g., Methicillin resistant staph) — An infection in which bacteria have developed a resistance to the effective actions of an antibiotic. Check this item only if there is supporting documentation in the clinical record (including transmittal records of new admissions and recent transfers from other institutions).

Clostridium difficile (C.diff) — Diarrheal infection caused by the Clostridium difficile bacteria. Check this item only if there is supporting documentation in the clinical record of new admissions and recent transfers (e.g., hospital referral or discharge summary, laboratory report).

Conjunctivitis— Inflammation of the mucous membranes lining the eyelids. May be of bacterial, viral, allergic, or traumatic origin.

HIV infection — Check this item only if there is supporting documentation or the resident (or surrogate decision-maker) informs you of the presence of a positive blood test result for the Human Immunodeficiency Virus or diagnosis of AIDS.

Pneumonia — Inflammation of the lungs; most commonly of bacterial or viral origin.

Respiratory infection — Any upper or lower (e.g., bronchitis) respiratory infection other than pneumonia.

Septicemia— Morbid condition associated with bacterial growth in the blood.

Sexually transmitted diseases — Check this item only if there is supporting documentation of a current diagnosis of gonorrhea, or syphilis. DO NOT include HIV in this category.

Tuberculosis — Includes residents with active tuberculosis or those who have converted to PPD positive tuberculin status and are currently receiving drug treatment (e.g., isoniazid (INH), ethambutol, rifampin, cycloserine) for tuberculosis.

Urinary tract infection — Includes chronic and acute symptomatic infection(s) in the last 30 days. Check this item only if there is current supporting documentation and significant laboratory findings in the clinical record.

Viral hepatitis — Inflammation of the liver of viral origin. This category includes diagnoses of hepatitis A, hepatitis B, hepatitis non-A non-B, and hepatitis C.

Wound infection — Infection of any type of wound (e.g., surgical; traumatic; pressure) on any part of the body.

Process: Consult transfer documentation and the resident's clinical record (including current physician treatment orders and nursing care plans). Accept statements by the resident that seem to have clinical validity. Consult with physician for confirmation and initiate necessary physician documentation.

Physician involvement in this part of the assessment process is crucial.

Coding: Check an item only if the infection has a relationship to current ADL status, cognitive status, mood and behavior status, medical treatment, nursing monitoring, or risk of death. Do not record any conditions that have been resolved and no longer affect the resident's functional status or care plan. For example, do not check "tuberculosis" if the resident had TB several years ago unless the TB is either currently being controlled with medications or is being regularly monitored to detect a recurrence.

Check all that apply. If none of the conditions apply, check *NONE OF ABOVE*. If you have more detailed information available in the clinical record for a more definitive diagnosis than is provided in the list in Section I2 check the appropriate box in I2 and enter the more detailed information (with ICD-9-CM code) under I3.

ICD-9-CM Codes for Diseases Listed in Section I2

ICD-9-CM Code	Disease Condition
INFECTION	
041.9 or 041.11 or 041.19	Antibiotic resistant infection (e.g., methicillin resistant staph)
040.0	Clostridium difficile (C.diff)
372.30	Conjunctivitis
042	HIV infection
486	Pneumonia (organism unspecified)
038.9	Septicemia (not otherwise specified)
099.9	Sexually transmitted diseases (Venereal diseases) (unspecified)
011.90	Tuberculosis (pulmonary unspecified)
599.0	Urinary tract infection (site not specified)
070.9	Viral hepatitis (unspecified, without mention of hepatic coma)
958.3 or 998.5	Wound infection

ICD-9-CM: The International Classification of Diseases – 9th Revision – Clinical Modification. Ann Arbor, Michigan: Edward Brothers, Inc., October, 1989.

3. Other Current Diagnoses and ICD-9-CM Codes

Intent: To identify conditions not listed in Item I1 and I2 that affect the resident's current ADL status, mood and behavioral status, medical treatments, nursing monitoring, or risk of death. Also, to record more specific designations for general disease categories listed under I1 and I2.

Coding: Enter the description of the diagnoses on the lines provided. For each diagnosis, an ICD-9-CM code must be entered in the boxes to the right of the line. If this information is not available in the medical records, consult the most recent version of the full set of volumes of ICD-9-CM codes.

The person assigned to enter these codes should be trained in the ICD-9-CM assignment system. The task is best completed by a member of the medical record staff or the facility's medical record consultant. The person entering the ICD-9-CM codes must also enter his or her signature under MDS item R2, indicating that these codes were entered. The most recently updated version of the International Classification of Diseases - 9th Revision - Clinical Modification (ICD-9-CM) must be used. Volumes 1 and 2 of ICD-9-CM can be ordered from the Superintendent of Documents, U.S. Government Printing Office, Washington, D.C. 20402. Specify order number S/N 9176--014-000000-1. Facilities do not need to order Volume 3, which classifies surgical, diagnostic, and nonsurgical procedures.

SECTION J.
HEALTH CONDITIONS

1. Problem Conditions

To record specific problems or symptoms that affect or could affect the resident's health or functional status, and to identify risk factors for illness, accident, and functional decline.

INDICATORS OF FLUID STATUS — It is often difficult to recognize when a frail, chronically ill elder is experiencing fluid overload that could precipitate congestive heart failure, or alternatively dehydration. Ways to monitor the problem, particularly in residents who are unable to recognize or report the common symptoms of fluid variation, are as follows:

Definition: **Weight gain or loss of 3 or more pounds within a 7-day period** — This can only be determined in residents who are weighed in the same manner at least weekly. However, the majority of residents will not require weekly or more frequent weights, and for these residents you will be unable to determine whether there has been a 3 or more pound gain or loss. When this is the case, leave this item blank.

Inability to lie flat due to shortness of breath — resident is uncomfortable lying supine. Resident requires more than one pillow or having the head of the bed mechanically raised in order to get enough air. This symptom often occurs with fluid overload. If the resident has shortness of breath when not lying flat, also check item J11 "Shortness of breath." If the resident does not have shortness of breath when upright (e.g., O.K. when using two pillows or sitting up) do not check item J11.

Dehydrated; output exceeds intake — check this item if the resident has 2 or more of the following indicators.

- Resident usually takes in less than the recommended 2500 ml of fluids daily (water or liquids in beverages, and water in food).
- Resident has clinical signs of dehydration.
- Resident's fluid loss exceeds the amount of fluids he or she takes in (e.g., loss from vomiting, fever, diarrhea that exceeds fluid replacement).

Insufficient fluid; did NOT consume all/almost all liquids provided during last 3 days — Liquids can include water, juices, coffee, gelatins, and soups.

OTHER

Delusions — Fixed, false beliefs not shared by others that the resident holds even when there is obvious proof or evidence to the contrary (e.g., belief he or she is terminally ill; belief that spouse is having an affair; belief that food served by the facility is poisoned).

Dizziness/vertigo — The resident experiences the sensation of unsteadiness, that he or she is turning, or that the surroundings are whirling around.

Edema — Excessive accumulation of fluid in tissues, either localized or systemic (generalized). Includes all types of edema (e.g., dependent, pulmonary, pitting).

Fever — Rectal temperatures above 100°Fahrenheit (38°Celsius) are considered significant in an elderly nursing home population. Many frail elders have normally low rectal baseline temperatures (e.g., 96° to 99°F). A fever is present when the resident's temperature (°F) is 2.4 degrees greater than the baseline temperature.

Hallucinations — False perceptions that occur in the absence of any real stimuli. A hallucination may be auditory (e.g., hearing voices), visual (e.g., seeing people, animals), tactile (e.g., feeling bugs crawling over skin), olfactory (e.g., smelling poisonous fumes), or gustatory (e.g., having strange tastes).

Internal bleeding — Bleeding may be frank (such as bright red blood) or occult (such as guaiac positive stools). Clinical indicators include black, tarry stools, vomiting "coffee grounds", hematuria (blood in urine), hemoptysis (coughing up blood), and severe epistaxis (nosebleed).

Recurrent lung aspirations in last 90 days — Note the extended time frame. Often occurs in residents with swallowing difficulties or who receive tube feedings (ie. esophageal reflux of stomach contents). Clinical indicators include productive cough, shortness of breath, wheezing. It is not necessary that there be X-ray evidence of lung aspiration for this item to be checked.

Shortness of breath — Difficulty breathing (dyspnea) occurring at rest, with activity, or in response to illness or anxiety. If the resident has shortness of breath while lying flat, also check item J1b ("Inability to lie flat due to shortness of breath.").

Syncope (fainting) — Transient loss of consciousness, characterized by unresponsiveness and loss of postural tone with spontaneous recovery.

Unsteady gait — A gait that places the resident at risk of falling. Unsteady gaits take many forms. The resident may appear unbalanced or walk with a sway. Other gaits may have uncoordinated or jerking movements. Examples of unsteady gaits may include fast gaits with large, careless movements; abnormally slow gaits with small shuffling steps; or wide-based gaits with halting, tentative steps.

Vomiting — Regurgitation of stomach contents; may be caused by any etiology (e.g., drug toxicity; influenza; psychogenic).

Process: Ask the resident if he or she has experienced any of the listed symptoms in the last seven days. Review the clinical records (including current nursing care plan) and consult with facility staff members and the resident's family if the resident is unable to respond. A resident may not complain to staff members or others, attributing such symptoms to "old age." Therefore, it is important to ask and observe the resident, directly if possible, since the health problems being experienced by the resident can often be remedied.

Coding: Check all conditions that occurred within the past seven days unless otherwise indicated (i.e. lung aspirations in the last 90 days). If no conditions apply, check *NONE OF ABOVE*.

2. Pain Symptoms

Intent: To record the frequency and intensity of signs and symptoms of pain. For care planning purposes this item can be used to identify indicators of pain as well as to monitor the resident's response to pain management interventions.

Definition: **Pain** — For MDS assessment purposes, pain refers to any type of physical pain or discomfort in any part of the body. Pain may be localized to one area, or may be more generalized. It may be acute or chronic, continuous or intermittent (comes and goes), or occur at rest or with movement. The pain experience is very subjective; pain is whatever the resident says it is.

Shows evidence of pain — depends on the observation of others (i.e., cues), either because the resident does not verbally complain, or is unable to verbalize.

Process: Ask the resident if he or she has experienced any pain in the last seven days. Ask him/her to describe the pain. If the resident states he or she has pain, take his or her word for it. Pain is a subjective experience. Also observe the resident for indicators of pain. Indicators include moaning, crying, and other vocalizations; wincing or frowning and other facial expressions; or body posture such as guarding/protecting an area of the body, or lying very still; or decrease in usual activities.

In some residents, the pain experience can be very hard to discern. For example, in residents who have dementia and cannot verbalize that they are feeling pain, symptoms of pain can be manifested by particular behaviors such as calling out for help, pained facial expressions, refusing to eat, or striking out at a nurse assistant who tries to move them or touch a body part. Although such behaviors may not be solely indicative of pain, but rather may be indicative of multiple problems, code for the frequency and intensity of symptoms if in your clinical judgement it is possible that the behavior could be caused by the resident experiencing pain.

Ask nurse assistants and therapists who work with the resident if the resident had complaints or indicators of pain the last week.

Coding: Code for the highest level of pain present in the last seven days. If the resident has no pain, code "0", (No pain) and then Skip to item J4.

a. **Frequency** — How often the resident complains or shows evidence of pain.

Codes: **0. No pain (Skip to item J4)**
1. Pain less than daily
2. Pain daily

b. **Intensity** — The severity of pain as described or manifested by the resident.

Codes: **1. Mild pain** — Although the resident experiences some ("a little") pain he or she is usually able to carry on with daily routines, socialization, or sleep.

2. Moderate pain — Resident experiences "a medium" amount of pain.

3. Times when pain is horrible or excruciating — Worst possible pain. Pain of this type usually interferes with daily routines, socialization, sleep.

Use your best clinical judgement when coding. If you have difficulty determining the exact frequency or intensity of pain, code for the more severe level of pain. ***Rationale***: Residents having pain will usually require further evaluation to determine the cause and to find interventions that promote comfort. You never want to miss an opportunity to relieve pain.

Pain control often enables rehabilitation, greater socialization and activity involvement.

Examples	Pain Frequency	Pain Intensity
Mrs. G, a resident with poor short-and-long term memory and moderately impaired cognitive function asked the charge nurse for "a pill to make my aches and pains go away" once a day during the last 7 days. The medication record shows that she received Tylenol every evening. The charge nurse states that Mrs. G usually rubs her left hip when she asks for a pill. However, when you ask her about pain, Mrs. G tells you that she is fine and never has pain. ***Rationale for coding*:** It appears that Mrs. G has forgotten that she has reported having pain during the last 7 days. Best clinical judgement calls for coding that reflects that Mrs. G has mild, daily pain.	2	1
Mr. T is cognitively intact. He is up and about and involved in self-care, social and recreational activities. During the last week he has been cheerful, engaging and active. When checked by staff at night, he appears to be sleeping. However, when you ask him how he's doing, he tells you that he has been having horrible cramps in his legs every night. He's only been resting, but feels tired upon arising. ***Rationale for coding*:** Although Mr. T may look comfortable to staff, he reports to you that he has terrible cramps. Best clinical judgement for coding this "screening" item for pain would be to record codes that reflect what Mr. T tells you. It is highly likely that Mr. T warrants a further evaluation.	2	3

3. Pain Site

Intent: To record the location of physical pain as described by the resident, or discerned from objective physical and laboratory tests. Sometimes is difficult to pinpoint the exact site of pain, particularly if the resident is unable to describe the quality and location of pain in detail. Likewise, it will be difficult to pinpoint the exact site if the resident has not had physical or laboratory tests to evaluate the pain. In order to begin to develop a responsive care plan for promoting comfort, the intent of this item is to help residents and caregivers begin a pain evaluation by attempting to target the site of pain.

Definition: **Back pain** — Localized or generalized pain in any part of the neck or back.

Bone pain — Commonly occurs in metastatic disease. Pain is usually worse during movement but can be present at rest. May be localized and tender but may also be quite vague.

Chest pain while doing usual activities — The resident experiences any type of pain in the chest area, which may be described as burning, pressure, stabbing, vague discomfort, etc. "Usual activities" are those that the resident engages in normally. For example, the resident's usual activities may be limited to minor participation in dressing and grooming, short walks from chair to toilet room.

Headache — The resident regularly complains or shows evidence (clutching or rubbing the head) of headache.

Hip pain — Pain localized to the hip area. May occur at rest or with physical movement.

Incisional pain — The resident complains or shows evidence of pain at the site of a recent surgical incision.

Joint pain (other than hip) — The resident complains or shows evidence of discomfort in one or more joints either at rest or with physical movement.

Soft tissue pain — Superficial or deep pain in any muscle or non-bony tissue. Examples include abdominal cramping, rectal discomfort, calf pain, wound pain.

Stomach Pain — The resident complains or shows evidence of pain or discomfort in the left upper quadrant of the abdomen.

Other — Includes either localized or diffuse pain of any other part of the body. Examples include general "aches and pains," etc.

Process: Ask the resident and observe for signs of pain. Consult staff members. Review the clinical record. Use your best clinical judgement.

Coding: Check all that apply during the last 7 days. If the resident has mouth pain check item K1c in Section K, "Oral/Nutritional Status."

4. Accidents

Intent: To determine the resident's risk of future falls or injuries. Falls are a common cause of morbidity and mortality among elderly nursing home residents. Residents who have sustained at least one fall are at risk of future falls. About half of all residents fall each year, with serious injury resulting from 6 to 10 percent of falls. Hip fractures account for approximately one-half of all serious injuries.

Definition: **Fell** — Note time frames (past 30 days and past 31-180 days).

Hip fracture in last 80 days — Note time frame (last 180 days).

Other fracture in last 180 days — Any fracture other than a hip fracture. Note time frame (last 180 days).

Process: **New admissions** — Consult with the resident and the resident's family. Review transfer documentation.

Current residents — Review the resident's records (including incident reports, current nursing care plan, and monthly summaries). Consult with the resident. Sometimes, a resident will fall, and believing that he or she "just tripped," will get up and not report the event to anyone. Therefore, do not rely solely on the clinical records but also ask the resident directly if he or she has fallen during the indicated time frame.

Coding: Check all conditions that apply. If no conditions apply, check *NONE OF ABOVE.*

5. Stability of Conditions

Intent: To determine if the resident's disease or health conditions present over the last seven days are acute, unstable, or deteriorating.

Definition: **Fluctuating, precarious, deteriorating** — Denotes the changing and variable nature of the resident's condition. For example, a resident may experience a variable response to the intensity of pain and the analgesic effect of pain medications. On "good days" over the last seven days, he or she will participate in ADLs, be in a good mood, and enjoy preferred leisure activities. On "bad days," he or she will be dependent on others for care, be agitated, cry, etc. Likewise, this category reflects the degree of difficulty in achieving a balance between treatments for multiple conditions.

Acute episode — Resident is symptomatic for an acute health condition (e.g., new myocardial infarction; adverse drug reaction; influenza), a recurrent (acute) condition (e.g., aspiration pneumonia; urinary tract infection) or an acute phase of a chronic disease (e.g., shortness of breath, edema, and confusion in a resident with congestive heart disease; acute joint pain and swelling in a resident who has had arthritis for many years). An acute episode is usually of sudden onset, has a time-limited course, requires physician evaluation and a significant increase in licensed nursing monitoring.

End-stage disease — In one's best clinical judgement, the resident with any end-stage disease has only six or fewer months to live. This judgment should be substantiated by a well documented disease diagnosis and deteriorating clinical course.

Process: Observe the resident. Consult staff members, especially the resident's physician. Review the resident's clinical record.

Coding: Check all that apply during last seven days. If none apply, check *NONE OF ABOVE.*

Examples

Mrs. M is diabetic. She requires daily or more frequent blood sugar tests in conjunction with administering sliding-scale insulin dosages. She has been confused on one occasion in the past week when she was hypoglycemic. **Check "a" for unstable — fluctuating, precarious, or deteriorating.**

If Mrs. M (above) were also to have pneumonia and fever during her assessment period, **check "a" for unstable and "b" for acute**.

Ms. F had been doing well and was ready for discharge to her apartment in elderly housing until she came down with the flu. Currently she has a low grade fever, general aches and pains, and respiratory symptoms of productive cough and nasal congestion. Although she has taken to bed for a few days she has had no change in ADL function, mood, etc. and is looking forward to discharge in a few days. **Check "b" for acute.**

Mrs. T was admitted to the unit with a diagnosis of chronic congestive heart failure. During the past few months she has had 3 hospital admissions for acute CHF. Her heart has become significantly weaker despite maximum treatment with medications and oxygen. Her physician has discussed her deteriorating condition with her and her family and has documented that her prognosis for survival in the next couple of months is poor. **Check "c" for end-stage disease.**

(continued on next page)

Examples (continued)

Mr. R is a diabetic who receives a daily dose of NPH insulin 20 units sc QAM. He requires only monthly blood sugar determinations for follow-up, and has no current acute illness. **Check "d" for *NONE OF ABOVE*.**

SECTION K. ORAL/NUTRITIONAL STATUS

1. Oral Problems

Intent: To record any oral problems present in the last seven days.

Definition: **Chewing problem** — Inability to chew food easily and without pain or difficulties, regardless of cause (e.g., resident uses ill-fitting dentures, or has a neurologically impaired chewing mechanism, or has temporomandibular joint pain, or a painful tooth).

Swallowing problem — Dysphagia. Clinical manifestations include frequent choking and coughing when eating or drinking, holding food in mouth for prolonged periods of time, or excessive drooling.

Mouth pain — Any pain or discomfort associated with any part of the mouth, regardless of cause. Clinical manifestations include favoring one side of the mouth while eating, refusing to eat, refusing food or fluids of certain temperatures (hot or cold).

Process: Ask the resident about difficulties in these areas. Observe the resident during meals. Inspect the mouth for abnormalities that could contribute to chewing or swallowing problems or mouth pain.

Coding: Check all that apply. If none apply, check *NONE OF ABOVE*.

2. Height and Weight

Intent: To record a current height and weight in order to monitor nutrition and hydration status over time; also, to provide a mechanism for monitoring stability of weight over time. For example, a resident who has had edema can have an intended and expected weight loss as a result of taking a diuretic. Or weight loss could be the result of poor intake, or adequate intake accompanied by recent participation in a fitness program.

a. **Height**

Process: **New admissions** — Measure height in inches.

Current resident — Check the clinical records. If the last height recorded was more than one year ago, measure the resident's height again.

Coding: Round height upward to nearest whole inch. Measure height consistently over time in accord with standard facility practice (shoes off, etc.)

b. **Weight**

Process: Check the clinical records. If the last recorded weight was taken more than one month ago or weight is not available, weigh the resident again. If the resident's weight was taken more than once during the preceding month, record the most recent weight.

Coding: Round weight upward to the nearest whole pound. Measure weight consistently over time in accord with standard facility practice (after voiding, before meal, etc.).

3. Weight Change

Intent: To record variations in the resident's weight over time.

a. **Weight Loss**

Definition: **Weight loss in percentages** (e.g., 5% or more in last 30 days, or 10% or more in last 180 days).

Process: **New admission** — Ask the resident or family about weight changes over the last 30 and 180 days. Consult physician, review transfer documentation and compare with admission weight. Calculate weight loss in percentages during the specified time periods.

Current resident — Review the clinical records and compare current weight with weights of 30 and 180 days ago. Calculate weight loss in percentages during the specified time periods.

Coding: Code "0" for No or "1" for Yes. If there is no weight to compare to, enter NA or a circled dash ⊖.

b. Weight Gain

Definition: **Weight gain in percentages** (i.e., 5% or more in last 30 days, or 10% or more in last 180 days).

Process: **New admission** — Ask the resident or family about weight changes over the last 30 and 180 days. Consult physician, review transfer documentation and compare with admission weight. Calculate weight gain during the specified time periods.

Current resident — Review the clinical records and compare current weight with weights of 30 and 180 days ago. Calculate weight gain during the specified time periods.

Coding: Code "0" for No or "1" for Yes. If there is no weight to compare to, enter NA or a circled dash ⊖ .

4. Nutritional Problems

Intent: To identify specific problems, conditions, and risk factors for functional decline present in the last seven days that affect or could affect the resident's health or functional status. Such problems can often be reversed and the resident can improve.

Definition: **Complains about the taste of many foods** — The sense of taste can change as a result of health conditions or medications. Also, complaints can be culturally based — e.g., someone used to eating spicy foods may find nursing home meals bland.

Regular or repetitive complaints of hunger — On most days (at least 2 out of 3), resident asks for more food or repetitively complains of feeling hungry (even after eating a meal).

Leaves 25% or more of food uneaten at most meals — Eats less than 75 percent of food (even when substitutes are offered) at least 2 out of 3 meals a day.

Process: Consult resident's records (including current nursing care plan), dietary/fluid intake flow sheets, dietary progress notes/assessments. Consult with direct-care staff and consulting dietician. Ask the resident if he or she experienced any of these symptoms in the last seven days. Sometimes a resident will not complain to staff members because he or she attributes symptoms to "old age." Therefore, it is important to ask the resident directly. Observe the resident while eating. If he or she leaves food or picks at it, ask "Why are you not eating?" Note if resident winces or makes faces while eating.

Coding: Check all conditions that apply. If no conditions apply, check *NONE OF ABOVE.*

5. Nutritional Approaches

Definition: **Parenteral/IV**— Intravenous (IV) fluids or hyperalimentation given continuously or intermittently. This category also includes administration of fluids via IV lines with fluids running at KVO (keep vein open), or via heparin locks. This category does not include administration of IV medications. If the resident receives IV medications, check item P1c in "Special Treatments and Procedures".

Feeding tube — Presence of any type of tube that can deliver food/nutritional substances/fluids/medications directly into the gastrointestinal system. Examples include, but are not limited to, nasogastric tubes, gastrostomy tubes, jejunostomy tubes, percutaneous endoscopic gastrostomy (PEG) tube.

Mechanically altered diet — A diet specifically prepared to alter the consistency of food in order to facilitate oral intake. Examples include soft solids, pureed foods, ground meat. Diets for residents who can only take liquids that have been thickened to prevent choking are also included in this definition.

Syringe (oral feeding) — Use of syringe to deliver liquid or pureed nourishment directly into the mouth.

Therapeutic diet — A diet ordered to manage problematic health conditions. Examples include calorie-specific, low-salt, low-fat lactose, no added sugar, and supplements during meals.

Dietary supplement between meals — Any type of dietary supplement provided between scheduled meals (e.g., high protein/calorie shake, or 3 p.m. snack for resident who receives q.a.m. dose of NPH insulin). Do not include snacks that everyone receives as part of the unit's daily routine.

Plate guard, stabilized built-up utensils, etc. — Any type of specialized, altered, or adaptive equipment to facilitate the resident's involvement in self-performance of eating.

On planned weight change program — Resident is receiving a program of which the documented purpose and goal are to facilitate weight gain or loss (e.g., double portions; high calorie supplements; reduced calories; 10 grams fat).

Coding: Check all that apply. If none apply, check *NONE OF ABOVE.*

6. Parenteral or Enteral Intake — Skip to Section L if neither item K5a nor K5b is checked.

Intent: To record the proportion of calories received, and the average fluid intake, through parenteral or tube feeding in the last seven days.

a. CALORIE INTAKE

Definition: **Proportion of total calories received** — the proportion of all calories during the last seven days ingested that the resident actually received (not ordered) by parenteral or tube feedings. Determined by calorie count.

Process: Review Intake record. If the resident took no food or fluids by mouth, or took just sips of fluid, stop here and code "4" (76%-100%). If the resident had more substantial oral intake than this, consult with the dietician who can derive a calorie count received from parenteral or tube feedings.

Coding: **Code for the best response.**

0. None
1. 1% to 25%
2. 26% to 50%
3. 51% to 75%
4. 76% to 100%

Example of Calculation for Proportion of Total Calories from IV or Tube Feeding

Mr. H has had a feeding tube since his surgery. He is currently more alert, and feeling much better. He is very motivated to have the tube removed. He has been taking soft solids by mouth, but only in small to medium amounts. For the past week he has been receiving tube feedings for nutritional supplementation. As his oral intake improves, the amount received by tube will decrease. The dietician has totalled his calories per day as follows:

Step #1:	**Oral**		**Tube**
Sun.	500	+	2000
Mon.	250	+	2250
Tues.	250	+	2250
Wed.	350	+	2250
Thurs.	500	+	2000
Fri.	800	+	1800
Sat.	800	+	1800
TOTAL	3450	+	14350

Step #2: Total calories = 3450 + 14350 = 17800

Step #3: Calculate percentage of total calories by tube feeding.

$\frac{14350}{17800} \times \frac{x}{100}$ [multiply total tube amount by 100, then divide by total calories]

1435000 divided by 17800 = 80.6% of total calories received by tube.

Step #4: **Code "4" for 76% to 100%**

b. AVERAGE FLUID INTAKE

Definition: Average fluid intake per day by IV or tube feeding in last seven days refers to the actual amount of fluid the resident received by these modes (not the amount ordered).

Process: Review the Intake and Output record from the last seven days. Add up the total amount of fluid received each day by IV and/or tube feedings only. Divide the week's total fluid intake by 7. This will give you the average of fluid intake per day.

Coding: Code for the average number of cc's of fluid the resident received per day by IV or tube feeding.

Codes:
0. None
1. 1 to 500 cc/day
2. 501 to 1000 cc/day
3. 1001 to 1500 cc/day
4. 1501 to 2000 cc/day
5. 2001 to or more cc/day

Example of Calculation for Average Daily Fluid Intake

Ms. A has swallowing difficulties secondary to Huntington's disease. She is able to take oral fluids by mouth with supervision, but not enough to maintain hydration. She received the following daily fluid totals by supplemental tube feedings (including water, prepared nutritional supplements, juices) during the last 7 days.

Step #1:

Sun.	1250 cc
Mon.	775 cc
Tues.	925 cc
Wed.	1200 cc
Thurs.	1200 cc
Fri.	1200 cc
Sat.	1000 cc
TOTAL	7550

Step #2:
7550 divided 7 = 1078.6 cc

Step #3:
Code "3" for 1001 to 1500 cc/day

SECTION L. ORAL/DENTAL STATUS

1. Oral Status and Disease Prevention

Intent: To document the resident's oral and dental status as well as any problematic conditions.

Definition: **Carious** — Pertains to tooth decay and disintegration (cavities).

Process: Ask the resident, and examine the resident's mouth. Ask direct care staff if they have noticed any problems. Review the clinical record.

Coding: Check all that apply. If none apply, check *NONE OF ABOVE*.

SECTION M. SKIN CONDITION

To determine the condition of the resident's skin, identify the presence, stage, type, and number of ulcers, and document other problematic skin conditions. Additionally, to document any skin treatments for active conditions as well as any protective or preventive skin or foot care treatments the resident has received in the last seven days.

1. Ulcer (due to any cause)

Intent: To record the number of ulcers, of any type at each ulcer stage, on any part of the body.

Definition: **Stage 1.** A persistent area of skin redness (without a break in the skin) that does not disappear when pressure is relieved.

Stage 2. A partial thickness loss of skin layers that presents clinically as an abrasion, blister, or shallow crater.

Stage 3. A full thickness of skin is lost, exposing the subcutaneous tissues. Presents as a deep crater with or without undermining adjacent tissue.

Stage 4. A full thickness of skin and subcutaneous tissue is lost, exposing muscle or bone.

Process: Review the resident's record and consult with the nurse assistant about the presence of an ulcer. Examine the resident and determine the stage and number of any ulcers present. Without a full body check, an ulcer can be missed.

Assessing a Stage 1 ulcer requires a specially focused assessment for residents with darker skin tones to take into account variations in ebony-colored skin. To recognize Stage 1 ulcers in ebony complexions, look for: (1) any change in the feel of the tissue in a high-risk area; (2) any change in the appearance of the skin in high-risk areas, such as the "orange-peel" look; (3) a subtle purplish hue; and (4) extremely dry, crust-like areas that, upon closer examination, are found to cover a tissue break.

Coding: Record the number of ulcers at each stage on the resident's body, in the last 7 days, regardless of the ulcer cause. If necrotic eschar is present, prohibiting accurate staging, code the ulcer as Stage "4" until the eschar has been debrided (surgically or mechanically) to allow staging. If there are no ulcers at a particular stage, record "0" (zero) in the box provided. If there are more than 9 ulcers at any one stage, enter "9" in the appropriate box.

Example

Mrs. L has end-stage metastatic cancer and weighs 75 pounds. She has a Stage 3 ulcer over her sacrum and two Stage 1 ulcers over her heels.

Stage	Code
a. 1	2
b. 2	0
c. 3	1
d. 4	0

2. Type of Ulcer

Intent: To record the highest stage for two types of ulcers, Pressure and Stasis, that were present in the last 7 days.

Definition: **Pressure ulcer** — Any lesion caused by pressure resulting in damage of underlying tissues. Other terms used to indicate this condition include bed sores and decubitus ulcers.

Stasis ulcer — An open lesion, usually in the lower extremities, caused by decreased blood flow from chronic venous insufficiency; also referred to as a venous ulcer or ulcer related to peripheral vascular disease (PVD).

Process: Review the resident's record. Consult with the physician regarding the cause of the ulcer(s).

Coding: Using the ulcer staging scale in item M1 record the highest ulcer stage for pressure and stasis ulcers present in the last 7 days. Remember that there are other types of ulcers than the two listed in this item (e.g., ischemic ulcers). An ulcer recorded in item M1 may not necessarily be recorded in item M2. (See last example below).

Example

Mr. C has diabetes and poor circulation to his lower extremities. Last month Mr. C spent 2 weeks in the hospital where he had a left below the knee amputation (BKA) for treatment of a gangrenous foot. His hospital course was complicated by delirium (acute confusion) and he spent most of his time on bedrest. Nurses remarked that he would only stay lying on his back. He had only an eggcrate mattress on his bed to relieve pressure. A water mattress and air mattress were both tried but aggravated his agitation. He was readmitted to the nursing home 3 days ago with a Stage II pressure ulcer over his sacrum and a Stage I pressure ulcer over his right heel and both elbows. No other ulcers were present.

Type of Ulcer	Code (highest stage)
a. Pressure ulcer	2
b. Stasis ulcer	0

***Rationale for coding*:** Mr. C has 4 pressure ulcers, the highest stage of which is Stage 2.

Mrs. B has a blockage in the arteries of her right leg causing impaired arterial circulation to her right foot (ischemia). She has only 1 ulcer, a Stage 3 ulcer on the dorsal surface (top) of her right foot.

Type of Ulcer	Code (highest stage)
a. Pressure ulcer	0
b. Stasis ulcer	0

***Rationale for coding*:** Mrs. B's ulcer is an ischemic ulcer rather than caused by pressure or venous stasis.

3. History of Resolved/Cured Ulcers

Intent: To determine if the resident previously had an ulcer that was resolved or cured during the past 90 days. Identification of this condition is important because it is a risk factor for development of subsequent ulcers.

Process: Review clinical records, including the last Quarterly Assessment

Coding: Code "0" for No or "1" for Yes.

4. Other Skin Problems or Lesions Present

Intent: To document the presence of skin problems other than ulcers, and conditions that are risk factors for more serious problems.

Definition: **Abrasions, bruises** — Includes skin scrapes, ecchymoses, localized areas of swelling, tenderness and discoloration.

Burns (second or third degree) — Includes burns from any cause (e.g., heat, chemicals) in any stage of healing. This category does not include first degree burns (changes in skin color only).

Rashes — Includes inflammation or eruption of the skin that may include change in color, spotting, blistering, etc. and symptoms such as itching, burning, or pain. Record rashes from any cause (e.g., heat, drugs, bacteria, viruses, contact with irritating substances such as urine or detergents, allergies, etc.). Intertrigo refers to rashes (dermatitis) within skin folds.

Skin desensitized to pain or pressure — The resident is unable to perceive sensations of pain or pressure.

Review the resident's record for documentation of impairment of this type. An obvious example of a resident with this problem is someone who is comatose. Other residents at high risk include those with quadriplegia, paraplegia, hemiplegia or hemiparesis, peripheral vascular disease and neurological disorders. In the absence of documentation in the clinical record, sensation can be tested in the following way:

- To test for pain, use a new, disposable safety pin or wooden "orange stick" (usually used for nail care). Always dispose of the pin or stick after each use to prevent contamination.

- Ask the resident to close his or her eyes. If the resident cannot keep his or her eyes closed or cannot follow directions to close eyes, block what you are doing (in local areas of legs and feet) from view with a cupped hand or towel.

- Lightly press the pointed end of the pin or stick against the resident's skin. Do not press hard enough to cause pain, injury, or break in the skin. Use the pointed and blunt ends of the pin or stick alternately to test sensations on the resident's arms, trunk, and legs. Ask the resident to report if the sensation is "sharp" or "dull."

- Compare the sensations in symmetrical areas on both sides of the body.

- If the resident is unable to feel the sensation, or cannot differentiate sharp from dull, the area is considered desensitized to pain sensation.

- For residents who are unable to make themselves understood or who have difficulty understanding your directions, rely on their facial expressions (e.g., wincing, grimacing, surprise), body motions (e.g., pulling the limb away, pushing the examiner) or sounds (e.g., "Ouch!") to determine if they can feel pain.

- Do not use pins with agitated or restless residents. Abrupt movements can cause injury.

Skin tears or cuts (other than surgery) — Any traumatic break in the skin penetrating to subcutaneous tissue. Examples include skin tears, lacerations, etc.

Surgical wounds — Includes healing and non-healing, open or closed surgical incisions, skin grafts or drainage sites on any part of the body. This category does not include healed surgical sites or stomas.

Process: Ask the resident if he or she has any problem areas. Examine the resident. Ask nurse assistant. Review the resident's record.

Coding: Check all that apply. If there is no evidence of such problems in the last seven days, check *NONE OF ABOVE.*

5. Skin Treatments

Intent: To document any specific or generic skin treatments the resident has received in the past seven days.

Definition: **Pressure relieving device(s) for chair** — Includes gel, air (e.g., Roho), or other cushioning placed on a chair or wheelchair. Do not include egg crate cushions in this category.

Pressure relieving device(s) for bed — Includes air fluidized, low airloss therapy beds, flotation, water, or bubble mattress or pad placed on the bed. Do not include egg crate mattresses in this category.

Turning/repositioning program — Includes a continuous, consistent program for changing the resident's position and realigning the body.

Nutrition or hydration intervention to manage skin problems — Dietary measures received by the resident for the purpose of preventing or treating specific skin conditions — e.g., wheat-free diet to prevent allergic dermatitis, high calorie diet with added supplements to prevent skin breakdown, high protein supplements for wound healing.

Ulcer care — Includes any intervention for treating an ulcer at any ulcer stage. Examples include use of dressings, chemical or surgical debridement, wound irrigations, and hydrotherapy.

Surgical wound care — Includes any intervention for treating or protecting any type of surgical wound. Examples of care include topical cleansing, wound irrigation, application of antimicrobial ointments, dressings of any type, suture removal, and warm soaks or heat application.

Application of dressings (with or without topical medications) other than to feet — Includes dry gauze dressings, dressings moistened with saline or other solutions, transparent dressings, hydrogel dressings, and dressings with hydrocolloid or hydroactive particles.

Application of ointments/medications (other than to feet) — Includes ointments or medications used to treat a skin condition (e.g., cortisone, antifungal preparations, chemotherapeutic agents, etc.). This definition does not include ointments used to treat non-skin conditions (e.g., nitropaste for chest pain).

Other preventative or protective skin care (other than to feet) — Includes application of creams or bath soaks to prevent dryness, scaling; application of protective elbow pads (e.g., down, sheepskin, padded, quilted).

Process: Review the resident's records. Ask the resident and nurse assistant.

Coding: Check all that apply. If none apply in the past seven days, check *NONE OF ABOVE*

6. Foot Problems and Care

Intent: To document the presence of foot problems and care to the feet during the last seven days.

Definition: **Open lesions on the foot** — Includes cuts, ulcers, fissures.

Nails or callouses trimmed during the last 90 days — Pertains to care of the feet. Includes trimming by nurse or any health professional, including a podiatrist.

Received preventative or protective foot care — Includes any care given for the purpose of preventing skin problems on the feet, such as diabetic foot care, foot soaks, protective booties (e.g., down, sheepskin, padded, quilted), special shoes, orthotics, application of toe pads, toe separators, etc.

Application of dressings with or without topical medications — Includes dry gauze dressings, dressings moistened with saline or other solutions, transparent dressings, hydrogel dressings, and dressings with hydrocolloid or hydroactive particles.

Process: Ask the resident and nurse assistant. Inspect the resident's feet. Review the resident's clinical records.

Coding: Check all that apply. If none apply in the past seven days, check *NONE OF ABOVE*

SECTION N. ACTIVITY PURSUIT PATTERNS

Intent: To record the amount and types of interests and activities that the resident currently pursues, as well as activities the resident would like to pursue that are not currently available at the facility.

Definition: Activity pursuits. Refers to any activity other than ADLs that a resident pursues in order to enhance a sense of well-being. These include activities that provide increased self-esteem, pleasure, comfort, education, creativity, success, and financial or emotional independence.

1. Time Awake

Intent: To identify those periods of a typical day (over the last seven days) when the resident was awake all or most of the time (i.e., no more than one hour nap during any such period). For careplanning purposes this information can be used in at least two ways:

- The resident who is awake most of the time could be encouraged to become more mentally, physically, and/or socially involved in activities (solitary or group).
- The resident who naps a lot may be bored or depressed and could possibly benefit from greater activity involvement.

Process: Consult with direct care staff, the resident, and the resident's family.

Coding: Check all periods when resident was awake all or most of the time. Morning is from 7 am (or when resident wakes up, if earlier or later than 7 am) until noon. Afternoon is from noon to 5 pm. Evening is from 5 pm to 10 pm (or bedtime, if earlier). **If resident is comatose, this is the only Section N item to code, skip all other Section N items and go to Section O.**

2. Average Time Involved in Activities

Intent: To determine the proportion of available time that the resident was actually involved in activity pursuits as an indication of his or her overall activity-involvement pattern. This time refers to free time when the resident was awake and was not involved in receiving nursing care, treatments, or engaged in ADL activities and could have been involved in activity pursuits and Therapeutic Recreation.

Process: Consult with direct care staff, activities staff members, the resident, and the resident's family. Ask about time involved in different activity pursuits.

Coding: In coding this item, exclude time spent in receiving treatments (e.g., medications, heat treatments, bandage changes, rehabilitation therapies, or ADLs). Include time spent in pursuing independent activities (e.g., watering plants, reading, letter-writing); social contacts (e.g., visits, phone calls) with family, other residents, staff, and volunteers; recreational pursuits in a group, one-on-one or an individual basis; and involvement in Therapeutic Recreation.

3. Preferred Activity Settings

Intent: To determine activity circumstances/settings that the resident prefers, including (though not limited to) circumstances in which the resident is at ease.

Process: Ask the resident, family, direct care staff, and activities staff about the resident's preferences. Staff's knowledge of observed behavior can be helpful, but only provides part of the answer. Do not limit preference list to areas to which the resident now has access, but try to expand the range of possibilities for the resident.

> **Example**
>
> Ask the resident, "Do you like to go outdoors? Outside the facility (to a mall)? To events downstairs?" Ask staff members to identify settings that resident frequents or where he or she appears to be most at ease.

Coding: Check all responses that apply. If the resident does not wish to be in any of these settings, check *NONE OF ABOVE*.

4. General Activity Preferences (adapted to resident's current abilities)

Intent: Determine which activities of those listed the resident would prefer to participate in (independently or with others). Choice should not be limited by whether or not the activity is currently available to the resident, or whether the resident currently engages in the activity.

Definition: **Exercise/sports** — Includes any type of physical activity such as dancing, weight training, yoga, walking, sports (e.g., bowling, croquet, golf, or watching sports).

Music — Includes listening to music or being involved in making music (singing, playing piano, etc.)

Reading/writing — Reading can be independent or done in a group setting where a leader reads aloud to the group or the group listens to "talking books." Writing can be solitary (e.g., letter-writing or poetry writing) or done as part of a group program (e.g., recording oral histories). Or a volunteer can record the thoughts of a blind, hemiplegic, or apraxic resident in a letter or journal.

Spiritual/religious activities — Includes participating in religious services as well as watching them on television or listening to them on the radio.

Gardening or plants — Includes tending one's own or other plants, participating in garden club activities, regularly watching a television program or video about gardening.

Talking or conversing — Includes talking and listening to social conversations and discussions with family, friends, other residents, or staff. May occur individually, in groups, or on the telephone; may occur informally or in structured situations.

Helping others — Includes helping other residents or staff, being a good listener, assisting with unit routines, etc.

Process: Consult with the resident, the resident's family, activities staff members, and nurse assistants. Explain to the resident that you are interested in hearing about what he or she likes to do or would be interested in trying. Remind the resident that a discussion of his or her likes and dislikes should not be limited by perception of current abilities or disabilities. Explain that many activity pursuits are adaptable to the resident's capabilities. For example, if a resident says that he used to love to read and misses it now that he is unable to see small print, explain about the availability of taped books or large print editions.

For residents with dementia or aphasia, ask family members about resident's former interests. A former love of music can be incorporated into the care plan (e.g., bedside audiotapes, sing-a-longs). Also observe the resident in current activities. If the resident appears content during an activity (e.g., smiling, clapping during a music program) check the item on the form.

Coding: Check each activity preferred. If none are preferred, check *NONE OF ABOVE.*

5. Prefers Change in Daily Routine

Intent: To determine if the resident has an interest in pursuing activities not offered at the facility (or on the nursing unit), or not made available to the resident. This includes situations in which an activity is provided but the resident would like to have other choices in carrying out the activity (e.g., the resident would like to watch the news on TV rather than the game shows and soap operas preferred by the majority of residents; or the resident would like a Methodist service rather than the Baptist service provided for the majority of residents). Residents who resist attendance/involvement in activities offered at the facility are also included in this category in order to determine possible reasons for their lack of involvement.

Process: Review how the resident spends the day. Ask the resident if there are things he or she would enjoy doing (or used to enjoy doing) that are not currently available or, if available, are not "right" for him or her in their current format. If the resident is unable to answer, ask the same question of a close family member, friend, activity professional, or nurse assistant. Would the resident prefer slight or major changes in daily routines, or is everything OK?

Coding: For each of the items, code for the resident's preferences in daily routines using the codes provided.

0. **No change** — Resident is content with current activity routines.

1. **Slight change** — Resident is content overall but would prefer minor changes in routine (e.g., a new activity, modification of a current activity).

2. **Major change** — Resident feels bored, restless, isolated, or discontent with daily activities or resident feels too involved in certain activities, and would prefer a significant change in routine.

Example

Mrs. B is regularly involved in several small group activities. She also has expressed a preference for music. However, she has consistently refused to go to group sing-alongs when the activity staff offer to bring her. She says she doesn't like big groups and prefers to relax and listen to classical music in her room. She wishes she had a radio or tape player to do this.

		Code
a.	Type of activities in which resident is currently involved	1 (Slight change)
b.	Extent of resident involvement in activities.	1 (Slight change)

SECTION O. MEDICATIONS

1. Number of Medications

Intent: To determine the number of different medications (over-the-counter and prescription drugs) the resident has received in the past seven days.

Process: Count the number of different medications (not the number of doses or different dosages) administered by any route (e.g., oral, IV, injections, patch) at any time during the last seven days. Include any routine, prn, and stat doses given. "Medications" can also include topical preparations, ointments, creams used in wound care (e.g., Elase), eyedrops, vitamins, and suppositories. Include any medication that the resident administers to self, if known. If the resident takes both the generic and brand name of a single drug, count as only one medication. If the resident received a long-acting antipsychotic medication prior to the assessment period (e.g., if a fluphenazine deconoate or haloperidol deconoate is given once a month) count as one drug.

Coding: Write the appropriate number in the answer box. Count only those medications actually administered and received by the resident over the last seven days. Do not count medications ordered but not given.

Example
Resident was given Digoxin 0.25 mg po on Tuesday and Thursday and Digoxin 0.125 mg po on Monday, Wednesday, and Friday. Although the dosage is different for different days of the week, the medication is the same. **Code "1" (one medication received).**

2. New Medications

Intent: To record whether the resident is currently receiving medications that were initiated in the last 90 days.

Coding: Code "1" if the resident received (and continues to receive) new medications in the last 90 days. Code "0" if the resident did not receive any new medications in the past 90 days. If the resident received new medication(s) in the last 90 days but they were discontinued prior to this assessment period, code "0" (no new medication).

3. Injections

Intent: To determine the number of days during the past seven days that the resident received any type of medication, antigen, vaccine, by subcutaneous, intramuscular or intradermal injection. Although antigens and vaccines are considered "biologicals" and not medication per se, it is important to track when they are given to monitor for localized or systemic reactions. This category does not include intravenous (IV) fluids or medications. If the resident received IV fluids, record in Item K5a, Parenteral/IV. If IV medications were given, record in Item P1c, IV medications.

Coding: Record the number of DAYS in the answer box.

Example

During the last seven days, Mr. T received a flu shot on Monday, a PPD test (for tuberculosis) on Tuesday, a Vitamin B_{12} injection on Wednesday. **Code "3" for Resident received injections on three days during the last seven days.**

4. Days Received the Following Medication

Intent: To record the number of days that the resident received each type of medication listed (antipsychotics, antianxiety, antidepressants, hypnotics, diuretics) in the past seven days. See Appendix E for list of drugs by category. Includes any of these medications given to the resident by any route (po, IM, or IV) in any setting (e.g., at the nursing home, in a hospital emergency room).

Process: Review the resident's clinical record for documentation that a medication was received by the resident during the past seven days. In the case of a new admission, review transmittal records.

Coding: Enter the number of days each of the listed types of medications was received by the resident during the past seven days. In the case of a new admission, if it is clearly documented that the resident received any type of medication (listed in this item) at the sending facility, record the number of days each listed medication was received during the past seven days. If transmittal records are not clear or do not reference that the resident received one of these medications, record "0" (not used) in the corresponding box. If the resident did not use any medications from a drug category, enter "0". If the resident uses long-lasting drugs that are taken less often than weekly (e.g., Prolixin (Fluphenazine deconoate) or Haldol (Haloperidol deconoate) given every few weeks or monthly) enter "1."

Example 1

Medication Record for Mrs. P

- Haldol 0.5 mg po BID p.r.n.: Received once a day on Monday, Wednesday, and Thursday [Note: Haldol = Antipsychotic drug]

- Ativan 1 mg po QAM: Received every day [Note: Ativan = Antianxiety drug]

- Restoril 15 mg po QHS p.r.n.: Received at H.S. on Tuesday and Wednesday only [Note: Restoril = Hypnotic]

- Mrs. P became severely short of breath in the middle of the night during the last seven days. She was transferred (but not admitted) to the emergency room (ER) at the local hospital. Upon her return to the nursing home the ER transmittal record stated that she had received 1 dose of IV Lasix [Note: Lasix = Diuretic].

Coding

Medication	No. of days received
a. Antipsychotic:	"3" (days)
b. Antianxiety:	"7" (days)
c. Antidepressant:	"0" (days)
d. Hypnotic:	"2" (days)
e. Diuretic:	"1" (days)

Example 2

Mr. S was admitted to the nursing home on 9/12/94 (Date of Entry) from an acute care hospital. The clinical staff established that 9/16/94 would be the MDS assessment reference date (last day of MDS observation period). By establishing 9/16/94 as the reference date, the observation period of 7 days extended back to 9/10/94 when Mr. S was still in the hospital. His hospital discharge summary mentioned that Mr. S was started on a daily dose of Prozac (an antidepressant) on 8/20. The hospital discharge summary was too sketchy to accurately determine if Mr. S received other medications during his hospital stay. Since admission to the nursing home Mr. S continues to receive the same dose of Prozac.

Coding

Medication	No. of days received
a. Antipsychotic:	"0" (days)
b. Antianxiety:	"0" (days)
c. Antidepressant:	"7" (days)
d. Hypnotic:	"0" (days)
e. Diuretic:	"0" (days)

SECTION P. SPECIAL TREATMENTS AND PROCEDURES

1. Special Treatments, Procedures, and Programs

Intent: To identify any special treatments, therapies, or programs that the resident received in the specified time period.

a. SPECIAL CARE

TREATMENTS — The following treatments may be received by a nursing facility resident either at the facility, as a hospital out-patient, or in-patient basis, etc. Check the appropriate MDS item regardless of where the resident received the treatment.

Definition: **Chemotherapy** — Includes any type of chemotherapy (anticancer drug) given by any route.

Dialysis — Includes peritoneal or renal dialysis that occurs at the nursing facility or at an other facility.

IV Medication — Includes any drug or biological (e.g., contrast material) given by intravenous push or drip through a central or peripheral port. Does not include a saline or heparin flush to keep a heparin lock patent, or IV fluids without medication.

Intake/output — The measurement and evaluation of all fluids the resident received and/or excreted for at least three consecutive shifts (i.e., 24 hours).

Monitoring acute medical condition — Includes observation by a licensed nurse for ANY acute physical or psychiatric illness.

Ostomy care — This item refers only to care that requires nursing assistance. Do not include tracheostomy care. Code tracheostomy care by checking item P1j.

Oxygen therapy — Includes continuous or intermittent oxygen via mask, cannula, etc.

Radiation — Includes radiation therapy or having a radiation implant.

Suctioning — Includes nasopharyngeal or tracheal aspiration.

Tracheostomy care — Includes cleansing of tracheostomy and cannula.

Transfusions — Includes transfusions of blood or any blood products (e.g., platelets).

Ventilator or respirator — Assures adequate ventilation in residents who are, or who may become, unable to support their own respiration. Includes any type of electrically or pneumatically powered closed system mechanical ventilatory support devices. Any resident who was in the process of being weaned off of the ventilator or respirator in the last 14 days should be coded under this definition.

PROGRAMS — The following programs refer to those received within a nursing facility ONLY.

Alcohol/drug treatment program — A comprehensive interdisciplinary program within an entire or contiguous unit, wing, or floor where interventions are designed specifically for the treatment of alcohol or drug addictions.

Alzheimer's/dementia special care unit — Any identifiable part of the nursing facility, such as an entire or a contiguous unit, wing, or floor where staffing patterns and resident care interventions are designed specifically for cognitively impaired residents who may or may not have a specific diagnosis of Alzheimer's disease.

Hospice care — The resident is identified as being in a program for terminally ill persons where services are necessary for the palliation and management of terminal illness and related conditions.

Pediatric unit — Any identifiable part of the nursing facility, such as an entire or contiguous unit or wing where staffing patterns and resident care interventions are designed specifically for persons aged 22 or younger.

Respite care — Resident's care program involves a short-term stay in the facility for the purpose of providing relief to a nursing home-eligible resident's primary home based caregiver(s). Following this planned short stay, it is anticipated that the resident will return to his or her home in the community.

Training in skills required to return to the community — Resident is regularly involved in individual or group activities with a licensed skilled professional to attain goals necessary for community living (e.g., medication management, housework, shopping, using transportation, activities of daily living).

Process: Review the resident's clinical record.

Coding: Check all treatments and procedures that were received during the last 14 days. If no items apply in the last 14 days, check NONE OF ABOVE.

b. THERAPIES

Therapies that occurred after admission to the nursing home, were ordered by a physician, and were performed by a qualified therapist (i.e., one who meets state credentialing requirements or in some instances, under such a person's direct supervision).

The therapy treatment may occur either inside or outside the facility. Includes **only** therapies based on a therapist's assessment and treatment plan that is documented in the resident's clinical record.

Intent: To record the (A) number of days and (B) total number of minutes each of the following therapies was administered (for at least 15 minutes a day) in the last 7 days.

Definition: **Speech-language pathology, audiology services** — Services that are provided by a qualified speech-language pathologist.

Occupational therapy — Therapy services that are provided or directly supervised by a qualified occupational therapist. A qualified occupational therapy assistant may provide therapy but not supervise others (aides or volunteers) giving therapy. Include services provided by a qualified occupational therapy assistant who is employed by (or under contract to) the nursing facility only if he or she is under the direction of a qualified occupational therapist.

Physical therapy — Therapy services that are provided or directly supervised by a qualified physical therapist. A qualified physical therapy assistant may provide therapy but not supervise others (aides or volunteers) giving therapy. Include service provided by a qualified physical therapy assistant who is employed by (or under contract to) the nursing facility only if he or she is under the direction of a qualified physical therapist.

Respiratory therapy — Included are coughing, deep breathing, heated nebulizers, aerosol treatments, and mechanical ventilation, etc., which must be provided by a qualified professional (i.e., trained nurse, respiratory therapist). Does not include hand held medication dispensers. Count only the time that the qualified professional spends with the resident.

Psychological therapy — Therapy given by any licensed mental health professional, such as a psychiatrist, psychologist, psychiatric nurse, or psychiatric social worker.

Process: Review the resident's clinical record and consult with each of the qualified therapists.

Coding: **Box A:** In the first column, enter the number (#) of days the therapy was administered for 15 minutes or more in the last seven calendar days. Enter "0" if none.

Box B: In the second column, enter the total number (#) of minutes the particular therapy was provided in the last seven days even if you entered "0" in Box A (e.g., less than 15 minutes of therapy provided). The time should include only the actual treatment time (not time waiting or writing reports). Enter"0" if none.

Example

Following a stroke Mrs. F was admitted to the nursing home in stable condition for rehabilitation therapies. Since admission she has been receiving speech therapy twice weekly for 30-minute sessions, occupational therapy twice weekly for 30-minute sessions, and physical therapy twice a day (30 minute sessions) for 5 days and respiratory therapy for 10 minutes per day on each of the last 7 days. During the last seven days Mrs. F has participated in all of her scheduled sessions.

Coding	A	B
a. Speech-language pathology, audiology services	2	60
b. Occupational therapy	2	60
c. Physical therapy	5	300
d. Respiratory therapy	0	70
e. Psychological therapy	0	0

2. Intervention Programs for Mood, Behavior, Cognitive Loss

Definition: **Special behavior symptom evaluation program** — A program of ongoing, comprehensive, interdisciplinary evaluation of behavioral symptoms (such as the symptoms described in item E4). The purpose of such a program is to attempt to understand the "meaning" behind the resident's behavioral symptoms in relation to the resident's health and functional status, and social and physical environment. The ultimate goal of the evaluation is to develop and implement a plan of care that serves to reduce distressing symptoms.

Evaluation by a licensed mental health specialist in the last 90 days — An assessment of a mood, behavior disorder, or other mental health problem by a qualified clinical professional such as a psychiatrist, psychologist, psychiatric nurse, or psychiatric social worker, depending on State practice acts. Do not check this item for routine visits by the facility social worker. Evaluation may take place at the nursing home, private office, clinic, community mental health center, etc.

Group therapy — Resident regularly attends sessions at least weekly. Therapy is aimed at helping to reduce loneliness, isolation, and the sense that one's problems are unique and difficult to solve. The session may take place either at the nursing home (e.g., support group run by the facility's social worker) or outside the facility (e.g., group program at community mental health center, Alcoholics Anonymous meeting at a local church, Parkinson's Disease support group at local hospital). This item does not include group recreational or leisure activities.

Resident-specific deliberate changes in the environment to address mood/behavior/cognitive patterns — Adaptation of the milieu focused on the resident's individual mood/behavior/cognitive pattern. Examples include placing a banner labeled "wet paint" across a closet door to keep the resident from repetitively emptying all the clothes out of the closet, or placing a bureau of old clothes in an alcove along a corridor to provide diversionary "props" for a resident who frequently stops wandering to rummage. The latter diverts the resident from rummaging through belongings in other residents' rooms along the way.

Reorientation — Individual or group sessions that aim to reduce disorientation in confused residents. Includes environmental cueing in which all staff involved with the resident provide orienting information and reminders.

Process: Review the resident's clinical record for documentation of intervention programs. These interventions also should be documented in the care plan.

Coding: Check all that apply. If none apply, check *NONE OF ABOVE.*

3. Nursing Rehabilitation/Restorative Care

Intent: To determine the extent to which the resident receives nursing rehabilitation or restorative services from other than specialized therapy staff (e.g., occupational therapist, physical therapist, etc.). Rehabilitative or restorative care refers to nursing interventions that promote the resident's ability to adapt and adjust to living as independently and safely as is possible. This concept actively focuses on achieving and maintaining optimal physical, mental, and psychosocial functioning.

Skill practice in such activities as walking and mobility, dressing and grooming, eating and swallowing, transferring, amputation care, and communication can improve or maintain function in physical abilities and ADLs and prevent further impairment.

Definition: **Rehabilitation/restorative care** — Included are nursing interventions that assist or promote the resident's ability to attain his or her maximum functional potential. This item does not inclulde procedures or techniques carried out by or under the direction of qualified therapists, as identified in item P1b. In addition, **to be included in this section, a rehabilitation or restorative practice must meet all of the following additional criteria:**

- Measurable objectives and interventions must be documented in the care plan and in the clinical record.
- Evidence of periodic evaluation by licensed nurse must be present in the clinical record.
- Nurse assistants/aides must be trained in the techniques that promote resident involvement in the activity.
- These activities are carried out or supervised by members of the nursing staff. Sometimes under licensed nurse supervision, other staff and volunteers will be assigned to work with specific residents.
- This category does not include exercise groups with more than four residents per supervising helper or caregiver.

Range of motion — The extent to which, or the limits between which, a part of the body can be moved around a fixed point, or joint. Range of motion exercise is a program of passive or active movements to maintain flexibility and useful motion in the joints of the body.

Active range of motion — Exercises performed by a resident, with cueing or supervision by staff, that are planned, scheduled, and documented in the clinical record.

Splint or brace assistance — Assistance can be of 2 types: 1) where staff provide verbal and physical guidance and direction that teaches the resident how to apply, manipulate, and care for a brace or splint, or 2) where staff have a scheduled program of applying and removing a splint or brace, assess the resident's skin and circulation under the device, and reposition the limb in correct alignment. These sessions are planned, scheduled, and documented in the clinical record.

Training and skill practice — Activities including repetition, physical or verbal cueing, and task segmentation provided by any staff member or volunteer under the supervision of a licensed nurse.

Bed mobility — Activities used to improve or maintain the resident's self-performance in moving to and from a lying position, turning side to side, and positioning him or herself in bed.

Transfer — Activities used to improve or maintain the resident's self-performance in moving between surfaces or planes either with or without assistive devices.

Walking — Activities used to improve or maintain the resident's self-performance in walking, with or without assistive devices.

Dressing or grooming — Activities used to improve or maintain the resident's self-performance in dressing and undressing, bathing and washing, and performing other personal hygiene tasks.

Eating or swallowing — Activities used to improve or maintain the resident's self-performance in feeding one's self food and fluids, or activities used to improve or maintain the resident's ability to ingest nutrition and hydration by mouth.

Amputation/prosthesis care — Activities used to improve or maintain the resident's self-performance in putting on and removing a prosthesis, caring for the prosthesis, and providing appropriate hygiene at the site where the prosthesis attaches to the body (e.g., leg stump or eye socket).

Communication— Activities used to improve or maintain the resident's self-performance in using newly acquired functional communication skills or assisting the resident in using residual communication skills and adaptive devices.

Other — Any other activities used to improve or maintain the resident's self-performance in functioning. This includes, but is not limited to, teaching self-care for diabetic management, self-administration of medications, ostomy care, and cardiac rehabilitation.

Process: Review the clinical record and the current care plan. Consult with facility staff. Look for rehabilitation, restorative care schedule, assignment, and implementation record sheet on the nursing unit.

Coding: For the last seven days, enter the number of days on which the technique, procedure, or activity was practiced for a total of at least 15 minutes during the 24-hour period. The 15 minutes does not have to occur all at once. Remember that persons with dementia learn skills best through repetition that occurs multiple times per day. Review for each activity throughout the 24-hour period. Enter zero "0" if none.

Examples of Nursing Rehabilitation/Restoration

Mr. V has lost range of motion (ROM) in his right arm, wrist and hand due to a CVA experienced several years ago. He has moderate to severe loss of cognitive decision-making skills and memory. To avoid further ROM loss and contractures to his right arm, the occupational therapist fabricated a right resting handsplint and instructions for its application and removal. The nursing coordinator developed instructions for providing passive range of motion exercises to his right arm, wrist and hand 3 times per day. The nursing assistants and Mr. V's wife have been instructed on how and when to apply and remove the handsplint and how to do the passive ROM exercises. These plans are documented on Mr. V's care plan. The total amount of time involved each day in removing and applying the handsplint and completing the ROM exercises is 30 minutes. The nursing assistants report that there is less resistance in Mr. V's affected extremity when bathing and dressing him. For both Splint or Brace assistance and Range of Motion (passive), **enter "7" as the number of days these nursing rehabilitative techniques were provided.**

Mrs. K was admitted to the nursing facility 7 days ago following repair to a fractured hip. Physical therapy was delayed due to complications and a weakened condition. Upon admission, she had difficulty moving herself in bed and required total assistance for transfers. To prevent further deterioration and increase her independence, the nursing staff implemented a plan on the second day following admission to teach her how to move herself in bed and transfer from bed to chair using a trapeze, the bedrails, and a transfer board. The plan was documented in Mrs. K's clinical record and communicated to all staff at the change of shift. The charge nurse documented in the nurses notes that in the five days Mrs. K has been receiving training and skill practice for bed mobility and transferring, her endurance and strength are improving, and she requires only extensive assistance for transferring. Each day the amount of time to provide this nursing rehabilitation intervention has been decreasing so that for the past five days, the average time is 45 minutes. **Enter "5" as the number of days training and skill practice for bed mobility and transfer was provided.**

Mrs. J had a CVA less than a year ago resulting in left-sided hemiplegia. Mrs. J has a strong desire to participate in her own care. Although she cannot dress herself independently, she is capable of participating in this activity of daily living. Mrs. J's overall care plan goal is to maximize her independence in ADL's. A plan, documented on the care plan, has been developed to teach Mrs. J how to put on and take off her blouse with no physical assistance from the staff. All of her blouses have been adapted for front closure with velcro. The nursing assistants have been instructed in how to verbally guide Mrs. J as she puts on and takes off her blouse. It takes approximately 20 minutes per day for Mrs. J to complete this task (dressing and undressing). **Enter "7" as the number of days training and skill practice for dressing and grooming was provided.**

(continued on next page)

Examples of Nursing Rehabilitation/Restoration (continued)

Using a quad cane and a short leg brace, Mrs. D is receiving training and skill practice in walking. Together, Mrs. D and the nursing staff have set progressive walking distance goals. The nursing staff have received instruction on how to provide Mrs. D with the instruction and guidance she needs to achieve the goals. She has three scheduled times each day where she learns how to apply her short leg brace followed by walking. Each teaching and practice episode for brace application and walking, supervised by a nursing assistant, takes approximately 15 minutes. **Enter "7" as the number of days for splint and brace assistance and training and skill practice in walking were provided**.

Experiencing a slow recovery from Guillain Barre syndrome, Mr. B is receiving daily training and skill practice in swallowing. Along with specially designed cups and appropriate food consistency, the documented plan of care to improve his ability to swallow involves proper body positioning, consistent verbal instructions, and jaw control techniques. Mr. B requires close monitoring when given food and fluids as he is at risk for choking and aspiration. Therefore, only licensed nurses provide this nursing rehabilitative intervention. It takes approximately 35 minutes each meal for Mr. B to finish his food and liquids. He receives supplements via a gastrostomy tube if her does not achieve the prescribed fluid and caloric intake by mouth. **Enter "7" as the number of days training and skill practice in swallowing was provided.**

Mr. W's cognitive status has been deteriorating progressively over the past several months. Despite deliberate nursing restoration, attempts to promote his independence in feeding himself, he will not eat unless he is fed. Because Mr. W did not receive nursing rehabilitation/restoration for eating in the last 7 days, **enter "0" as the number of days training and skill practice for eating was provided.**

Mrs. E has amyotrophic lateral sclerosis. She no longer has the ability to speak or even to nod her head "yes" and "no". Her cognitive skills remain intact, she can spell, and she can move her eyes in all directions. The speech language pathologist taught both Mrs. E and the nursing staff to use a communication board so that Mrs. E. could communicate with staff. The communication board has proven very successful and the nursing staff, volunteers and family members are reminded by a sign over Mrs. E's bed that they are to provide her with the board to enable her to communicate with them. This is also documented in Mrs. E's care plan. Because the teaching and practice in using the communication board had been completed two weeks ago and Mrs. E is able to use the board to communicate successfully, she no longer receives skill and practice training in communication. **Enter "0" as the number of days training and skill practice in communication was provided.**

4. Devices and Restraints

Intent: To record the frequency, over the last seven days, with which the resident was restrained by any of the devices listed below at any time during the day or night.

Definition: This category includes the use of any device (e.g., physical or mechanical device, material, or equipment attached or adjacent to the resident's body) that the resident cannot easily remove and that restricts freedom of movement or normal access to his or her body.

- **Full bed rails** — Full rails may be one or more rails along both sides of the resident's bed that block three-quarters to the whole length of the mattress from top to bottom. This definition also includes beds with one side placed against the wall (prohibiting the resident from entering and exiting on that side) and the other side blocked by a full rail (one or more rails). A veil screen (used in pediatric units) is included in this category.

- **Other types of bed rails used** (e.g., one-side half rail, one-side full rail, two-sided half rails).

- **Trunk restraint** — Includes any device or equipment or material that the resident cannot easily remove (e.g., vest or waist restraint).

- **Limb restraint** — Includes any device or equipment or material that the resident cannot easily remove, that restricts movement of any part of an upper extremity (i.e., hand, arm) or lower extremity (i.e., foot, leg).

- **Chair prevents rising** — Any type of chair with locked lap board or chair that places resident in a recumbent position that restricts rising or a chair that is soft and low to the floor (e.g., bean bag chair). Includes "comfort cushions" (e.g., lap buddy), "merry walkers."

Process: Check the resident's clinical records and restraint flow sheets. Consult nursing staff. Observe the resident.

Coding: For each device type, enter:

0. Not used in last seven days
1. Used, but used less than daily in last seven days
2. Used on a daily basis in last seven days

5. Hospital Stay(s)

Intent: To record how many times the resident was admitted to the hospital with an overnight stay in the last 90 days or since the last assessment if less than 90 days [regardless of payment status for these days either by the hospital or by the nursing home]. If the resident is a new admission to the facility, this item includes admissions during the period prior to admission.

Definition: The resident was formally admitted by a physician as an in-patient with the expectation that he or she will stay overnight. It does not include day surgery, out-patient services, etc.

Process: Review the resident's record. If the resident is a new admission, ask the resident and resident's family. Sometimes transmittal records from recent hospital admissions are not readily available during a nursing home admission from the community.

Coding: Enter the number of hospital admissions in the box. Enter "0" if no hospital admissions.

Examples

Mrs. D, an insulin-dependent diabetic, was admitted to the nursing home yesterday from her own home. At home she had been having a lot of difficulty with insulin regulation since developing an ulcer on her left foot six weeks ago. During the last 90 days prior to admission, Mrs. D had two hospitalizations, for 3 and 5 days respectively. **Code "2" for two hospital admissions in the last 90 days.**

Mr. W has been a resident of the nursing facility for two years. He has a blood dyscrasia and receives transfusions at the local emergency room twice monthly. In the last month Mr. W was admitted to the hospital for 2 days after developing a fever during his blood transfusion. **Code "1" for one hospital admission in the last 90 days.**

6. Emergency Room (ER) Visit(s)

Intent: To record if during the last 90 days the resident visited a hospital emergency room (e.g., for treatment or evaluation) but was not admitted to the hospital for an overnight stay at that time. If the resident is a new admission to the facility, this item includes emergency room visits during the period prior to admission.

Definition: **Emergency room visit** — A visit to an emergency room not accompanied by an overnight hospital stay. Exclude prior scheduled visits for physician evaluation, transfusions, chemotherapy, etc.

Process: Review the resident's clinical record. For new admissions, ask the resident and the resident's family and review the transmittal record.

Coding: Enter the number of ER visits in the last 90 days (or since last assessment if less than 90 days). Enter "0" if no ER visits.

Examples

One evening, Mr. X complained of chest pain and shortness of breath. He was transferred to the local emergency room for evaluation. In the emergency room Mr. X was given IV Lasix, nitrates, and oxygen. By the time he stabilized, it was late in the evening and he was admitted to the hospital for observation. He was transferred back to the nursing home the next afternoon. **Code "0" for No ER visits.** The **rationale** for this coding is that although Mr. X was transferred to the emergency room, he was admitted to the hospital overnight. An overnight stay is not part of the definition of this item.

During the night shift, Mrs. F slipped and fell on her way to the bathroom. She complained of pain in her right hip and was transferred to the local emergency room for x-rays. The x-rays were negative for a fracture and Mrs. F was transferred back to the nursing home within several hours. **Code "1" for 1 ER visit.**

Once during the last 90 days, Mr. P's gastrostomy tube became dislodged and nursing home staff were unsuccessful in reinserting it after multiple attempts. Mr. P was then transferred to the local emergency room where the on-call physician reinserted the tube. **Code "1" for ER visit.**

7. Physician Visits

Intent: To record the **number of days** during the last 14-day period a physician has examined the resident (or since admission if less than 14 days ago). Examination can occur in the facility or in the physician's office. In some cases the frequency of physician's visits is indicative of clinical complexity.

Definition: **Physician** — Includes MD, osteopath, podiatrist, or dentist who is either the primary physician or consultant. Also include an authorized physician assistant, or nurse practitioner working in collaboration with the physician.

Physician exam — May be a partial or full exam at the facility or in the physician's office. This does not include exams conducted in an emergency room. If the resident was examined by a physician during an unscheduled emergency room visit, record the number of times this happened in the last 90 days in Item P6, "Emergency Room (Visits)".

Coding: Enter the number of days the physician examined the resident. If none, enter "0".

8. Physician Orders

Intent: To record the **number of days** during the last 14-day period (or since admission, if less than 14 days ago) in which a physician has changed the resident's orders. In some cases the frequency of physician's order changes is indicative of clinical complexity.

Definition: **Physician** — Includes MD, DO (osteopath), podiatrist, or dentist who is either the primary physician or a consultant. Also includes authorized physician assistant or nurse practitioner working in collaboration with the physician.

Physician orders — Includes written, telephone, fax, or consultation orders for new or altered treatment. Does NOT include admission orders, return admission orders, or renewal orders without changes.

Coding: Enter the number of days on which physician orders were changed. Do not include order renewals without change. If no order changes, enter "0".

9. Abnormal Lab Values

Intent: To document whether the resident had any abnormal laboratory values during the last 90 days. This item refers only to laboratory tests performed after admission to the nursing home. "Abnormal" refers to laboratory values that are abnormal when compared to standard values, not abnormal for the particular resident.

Example

An elevated prothrombin time in a resident receiving coumadin therapy is coded "1" for Yes (Abnormal) even though this may be the desired effect.

Process: Check medical records, especially laboratory reports.

Coding: Enter "0" if no abnormal value was noted in the record, and "1" if the resident has had at least one abnormal laboratory value.

SECTION Q. DISCHARGE POTENTIAL AND OVERALL STATUS

1. Discharge Potential

Intent: To identify residents who are potential candidates for discharge within the next three months. Some residents will meet the "potential discharge" profile at admission; others will move into this status as they continue to improve during the first few months of residency.

Definition: **Discharge** — Can be to home, another community setting, another care facility, or a residential setting. A prognosis of death should not be considered as an expected discharge.

Support person — Can be a spouse, family member, or significant other.

Process: For new and recent admissions, ask the resident directly. The longer the resident lives at the facility, the tougher it is to ask about preferences to return to the community. After one year of residency, many persons feel settled into the new lifestyle at the facility. Creating unrealistic expectations for a resident can be cruel. Use careful judgement. Listen to what the resident brings up (e.g., Calls out, "I want to go home"). Ask indirect questions that will give you a better feel for the resident's preferences. For example, say, "It's been about 1 year that we've known each other. How are things going for you here at (facility)".

Consult with primary care and social service staff, the resident's family, and significant others. Review clinical records. Discharge plans are often recorded in social service notes, nursing notes, or medical progress notes.

Coding:

a. **Resident expresses/indicates preference to return to the community.** Enter "0" for No or "1" for Yes.

b. **Resident has a support person who is positive towards discharge.** Enter "0" for No or "1" for Yes.

c. **Stay projected to be of a short duration** — Discharge projected within 90 days (do not include expected discharge due to death). Enter "0" for No, "1" for within 30 days, "2" for within 31-90 days, or "3" for discharge status uncertain.

Examples

Mrs. F is a 65 year old married woman who sustained a CVA 2 months ago. She was admitted to the nursing facility one week ago from a rehabilitation facility for further rehab, particularly for transfer, gait training, and wheelchair mobility. Mrs. F is extremely motivated to return home. Her husband is supportive and has been busy making their home "user friendly" to promote her independence. Their goal is to be ready for discharge within 2 months.

Discharge Potential	**Coding**
a. Resident expresses/indicates preference to return to the community.	1 (Yes)
b. Resident has a support person who is positive towards discharge.	1 (Yes)
c. Stay projected to be of a short duration — discharge projected within 90 days (do not include expected discharge due to death).	2 (Within 31-90 days)

Mrs. D is a 67 year old widow with end-stage metastatic cancer to bone with pathological fractures. Currently her major problems are pain control and confusion secondary to narcotics. Mrs. D periodically calls out for someone to take her home to her own bed. Her daughter is unwilling and unable to manage her hospice care at home. Because of the fractures, Mrs. D is totally dependent in all ADLs except eating (she can hold a straw).

Discharge Potential	**Coding**
a. Resident expresses/indicates preference to return to the community	1 (Yes)
b. Resident has a support person who is positive towards discharge	0 (No)
c. Stay projected to be of short duration — discharge projected within 90 days (do not include expected discharge due to death).	0 (No)

Rationale for coding:
Although Mrs. D is near death, you should apply a code of "0" (No). This MDS item instructs you "do not include expected discharge due to death."

Examples (continued)

Mr. S is a 70 year old married gentleman who was admitted to the facility 2 weeks ago from the hospital following surgical repair of a left hip fracture. Mr. S has a long history of alcoholism and cirrhosis of the liver. His daughter reports that when he is drinking he is abusive towards his wife of 40 years. Though he has a strong wish to return home, his wife states she can't take it anymore and doesn't want him to return home. He has basically worn out all his family options. Other social support options are being explored. At this time plans for discharge remain uncertain.

Discharge Potential		**Coding**
a.	Resident expresses/indicates preference to return to the community.	1 (Yes)
b.	Resident has a support person who is positive towards discharge.	0 (No)
c.	Stay projected to be of a short duration — discharge projected within 90 days (do not include expected discharge due to death).	3 (Uncertain)

2. Overall Change in Care Needs

Intent: To monitor the resident's overall progress at the facility over time. Document changes as compared to his or her status of 90 days ago (or since last assessment if less than 90 days ago). If the resident is a new admission to the facility, this item includes changes during the period prior to admission.

Definition: **Overall self-sufficiency** — Includes self-care performance and support, continence patterns, involvement patterns, use of treatments, etc.

Process: Review clinical record, transmittal records (if new admission or readmission), previous MDS assessments (including quarterly reviews), and care plan. Discuss with direct caregivers.

Coding: Record the number corresponding to the most correct response. Enter "0" for No change, "1" for Improved (receives fewer supports, needs less restrictive level of care), or "2" for Deteriorated (receives more support).

Examples

Mr. R is a 90 year old comatose gentleman admitted to the facility from a 6 months stay at another nursing facility to be closer to his wife's residence. His condition has remained unchanged for approximately 6 months. **Code "0" for No change.**

Mrs. T has a several year history of Alzheimer's disease. In the past four months her overall condition has generally improved. Although her cognitive function has remained unchanged, her mood is improved. She seems happier, less agitated, sleeps more soundly at night, and is more socially involved in daily activity programming. **Code "1" for Improved.**

Mr. D also has a several year history of Alzheimer's disease. Although for the past year he was quite dependent on others in most areas, he was able to eat and walk with supervision until recently. In the past 90 days he has become more dependent. He no longer feeds himself. Additionally, he fell 2 weeks ago and has been unable to learn how to use a walker. He requires a 2 person assist for walking even short distances. **Code "2" for Deteriorated.**

SECTION R. ASSESSMENT INFORMATION

1. Participation in Assessment

Intent: To record the participation of the resident, family and/or significant others in the assessment, and to indicate reason if the resident's assessment is incomplete.

Definition: **Family** — A spousal, kin (e.g., sibling, child, parent, nephew), or in-law relationship.

Significant other — May include close friend, lover, house mate, legal guardian, trust officer, or attorney. Significant other does not, however, include staff at the nursing facility.

Process: Preparing residents and family members to participate in the care-planning process begins with assessment. When staff members explain the assessment process to a resident, they should also explain that the outcome of assessment is care delivery guided by a care plan. Every assessment team member can establish an expectation of resident participation by asking for and respecting the resident's perspective during assessment.

Asking family members about their expectations of the nursing facility and their concerns during the assessment process can prove beneficial. Relatives may need to talk to a staff member or they may need information. Some family concerns and expectations can be appropriately addressed in the care-planning conference. Discussing these matters with the family during the assessment process can assist in maintaining a focus on the resident during the care-planning meeting.

Staff should consider some important aspects of resident and/or family participation in assessment and care planning. Attention to seating arrangements that will facilitate communication is necessary for several reasons:

- To keep the resident from feeling intimidated and/or powerless in front of professionals.

- To accommodate any communication impairments.

- To minimize any tendencies for family members to dominate the resident in the conference yet encourage them to support the resident if that is needed.

- To facilitate nonverbal support of the resident by staff with whom the resident is close.

Verbal communication should be directed to the resident, even when the resident is cognitively impaired. The terms used should be tailored to facilitate understanding by the resident. The resident's opinions, questions, and responses to the developing care plan should be solicited if they are not forthcoming.

Coding:

a) **Resident** — Enter zero "0" for No or "1" for Yes to indicate whether the resident participated in the assessment. This item should be completed last.

b) **Family** — Enter zero "0" for No or "1" for Yes to indicate whether the family participated; enter "2" for No family.

c) **Significant other** — Enter "0" for No or "1" for Yes to indicate whether a significant other participated; enter "2" for None if there is no significant other.

2. Signatures of Persons Completing the Assessment

Intent: Federal regulations at 42 CFR 483.20 (c) (1) and (2) require each individual who completes a portion of the assessment to sign and certify its accuracy. These regulations also require the RN Assessment Coordinator to sign and certify that the assessment is complete.

Process: Each staff member who completes any portion of the MDS must sign and date the MDS and indicate beside their signature which portions they completed. Two or more staff members can complete items within the same section of the MDS. The RN Assessment Coordinator must not sign and attest to completion of the assessment until all other assessors have finished their portions of the MDS. The RN Assessment Coordinator is not certifying the accuracy of portions of the assessment that were completed by other health professionals.

Coding: All persons completing part of this assessment, including the RN Assessment Coordinator, must sign their names in the appropriate locations. To the right of the name, enter title and the letters that correspond to sections of the MDS for which the assessor was responsible, and also enter the date on which the form is signed. Federal regulation requires the RN Assessment Coordinator to sign and thereby certify that the assessment is complete.

SECTION S.
STATE DEFINED SECTION

SECTION S IS RESERVED FOR ADDITIONAL STATE-DEFINED ITEMS. THERE IS NO SECTION S IN THE FEDERAL VERSION 2.0 MDS FORM. YOUR STATE MAY CHOOSE TO DESIGNATE A SECTION S.

SECTIONS T AND U ARE SUPPLEMENTAL SECTIONS FOR USE IN THE CASE-MIX AND QUALITY DEMONSTRATION STATES. COPIES OF THE SECTION T AND U FORMS ARE AT THE END OF THIS CHAPTER AND IN APPENDIX B.

SECTION T.
SUPPLEMENT ITEMS FOR MDS 2.0 IN CASE-MIX AND QUALITY DEMONSTRATION STATES

1. Special Treatments and Procedures

a. RECREATION THERAPY

Intent: To record the (A) number of days and (B) total number of minutes recreation therapy was administered (for at least 15 minutes a day) in the last 7 days.

Definition: **Recreation Therapy** -- Therapy ordered by a physician that provides therapeutic stimulation beyond the general activity program in a facility. The physician's order must include a statement of frequency, duration and scope of the treatment. Such therapy must be provided by a State licensed or nationally certified Therapeutic Recreation Specialist or Therapeutic Recreation Assistant. The therapeutic recreation assistant must work under the direction of a therapeutic recreation specialist.

Process: Review the resident's clinical record and consult with the qualified recreation therapists.

Coding: Box A: In the first column, enter the number (#) of days the therapy was administered for 15 minutes or more in the last seven days. Enter "0" if none.

Box B: In the second column, enter the total number (#) of minutes recreational therapy was provided in the last seven days. The time should include only the actual treatment time (not resident time waiting for treatment or therapist time documenting a treatment). Enter "0" if none.

b. ORDERED THERAPIES (item b, c, and d)

Skip this item unless this is a Medicare 5 day assessment, or initial admission assessment.

Intent: To recognize ordered and scheduled therapy services [physical therapy (PT), occupational therapy (OT) and speech pathology services (SP)] during the early days of the resident's stay. Often therapies are not initiated until after the end of the observation assessment period. This section provides an overall picture of the amount of therapy that a resident will likely receive through the fifteenth day from admission.

Process: For Item 1B: Review the resident's clinical record to determine if the physician has ordered one or more of the therapies to begin in first 14 days of stay. Therapies include physical therapy (PT), occupational therapy (OT), speech pathology services. If not, skip to item 3. If orders exist, consult with the therapists involved to determine if the initial evaluation is completed and therapy treatment(s) has been scheduled. If therapy treatment(s) will **not** be scheduled, skip to item 3.

If the resident is scheduled to receive at least one of the therapies, have the therapist(s) calculate the total number of days through the resident's fifteenth day since admission when at least one therapy service will be delivered. Then have the therapist(s) estimate the total PT, OT, and SP treatment minutes that will be delivered through the fifteenth day of admission.

Coding: **Item c**. Enter the number (#) of days at least one therapy service can be expected to have been delivered through the resident's fifteenth day of admission.

Item d. Enter the estimated **total** number of therapy minutes (across all therapies) it is expected the resident will receive through the resident's fifteenth day of admission.

Example of Ordered Therapies

Medicare 5 day assessment:
Mr. Z was admitted to the nursing home late Thursday afternoon. The physician's orders for both physical therapy and speech language pathology evaluation were obtained on Friday. Both therapy evaluations were completed on Monday and physical and speech therapy were scheduled to begin on Tuesday. Physical therapy was scheduled 5 days a week for 60 minutes each day. Speech therapy was scheduled for 3 days a week for 60 minutes each day. The RN Assessment Coordinator identified Monday as the end of the observation assessment period for this Medicare 5 day assessment. Within the 15 days from the resident's admission date (Thursday), the resident will receive 8 days of physical therapy (240 minutes) and 4 days of speech therapy (240 minutes) for a total of 480 minutes in the fifteen days.

Enter "8" in 2.c for the number of days that at least one therapy service is expected to be delivered.

Because physical therapy was scheduled more frequently than speech therapy, the total number of days of physical therapy would be used.

Enter "480" in 2.d for the estimated total number of minutes that both physical therapy and speech therapy are expected to be delivered.

(continued on next page)

Example of Ordered Therapies (continued)

Initial admission assessment:
Mrs. C was admitted to the facility Tuesday with an evaluation order for all three therapies. The physical therapist completed the evaluation for physical therapy and scheduled treatment to begin on Thursday, five days a week for 30 minutes each day. The occupational therapist completed the evaluation and scheduled therapy to begin on Monday, 3 days a week for one hour each day. The speech language pathologist's evaluation did not recommend speech therapy for the resident so speech therapy was not scheduled. The RN Assessment Coordinator identified Monday as the end of the observation assessment period, which was also the day for the initial admission assessment to be completed. Within the observation assessment period, the resident received 3 days of physical therapy for a total of 90 minutes. This was recorded in section P.1.b.c. of the MDS. The resident received one occupational therapy treatment for a total of 60 minutes which was also recorded in section P.1.b.b. However, to obtain a total picture of the resident's therapy regimen, section T.2.b-d was completed. It was expected that Mrs. C would receive 6 more days of physical therapy within the 15 days after the resident's admission for a total of 180 minutes and 3 more days of occupational therapy within the 15 days after the resident's admission for a total of 180 minutes.

Enter "6" in 2.c for the number of days that at least one therapy service is expected to be delivered.

Enter "360" in 2.d for the estimated total number of minutes that both physical therapy and occupational therapy is expected to be delivered.

2. Walking when most self-sufficient

Intent: Physical therapy treatment plans and nursing rehabilitation programs are often implemented to improve a resident's ability to walk. This includes residents with different problems (e.g. stroke, parkinsons disease, hip replacement) and at different stages of recovery (e.g. 1 week post-hip fracture versus 3 weeks post-hip fracture). It is important to monitor the gait pattern and walking progress for residents and how functional walking is integrated into the resident's activities of daily living on the nursing unit.

Four important walking components to be monitored are the **distance** a resident walks, the amount of **time** it takes to walk that distance, and the amount of **assistance** and **support** received. Assessment of the resident's ability to walk using these four components should be viewed in combination with information in Section G (walking in room, walking in corridor, locomotion on unit, balance test, functional range of motion, modes of locomotion and transfer, and rehabilitation potential); Section I (diagnoses that impact ability to walk such as cerebral palsy, hip fracture, stroke); and Section J (unsteady gait). This information will provide a picture of the resident's problems and level of functioning for comparison to the most self-sufficient walking episode. This information will assist all members of the interdisciplinary care team to differentiate the resident's "best walking effort" and the resident's usual walking performance. Discussions between the physical therapist working with the resident on walking and the RN Assessment Coordinator regarding these differences should lead to better coordination of care and foster continuity of physical therapy treatment for the resident on the nursing unit.

Assessment of the resident's most self-sufficient walking episode can be used to evaluate 1) the effectiveness of physical therapy and nursing rehabilitation, 2) the continued need for therapy and nursing rehabilitation, and 3) maintenance of walking ability after therapy or nursing rehabilitation was discontinued.

Complete item 2 when the following conditions are present. Otherwise, skip to item 3.

- **ADL self-performance score for TRANSFER (G.1.bA) is 0, 1, 2, or 3**

  AND
- **Resident receives physical therapy (P.1.b.c) involving gait training;**

  OR
- **Physical therapy is ORDERED for gait training (T.2.b)**

  OR
- **Resident is receiving nursing rehabilitation for walking (P.3.f)**

  OR
- **Physical therapy involving gait training has been discontinued within the past six months.**

Definition: **Most self-sufficient episode**--In the last seven days, the episode in which the resident used the LEAST amount of assistance and support while walking the longest and farthest **without sitting down.** The most self-sufficient episode can include physical help from others or assistive devices. Only episodes using a safe, functional gait should be used in determining the walking episode that was the most self-sufficient.

Assistive devices: Prostheses, different types of canes and walkers, crutches, splints, parallel bars, and pushing a wheel chair for support.

Examples for Most Self Sufficient Episode

Mrs. G had a hip replacement three weeks ago and was admitted to the nursing facility one week after the surgery. During the seven day assessment period of the initial comprehensive assessment, Mrs. G could only stand and transfer from bed to chair on the nursing unit with the assistance of one person. Physical therapy was initiated several days after admission for gait training. By the sixth day of admission, Mrs. G could walk two lengths of the parallel bars (20 feet) with stand by assistance from the therapist. The physical therapists and RN assessment coordinator conferred and together determined that Mrs. G's most self-sufficient walking episode took place in therapy using the parallel bars.

Following intensive physical therapy for gait training for weakness and paralysis from a stroke, Mr. T was discharged from physical therapy with the ability to walk using an appropriate and safe gait pattern, using a short leg brace and a quad cane. Mr. T's revised careplan includes a nursing rehabilitation program for walking. His walking rehabilitation program requires a nursing assistant to walk with Mr. T in the morning after breakfast and after dinner for 15 minute walking sessions using a measured "walking route" on the nursing unit. Mr. T's stamina during the walking sessions varied daily during the seven day assessment period. Sometimes he could only walk several feet before needing to sit down. On three occasions, Mr. T walked half the length of the corridor (75 feet) in 5 minutes without sitting down and using the gait pattern he was taught. This was his most self-sufficient walking episode.

During a brief meeting during morning report, the physical therapist, nursing staff on 2 South, and the RN assessment coordinator determined Mr. A's most self-sufficient walking episode during the last seven days. It was reported that Mr. A walked 50 feet in 7 minutes with a walker, cueing, and physical guidance on the nursing unit and walked 60 feet in 10 minutes with a walker and cueing for correct heel strike in physical therapy. The staff agreed that the walking episode in physical therapy was Mr. A's most self-sufficient episode.

Mrs. W requires weight bearing support (G.1.b.A=3) and the assistance of two persons (G.1.b.B=3) to transfer her from the bed to a chair. Due her overweight and overall weakness, the nursing staff cannot safely walk her on the nursing unit, therefore she received a code of "8-activity did not occur" for walking in room (G.1.c.A) and walking in corridor (G.1.d.A). However, Mrs. G is able to walk the length of the parallel bars with the assistance of two persons when she is in physical therapy which would be Mrs. G's most self-sufficient walking episode.

Process: There are four components to determining a resident's most *self-sufficient walking episode*: **distance, time, self-performance, and support**. During the seven day assessment period, it is likely that nursing and therapy staff will have had numerous opportunities to assess the resident's walking status. Staff are encouraged to use all of the assessment days to determine the resident's most self-sufficient walking episode. Needless to say, it is important that all staff observe the resident and contribute to the determination the resident's most self-sufficient walking episode during the seven day assessment period.

During each shift report, staff should be informed which residents are being assessed for their most self sufficient walking effort. This will remind staff to look for episodes when the resident does better than usual, to observe the distance the resident walks, check the time it takes for the resident to walk that distance, and note the support and assistance that the resident requires. For recently admitted residents receiving physical therapy for gait training, the most self sufficient walking episode will frequently occur during a physical therapy session. However, the best walking effort can occur on the nursing unit, off the unit, in therapy, or even outside the facility.

Distance walked: Determining the distance a resident walks involves knowing the distance between usual places the resident may walk (e.g. number of feet from the bed to the toilet room; number of feet from the resident's room to the dining room, day room, or nurses station). Some facilities may have a section of the corridor designated for walking residents that is measured for distance. Some facilities may be able to use floor tiles or ceiling tiles in determining the distance a resident walks. Take time to determine the distances associated with typical walking places in your facility and communicate these distances to staff. For example, if the distance from the resident's bed to a toilet room in your facility is 8 feet and the nursing assistant reported that the resident walked from the bed to the toilet room, it can be interpreted that the resident walked 8 feet during that walking episode.

Time walked: Staff should determine the time it takes a resident to walk a distance using a time piece with a second hand.

Self-performance in walking: This assessment item is similar to the self-performance ADL items in Section G, except this item refers **only to the ONE most self-sufficient walking episode** in the past seven days, rather than ALL of the walking episodes in the past seven days.

Walking support provided: This assessment item is OPPOSITE the ADL support items in Section G. In determining a resident's most self-sufficient walking episode, the episode with the LEAST amount of support used is identified. Section G requests scoring the MOST amount of support used for an ADL activity during any episode over the last 7 days.

Coding: **a. Furthest distance walked**--For the most self-sufficient episode using a safe and functional gait pattern, record the distance that the resident walked. Use the following codes:

0. 150 or more feet
1. 51-149 feet
2. 26-50 feet
3. 10-25 feet
4. Less than 10 feet

b. Time walked--For the same episode (T.3.a), record the time it took the resident to walk the distance. Use the following codes:

0. 1-2 minutes
1. 3-4 minutes
2. 5-10 minutes
3. 11-15 minutes
4. 16-30 minutes
5. 31 or more minutes

c. Self-performance in walking--For the same episode (T.3.a), record the amount of assistance the resident received during the walking episode. Use the following codes:

0. INDEPENDENT--No help or oversite provided while walking.
1. SUPERVISION--Oversight, encouragement, or cuing provided while walking.
2. LIMITED ASSISTANCE--Resident highly involved in walking; received physical help in guided maneuvering of limbs or other nonweight bearing assistance.
3. EXTENSIVE ASSISTANCE--Resident received weight bearing assistance while walking.

d. Walking support provided--For the same episode (T.3.a), record the amount of support the resident received during the walking episode. Use the following codes:

0. No setup or physical help from staff
1. Setup help only
2. One person physical assist
3. Two or more persons physical assist

e. Parallel bars used during walking--For the same episode(T.3.a), record if parallel bars were used. Code "0" if parallel bars were NOT used and "1" if parallel bars were used.

CODING EXAMPLES FOR WALKING WHEN MOST SELF SUFFICIENT

Mrs. D was admitted to the nursing facility 1 month ago for rehabilitation following a CVA. She has left sided hemiplegia and receives physical therapy 5 days a week for a 45 minute session twice daily. Mrs. D enjoys her PT sessions and puts forth her best efforts in walking when her therapist is present. During the last 7 days, Mrs. D's most self-sufficient episode was during a physical therapy session when she walked the length of the hallway outside the physical therapy room (approximately 50 feet) in 15 minutes without sitting down. Mrs. D used a short leg brace to prevent foot drop and a quad cane for support. The physical therapist walked beside Mrs. D, encouraging her and cueing her to pick up her left foot, but not providing physical support.

Code a (furthest distance walked) as "2"

Code b (longest time) as "3"

Code c (self-performance) as "1"

Code d (walking support provided) as "0"

****

Mr. G was admitted to the nursing facility following a lengthy hospitalization related to injuries sustained in a motor vehicle accident. Mr. G received physical therapy for 8 weeks to strengthen his lower extremities. Physical therapy was discontinued last week. Mr. G tires during the day, requiring more assistance with ambulation as the day progresses. During the morning, Mr. G walks from his bed to the toilet room (8 feet) with oversight from a staff person. It takes about 6 minutes for Mr. G to reach the toilet room. He uses a brace on his right leg and a walker which the staff put on for Mr. G.

During the night shift, Mr. G has much difficulty in bearing weight and manipulating his lower extremities. To walk to the toilet room, two nursing assistants are needed to provide weight-bearing support and to help Mr. G position his legs in taking steps. It takes approximately 6 minutes to reach the toilet room.

Code a (furthest distance) as "4"

Code b (longest time) as "2"

Code c (self-performance) as "1"

Code d (walking support provided) as "1"

SECTION U. MEDICATIONS

Nursing home residents are highly susceptible to adverse drug reactions and drug interactions. It is estimated that approximately 30% of all geriatric hospital admissions are due to drug-related problems. Polypharmacy is the use of two or more medications for no apparent reasons or for the same purpose. Polypharmacy also occurs when a medication is used to treat an adverse reaction from another medication. Polypharmacy can occur in nursing homes when there is no regular and careful monitoring of residents' prescribed medications.

Intent: This section will assist staff in identifying potential problems related to polypharmacy, drug reactions and interactions. Further, this section can also help staff to identify potential physical and emotional problems a resident may be experiencing. For example, reviewing and documenting the frequency a resident uses a PRN pain medication, sleeping medication, or laxative may lead the interdisciplinary team to do further assessment related to underlying causes associated with the use of PRN medications. Many of the RAPs and Triggers refer to assessment of medications in which this section would be very helpful.

In addition to using the medication information collected in Section U for resident care planning purposes, this section can be integrated into a facility's quality assurance program to monitor for quality care issues such as polypharmacy, overuse of different medications, and medication administration errors and omissions.

Finally, facilities in Case-mix Demonstration States are required to collect medication information. The drug-use data are linked to the assessment data for monitoring the quality and cost-efficiency of care in a Medicare/Medicaid payment system.

Definitions: Amount Administered--the number of tablets, capsules, suppositories, or amount of liquid (cc's, mls, units) **per dose** that is administered to a resident.

NDC--the National Drug Code (NDC) is a standardized system for coding medications. An individual NDC provides coded information on the drug name, dose, and form of the drug.

Medication Administration Record (MAR)--the part of the resident's clinical record that is used by the nurse administering medications to record the medication administered. The MAR typically is the form or document used specifying the medication, dose, frequency, and route for each medication that a resident is to receive on a scheduled or PRN basis.

Process: Recording all of the information required in this section can be done efficiently by having the following information: 1) current physician order sheets; 2) current Medication Administration Record (MAR), 3) NDC codes. Use the Medication Administration Record (MAR) as your **primary** document for identifying all medications administered in the last seven days. Check the physician's order sheet to determine if any medications had recently been ordered.

In some facilities, the pharmacist may complete some portions of Section U, particularly the NDC codes and the amount administered. The pharmacy may also be able to supply you with the NDC codes for the medications ordered for each resident. Talk to the pharmacist for your facility and engage their participation in assisting with the completion of this section. If the pharmacist does not complete any portions of the medication section of the MDS, you will need to consult the list of NDC codes. The manual provides the NDC codes for medications frequently used in nursing facilities. In addition, NDC codes can be found in the *Physicians Drug Reference (PDR)* or you may be able to obtain a list of NDC codes from your pharmacy.

Take special care to ensure that you have identified and recorded all medications that were administered in the last 7 days. Often residents can have several MAR pages, especially if medications have been discontinued and new ones ordered or if there are a lot of PRN medications ordered. Recheck the MAR at least twice to avoid missing any medications administered in the last seven days. Make sure you count medications that may have been discontinued, but were administered in the last seven days.

To accurately complete the NDC codes and amount administered, it will be necessary to look at the actual medications that are given to the resident. For example, some injectable medications can be provided in vials, ampules, or premeasured syringes.

If Section U is completed by the pharmacist or other nursing home personnel, these persons must certify its accuracy with their signature in section R.5. The RN Assessment Coordinator must review Section U to ensure that it is complete.

Coding: The coding instructions are extensive. Review them carefully. Study the examples. Complete the coding exercises at the end of this section.

1. **Medication Name and Dose Ordered**. Identify and record all medications that the resident <u>**received**</u> in the last seven days. Also identify and record any medications that may not have been given in the last seven days, but are part of the residents regular medication regimen (e.g. monthly B-12 injections). Do **not** record PRN medications that were **not** administered in the last seven days.

Record the name of the medication and dose that was ordered by the physician in column 1. Write the name of the medication and dose ordered *EXACTLY* as it appears on the MAR. For example, if the MAR indicates Acetaminophen 650 mg, **do not** write Acetaminophen 325 mg. 2 tabs--even if two 325 mg. tablets are administered to the resident.

Occasionally, dosages of medications may be changed during the seven day assessment period. The medication with dosage changes should be recorded separately.

EXAMPLE FOR MEDICATION NAME AND DOSE ORDERED

Medications as listed on MAR for assessment period of 8/11/94-8/17/94

A. Lasix 40 mg. daily p.o.
B. Acetaminophen 325 mg. 2 tabs q3-4 hrs PRN p.o. (given 3 times in last seven days)
C. B-12 1cc q month IM (given 8/8/94)
D. Isopto Carbachol 1.5% 2 drops OD TID
E. Robitussin-DM 5cc HS PRN p.o. (not given in last 7 days)
F. Motrin 300 mg. QID p.o. (discontinued 8/15/94)
G. Dilantin 300 mg. HS p.o. (ordered 8/15/94)
H. Theo-Dur 200 mg. BID p.o. (given 8/11-8/13/94 and then order discontinued)
I. Theo-Dur 200 mg TID p.o. (given 8/14-8/16/94 and then order discontinued)
J. Theo-Dur 400 mg BID p.o. (given 8/17)

1. Medication Name and Dose Ordered	2. RA	3. Freq	4. AA	5. PRN-n	6. NDC Codes
Lasix 40 mg.					
Acetaminophen 325 mg. 2 tabs					
B-12 1cc					
Isopto Carbachol 1.5% 2 drops					
Motrin 300 mg.					
Dilantin 300 mg.					
Theo-Dur 200 mg.					
Theo-Dur 200 mg.					
Theo-Dur 400 mg.					

*Note that Robitussin-DM was not recorded because it was not given in the last 7 days.

2. Route of Administration. Determine the Route of Administration (RA) used to administer each medication. The MAR and the physician's orders should identify the RA for each medication. Record the RA in column 2 using the following codes:

1=by mouth (PO)	5=subcutaneous (SQ)	8=inhalation
2=sub lingual (SL)	6=rectal (R)	9=enteral tube
3=intramuscular (IM)	7=topical	10=other
4=intravenous (IV)		

EXAMPLE FOR ROUTE OF ADMINISTRATION

Medications as listed on MAR for assessment period of 8/11/94-8/17/94

A. Mylanta 15 cc after meals p.o.
B. Zantac 150 mg. q 12 hrs. Per tube
C. Transderm nitro patch 2.5 1 patch daily
D. Humulin N 15 U before breakfast daily SQ
E. Lasix 80 mg. IV STAT
G. Acetaminophen suppository 650 mg. q 4 hrs. PRN (given on 2 occasions in last 7 days)

1. Medication Name and Dose Ordered	2. RA	3. Freq	4. AA	5.PRN-n	6. NDC Codes
Mylanta 15cc	1				
Zantac 150 mg.	9				
Transderm nitro patch 2.5 1 patch	7				
Humulin N 15 U	5				
Lasix 80 mg.	4				
Acetaminophen suppository 650 mg.	6				

3. Frequency. Determine the number of times per day, week, or month that each medication is given. Record the frequency in column 3 using the following codes:

PR=(PRN) as necessary	2D=(BID) two times daily (includes every 12 hrs)	QO=every other day
1H=(QH) every hour		4W=4 times each week
2H=(Q2H) every two hours	3D=(TID) three times daily	5W=five times each week
3H=(Q3H) every three hours	4D=(QID) four times daily	6W=six times each week
4H=(Q4H) every four hours	5D=five times daily	1M=(Q mo) once every month
6H=(Q6H) every six hours	1W=(Q week) once each wk	2M=twice every month
8H=(Q8H) every eight hours	2W=two times every week	C=continuous
1D=(QD or HS) once daily	3W=three times every week	O=other

Be careful to differentiate between similar frequencies. For example, some nursing facilities have a policy that antibiotics are to be administered around the clock. Therefore, if an antibiotic is ordered as T.I.D., the medication may actually be given q 8 hours. There is a different frequency code for T.I.D. (3D) and q 8 hrs (8H). In this case, the frequency code would be 8H (q 8 hrs.).

If insulin is given on a sliding scale, each different dose of insulin given is entered as a PRN medication.

EXAMPLE FOR FREQUENCY

Medications as listed on MAR for assessment period of 8/11/94-8/17/94

A. Ampicillin 250 mg. q 6 hrs x 10 days p.o. (8/10-8/20)
B. Beconase nasal inhaler 1 puff BID
C. Compazine suppository 5 mg. STAT
D. Lanoxin 0.25 mg. p.o. every other day. On alternate days, give Lanoxin 0.125 mg. p.o.
E. Peri-colace 2 capsules HS p.o.
F. Humulin N 15 U before breakfast daily SQ
G. Check blood sugar daily at 4 p.m. Sliding scale insulin: Humulin R 5 units if blood sugar 200-300; 10 units if over 300. (5 units given on 8/11/94 for BS of 255; 5 units given on 8/13/94 for BS of 233; 10 units given on 8/17/94 for BS of 305)

1. Medication Name and Dose Ordered	2. RA	3. Freq	4. AA	5.PRN-n	6. NDC Codes
Ampicillin 250 mg.	1	6H			
Beconase nasal inhaler 1 puff	8	2D			
Compazine suppository 5 mg.	6	PR			
Lanoxin 0.25 mg.	1	QO			
Lanoxin 0.125 mg.	1	QO			
Peri-colase 2 capsules	1	1D			
Humulin N 15 U	5	1D			
Humulin R 5U	5	PR			
Humulin R 10 U	5	PR			

4. Amount Administered (AA). Determine the amount of medication administered each time the medication was given. Amount administered **is not always** the dose. Rather, it is the number of tablets, capsules, suppositories, or amount of liquid (cc's, mls, units) **per dose** that is administered to a resident. For **tablets, capsules or suppositories**, enter the ***number*** of tablets or capsules that were given for each *administration* in column 4 (e.g. 1, 2, 1.5) For **liquids**, enter the ***number*** of cc's, mls, or units that were given for each *administration* in column 4 (e.g. 0. 5 ml, 2.5 cc, 10 units). For **topical medications** (e.g. creams, ointments, eye drops), **inhalation medications**, and **oral medications that are dissolved in water**, enter the numeric code **999** in column 4. If a half of tablet or half of cc is administered, enter it as a decimal (0.5) rather than a fraction.

EXAMPLE FOR AMOUNT ADMINISTERED (AA)

Medications as listed on MAR for assessment period of 8/11/94-8/17/94

A. Lanoxin 0.125 mg. daily p.o.
B. Haldol 1 mg. liquid q8 hrs PRN p.o. (received 2 times in last 7 days)
C. Ampicillin 250 mg. q 6 hrs liquid p.o.
D. Acetaminophen 650 mg. QID p.o. (pharmacy supplies two 325 mg. tablets)
E. Acetaminophen 325 mg. 3 tabs q3-4 hrs PRN for pain p.o. (received 5 times in last 7 days)
F. Humulin N 15 U before breakfast daily SQ
G. Check blood sugar daily at 4 p.m. Sliding scale insulin: Humulin R 5 units if blood sugar 200-300; 10 units if over 300. (5 units given on 8/11/94 for BS of 255; 5 units given on 8/13/94 for BS of 233; 10 units given on 8/17/94 for BS of 305)
H. Elase ointment to necrotic tissue on left heel TID
I. Diazepam 3 mg. HS p.o.
J. Dilantin 300 mg. HS p.o.
K. Metamucil powder 1 tbsp. in a.m. p.o.

1. Medication Name and Dose Ordered	2. RA	3. Freq	4. AA	5.PRN-n	6. NDC Codes
Lanoxin 0.125 mg.	1	1D	1		
Haldol 1 mg.	1	PR	.5cc		
Ampicillin 250 mg.	1	6H	5ml		
Acetaminophen 650 mg.	1	4D	2		
Acetaminophen 325 mg . 3 tabs	1	PR	3		
Humulin N 15 U	5	1D	15U		
Humulin R 5 U	5	PR	5U		
Humulin R 10 U	5	PR	10U		
Elase ointment	7	3D	999		
Diazepam 3 mg.	1	1D	1.5		
Dilantin 300 mg.	1	1D	3		
Metamucil powder 1 tbsp.	1	1D	999		

5. PRN-number of doses (PRN-n). The PRN-n column is only completed for medications that have a route of administration coded as PR. Record the **number of times** in the past seven days that each medication coded as PR was given. STAT medications are recorded as a PRN medication. Remember, if a PRN medication was **not** given in the past seven days, it should **not** be listed in Section U.

EXAMPLE FOR PRN-number (PRN-n)

Medications as listed on MAR for assessment period of 8/11/94-8/17/94

A. Mylanta 15 cc after meals PRN p.o. (administered 12 times in last 7 days)
B. Haldol 1 mg. liquid q8 hrs PRN p.o. (administered 2 times in last 7 days)
C. Hydrocortisone cream 1% PRN to back and chest (administered 5 times in last 7 days)
D. Lasix 80 mg. IV STAT
E. Check blood sugar daily at 4 p.m. Sliding scale insulin: Humulin R 5 units if blood sugar 200-300; 10 units if over 300. (5 units given on 8/11/94 for BS of 255; 5 units given on 8/13/94 for BS of 233; 10 units given on 8/17/94 for BS of 305
F. Nitroglycerin 0.3 mg 1 tab SL for chest pain; repeat 2 times at 5 minute intervals if pain is not relieved (given on 8/12/94 once and another five minutes following)

1. Medication Name and Dose Ordered	2. RA	3. Freq	4. AA	5.PRN-n	6. NDC Codes
Mylanta 15 cc	1	PR	15cc	12	
Haldol 1 mg .	1	PR	0.5cc	2	
Hydrocortisone cream 1%	7	PR	999	5	
Lasix 80 mg.	4	PR	8cc	1	
Humulin R 5 Units	5	PR	5U	2	
Humulin R 10 Units	5	PR	10U	1	
Nitroglycerin 0.3 mg.	2	PR	1	2	

6. National Drug Code (NDC). It is very important that all of the information about the medication (medication name, dose ordered, frequency, and amount administered) corresponds with the NDC code. A medication usually has more than one NDC code. The different types of NDC codes are based on the **strength** of the medication and the **form** of the medication (e.g. solution; tablets, ampules, syringes, ointment, cream, vial, spray, drops). For example, there are 21 NDC codes for morphine. If the resident was receiving 2 mg of morphine IM and the pharmacy sent it in an ampule form, the NDC code is 006411180; if the pharmacy sent the morphine in a vial, the NDC code is 006412343. If your pharmacist is involved in completing this section, the pharmacist would be able to provide the appropriate NDC code.

There will be occasions when a medication dosage will involve two NDC codes. For example, if Coumadin 3 mg. was ordered, the pharmacy would send a 1 mg. tablet and a 2 mg. tablet, each having a different NDC code. In cases such as this, use the NDC code for the largest dose (2 mg).

Code investigational drugs as 999999999. Code compounds (topical mixtures prepared by the pharmacist) as 888888888.

Record the NDC code in column 6. Begin writing in the left hand box entering one digit per box. There should be 9 numbers in the NDC code recorded in column 6. Recheck the number to be sure you have entered the digits correctly. Many NDC codes begin with one or more zeros. These zeros are important; do not omit them. If the NDC codes you are using have eleven (11) digits, disregard the last two digits as these are the package codes.

EXAMPLE FOR NDC CODES

Medications as listed on MAR for assessment period of 8/11/94-8/17/94

A. Lanoxin 0.125 mg. daily p.o.
B. Haldol 1 mg. liquid q8 hrs PRN p.o. (administered 2 times in last 7 days)
C. Ampicillin 250 mg. q 6 hrs. liquid p.o.
D. Acetaminophen 650 mg. QID p.o. (pharmacy supplies two 325 mg. tablets)
F. Humulin N 15 U before breakfast daily SQ
G. Check blood sugar daily at 4 p.m. Sliding scale insulin: Humulin R 5 units if blood sugar 200-300; 10 units if over 300. (5 units given on 8/11/94 for BS of 255; 5 units given on 8/13/94 for BS of 233; 10 units given on 8/17/94 for BS of 305).
H. Transderm Nitro 1 Patch QD
I. Lasix 80 mg. IV STAT
J. Diazepam 3 mg. HS p.o.
K. Dilantin 300 mg. HS p.o.

1. Medication Name and Dose Ordered	2.RA	3. Freq	4. AA	5.PRN-n	6. NDC Codes								
Lanoxin 0.125 mg.	1	1D	1		0	0	0	8	1	0	2	4	2
Haldol 1 mg.	1	PR	.5cc	2	0	0	0	4	5	0	2	5	0
Ampicillin 250 mg.	1	6H	5ml		0	0	0	4	7	2	3	0	2
Acetaminophen 650 mg.	1	4D	2		0	0	7	8	1	1	2	9	4
Humulin N 15 U	5	1D	15U		0	0	0	0	2	8	3	1	5
Humulin R 5 U	5	PR	5U	2	0	0	0	0	2	8	2	1	5
Humulin R 10 U	5	PR	10U	1	0	0	0	0	2	8	2	1	5
Transderm Nitro 1 patch	7	1D	999		0	0	0	8	3	2	0	2	5
Lasix 80 mg.	4	PR	8cc	1	0	0	0	3	9	0	0	6	3
Diazepam 3 mg.	1	1D	1.5		0	0	3	6	4	0	7	7	4
Dilantin 300 mg.	1	1D	3		0	0	0	7	1	0	3	6	2

Coding Exercises for Section U

Complete Section U for the following medications during a 7 day period (9/1/94-9/7/94):

1. Inderal 40 mg. BID p.o.
2. Sinemet 10/100 TID p.o.
3. Artificial Tears 1 drop OU QID
4. Anusol HC suppository 1 PRN (given 1 time in last seven days)
5. Amoxicillin 500 mg q 6 hrs per tube
6. Benylin cough syrup 2 tbs. PRN p.o. (given 10 times in last seven days)
7. Darvocet-N 100 2 tabs q 4-6 hrs PRN p.o. (given 5 times in last seven days)
8. Heparin lock flush 10 U daily
9. Ditropan syrup 2.5 mg daily p.o.
10. Nitrotransdermal .4 mg 1 patch daily
11. Novolin N 24 U before breakfast SQ
12. Check blood sugar before breakfast. Sliding scale insulin: Novolin R 10 units if blood sugar over 200. (10 units given on 2 days in last 7 days)
13. Questran 1 packet with each meal p.o.
14. Quinine sulfate 325 mg. HS
15. Coumadin 2.5 mg daily p.o. (discontinued 9/3/94)
16. Coumadin 5 mg. daily p.o. (ordered to start on 9/4/94)
17. Maalox 15 cc PRN for indigestion p.o. (not administered in last 7 days)

1. Medication Name and Dose Ordered	2. RA	3. Freq	4. AA	5.PRN-n	6. NDC Codes								

Compare your responses to the coding exercises with the responses on the next page.

1. Medication Name and Dose Ordered	2. RA	3. Freq	4. AA	5. PRN-n	6. NDC Codes										
Inderal 40 mg.	1	2D	1		0	0	0	4	6	0	4	2	4
Sinemet 10/100	1	3D	1		0	0	0	0	6	0	6	4	7
Artificial Tears 1 drop	7	4D	999		0	0	3	4	9	8	6	1	5
Anusol HC suppository 1	6	PR	1	1	0	0	0	7	1	1	0	8	8
Amoxicillin 500 mg	9	6H	10 ml		0	0	3	0	4	0	5	8	7
Benylin cough syrup 2 Tbs.	1	PR	30 cc	10	0	0	0	7	1	2	1	9	5
Darvocet-N 100 2 tabs	1	PR	2	5	0	0	0	0	2	0	3	6	3
Heparin lock flush 10 U	4	1D	1 ml		0	0	4	6	9	3	0	0	1
Ditropan syrup 2.5 mg	1	1D	2.5ml		0	0	0	8	8	1	3	7	3
Nitrotransdermal .4 mg.	7	1D	999		4	7	2	0	2	2	8	3	2
Novolin N 24 U	5	1D	24 U		0	0	0	0	3	1	8	3	4
Novolin R 10 U	5	PR	10 U	2	0	0	0	0	3	1	8	3	3
Questran 1 packet	1	3D	999		0	0	0	8	7	0	5	8	0
Quinine sulfate 325 mg.	1	1D	1		0	0	0	0	2	0	6	2	9
Coumadin 2.5 mg.	1	1D	1		0	0	0	5	6	0	1	7	6
Coumadin 5 mg.	1	1D	1		0	0	0	5	6	0	1	7	2

CHAPTER 4: PROCEDURES FOR COMPLETING THE RESIDENT ASSESSMENT PROTOCOLS (RAPs)

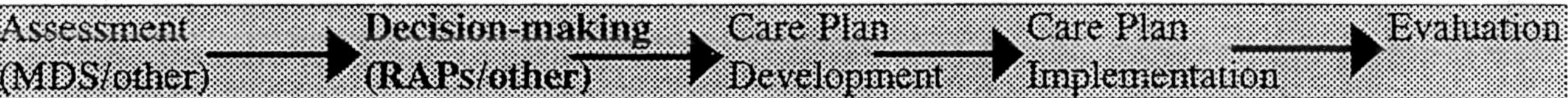

This chapter gives instructions on using the Resident Assessment Protocols (RAPs) to assess conditions identified by the Minimum Data Set (MDS) triggering mechanism. The goal of the RAPs is to guide the interdisciplinary team through a structured comprehensive assessment of a resident's functional status. Functional status differs from medical or clinical status in that the whole of a person's life is reviewed with the intent of assisting that person to function at his or her highest practicable level of well-being. Going through the RAI process will help staff set resident-specific objectives in order to meet the physical, mental and psychosocial needs of residents.

4.1 What are the Resident Assessment Protocols (RAPs)?

The MDS alone does not provide a comprehensive assessment. Rather, the MDS is used for preliminary screening to identify potential resident problems, strengths, and preferences. The RAPs are problem-oriented frameworks for additional assessment based on problem identification items (triggered conditions). They form a critical link to decisions about care planning. The RAP Guidelines provide guidance on how to synthesize assessment information within a comprehensive assessment. The Triggers target conditions for additional assessment and review, as warranted by MDS item responses; the RAP Guidelines help facility staff evaluate "triggered" conditions.

There are 18 RAPs in Version 2.0 of the RAI. The RAPs in the RAI cover the majority of areas that are addressed in a typical nursing home resident's care plan. The RAPs were created by clinical experts in each of the RAP areas.

The care delivery system in a facility is complex yet critical to successful resident care outcomes. It is guided by both professional standards of practice and regulatory requirements. The basis of care delivery is the process of assessment and care planning. Documentation of this process (to ensure continuity of care) is also necessary.

The RAI (MDS and RAPs) is an integral part of this process. It ensures that facility staff collect minimum, standardized assessment data for each resident at regular intervals. The main intent is to drive the development of an individualized plan of care based on the identified needs, strengths and preferences of the resident.

It is helpful to think of the RAI as a package. The MDS identifies actual or potential problem areas. The RAPs provide further assessment of the "triggered" areas; they help staff to look for causal or confounding factors (some of which may be reversible). Use the RAPs to analyze assessment findings and then "chart your thinking". It is important that the RAP documentation include the causal or unique risk factors for decline or lack of improvement. The plan of care then addresses these factors with the goal of promoting the resident's highest practicable level of functioning: 1) improvement where possible, or 2) maintenance and prevention of avoidable declines.

RAPs function as decision facilitators, which means they lead to a more thorough understanding of possible problem situations by providing educational insight and structure to the assessment process. The RAPs will give the interdisciplinary team a sound basis for the development of the resident's care plan. After the comprehensive assessment process is completed, the interdisciplinary team will be able to decide if:

- The resident has a troubling condition that warrants intervention, and addressing this problem is a necessary condition for other functional problems to be successfully addressed;
- Improvement of the resident's functioning in one or more areas is possible;
- Improvement is not likely, but the present level of functioning should be preserved as long as possible, with rates of decline minimized over time;
- The resident is at risk of decline and efforts should emphasize slowing or minimizing decline, and avoiding functional complications (e.g., contractures, pain); or
- The central issues of care revolve around symptom relief and other palliative measures during the last months of life.

OBRA 1987 mandated that facilities provide necessary care and services to help each resident attain or maintain their highest practicable well-being. Facilities must ensure that residents improve when possible and do not deteriorate unless the resident's clinical condition demonstrates that the decline was unavoidable.

4.2 How are the RAPs Organized?

There are four parts to each RAP:

Section I - The Problem gives general information about how a condition affects the nursing home population. The Problem statement often describes the focus or objectives of the protocol. It is important when reviewing a "triggered" RAP not to overlook information in the Problem section. Although **Section III - The Guidelines** contain the "detail", the Problem section should be reviewed for information relevant to the assessment.

Section II - The Triggers identify one or a combination of MDS item responses specific to a resident that alert the assessor to the resident's possible problems, needs, or strengths. The specific MDS response indicates that clinical factors are present that may or may not represent a condition that should be addressed in the care plan. Triggers merely "flag" conditions necessary for the interdisciplinary team members to consider in making care planning decisions.

When the resident's status on a particular MDS item(s) matches one of the "triggers" for a RAP, the RAP is "triggered" and a review (with the possibility of additional data gathering and assessment) is required using the RAP Guidelines.

Section III - The Guidelines present comprehensive information for evaluating factors that may cause, contribute to, or exacerbate the triggered condition. The Guidelines help facility staff decide if a triggered condition actually does limit the resident's functional status or if the resident is at particular risk of developing the condition.

If the condition is found to be a problem for the resident, the Guidelines will assist the interdisciplinary team in determining if the problem can be eliminated or reversed, or if special care must be taken to maintain a resident at his or her current level of functioning.

In addition to identifying causes or risk factors that contribute to the resident's problem, the Guidelines may assist the interdisciplinary team to:

- Find associated causes and effects. Sometimes a problem condition (e.g., falls) is associated with just one specific cause (e.g., new drug that caused dizziness). More often, a problem (e.g., falls) stems from a combination of multiple factors (e.g., new drug; resident forgot walker; bed too high, etc.).
- Determine if multiple triggered conditions are related.
- Suggest a need to get more information about a resident's condition from the resident, resident's family, responsible party, attending physician, direct care staff, rehabilitative staff, laboratory and diagnostic tests, consulting psychiatrist, etc.
- Determine if a resident is a good candidate for rehabilitative interventions.
- Identify the need for a referral to an expert in an area of resident need.
- Begin to formulate care plan goals and approaches.

Section IV - The RAP Key has two parts. The first part is a review of the items on the MDS that triggered a review of the RAP. The second part is a summary, but sometimes also provides a clarification of the information in the Guidelines section of the RAP. The RAP Key should be used as a reference, but does not take the place of the main body of the RAP.

There are 18 RAPs in the Resident Assessment Instrument, Version 2.0[1]:

Delirium
Cognitive Loss/Dementia
Visual Function
Communication
ADL Function /Rehabilitation
Urinary Incontinence and Indwelling Catheter
Psychosocial Well-Being
Mood State
Behavior Symptoms
Activities
Falls
Nutritional Status
Feeding Tubes
Dehydration/Fluid Maintenance
Dental Care
Pressure Ulcers
Psychotropic Drug Use
Physical Restraints

4.3 What does the RAP Process Involve?

There are various models for completing the RAP in-depth assessment process for a resident with a particular problem. Assessment of the resident in "triggered" RAP areas may be performed solely by the RN Coordinator (i.e., as the RAI must be completed or coordinated by an RN per the OBRA statute). Generally, the RAPs will be completed by various members of clinical disciplines as appropriate to the needs of individual residents. Facilities may also establish procedures in which certain RAPs are always reviewed by a particular discipline (e.g., the dietician completes the Nutritional Status and Feeding Tube RAPs, if triggered). The interdisciplinary team may also review RAP Guidelines in a joint manner and have the assessment process flow seamlessly into care planning. There are no mandates regarding the "process" of how facility staff use the RAPs. Rather, facility staff should be creative and experiment until they find "what works" most efficiently and effectively for them in achieving the desired outcome (i.e.,

[1] The names of the RAPs in Version 2.0 are unchanged from the original version, as are the RAP Guidelines. The triggers in almost all of the RAPs have been revised, however.

a sound and comprehensive assessment that is used to develop an individualized plan of care for each resident).

The RAP process includes the following steps:

1. Facility staff use the RAI triggering mechanism to determine which RAP problem areas require review and additional assessment. The triggered conditions are indicated in the appropriate column on the RAP Summary form.

2. Staff assess the resident in the areas that have been triggered and are guided by the RAPs and other assessment information as needed, to determine the nature of the problem and understand the causes specific to the resident.

3. Staff document key findings regarding the resident's status based on the RAP review. RAP assessment documentation should generally describe:

   — Nature of the condition (may include presence or lack of objective data and subjective complaints).

   — Complications and risk factors that affect the staff's decision to proceed to care planning.

   — Factors that must be considered in developing individualized care plan interventions.

   — Need for referrals or further evaluation by appropriate health professionals.

   Documentation about the resident's condition should support clinical decision-making regarding whether to proceed with a care plan for a triggered condition and the type(s) of care plan interventions that are appropriate for a particular resident.

   The decision to proceed to care planning should also be indicated in the appropriate column on the RAP Summary form.

4. Based on the review of assessment information, the interdisciplinary team decides whether or not the triggered condition affects the resident's functional status or well-being and warrants a care plan intervention.

5. The interdisciplinary team, in conjunction with the wishes of the resident, resident's family, and attending physician develop, revise, or continue the care plan based on this comprehensive assessment.

4.4 Identifying Need for Further Resident Assessment by Triggering RAP Conditions (RAP Process - Step 1)

A RAP may have several MDS items or sets of items that are defined as triggers. Only one of the trigger definitions must be present for a RAP to be triggered, although for many RAPs, each of the specific trigger items that are present must be investigated (e.g., address each of the potential side effects for the Psychotropic Drug Use RAP). Note that the concept of "automatic" and "potential" triggers used in the original version of the RAI has been eliminated. In Version 2.0, there are no "potential" triggers, or situations in which a symbol on the Trigger Legend does not require RAP review.

The **trigger definitions** can be found in:

- Section II of each RAP;
- The RAP Key found at the end of each RAP; and
- The RAP Trigger Legend.

The **Trigger Legend** is a **2 page form** that summarizes all of the triggers for the 18 RAPs. **It is not a required form that must be maintained in the resident's clinical record**. Rather, it is a worksheet that may be used by the interdisciplinary team members to determine which RAPs are triggered from a completed MDS form.

Many facilities use automated systems instead of the Trigger Legend form to trigger RAPs. The resulting set of triggered RAPs that is generated by your home's software program should be matched against the trigger definitions to make sure that triggered RAPs have been correctly identified.[2] HCFA has also developed test files for facility validation of a software program's triggering logic. It is the facility's responsibility to ensure that the software is triggering correctly. At a minimum, ask whether the triggered RAPs are what you would have expected. Did the software miss some RAPs you thought should have been triggered (do some of the RAPs seem to be missing); are there others triggered that you did not expect?

To identify the triggered RAPs using the Trigger Legend:

1. Compare the completed MDS with the Trigger Legend to determine which RAPs are "triggered" for review. Begin by looking at the **KEY** in the upper left corner of the Trigger Legend form.. Note that there are four possible ways for a RAP to trigger:

   The **first**, indicated by a **solid black circle**, is the predominant method and requires only one MDS item to trigger a RAP.

[2]This process should be performed on a sample of assessment records any time changes have been made in the MDS software.

The **second**, indicated by a **"2" within a solid circle**, requires two MDS items to trigger a RAP.

The **third**, indicated by an asterisk (*), requires one of three types of **psychotropic medications** (antipsychotic, antianxiety or antidepressant), and one other item in the Psychotropic Drug Use column indicated by a **solid black circle**.

The **fourth** is indicated by a **small case "a" within a circle**. This is a special ADL trigger that will focus the RAP review on rehabilitation or on the maintenance of current function.

Find the ADL -Rehabilitation Trigger A and the ADL-Maintenance Trigger B columns by scanning the top of the Trigger Legend form. Notice each ADL column title is marked with a circled "a".

If there are solid circles in both ADL columns, the ADL Maintenance column will take precedence.

2. Look at the two left columns of the Trigger Legend. These columns list the letter and number codes as well as the name of the MDS items to be considered. The third column lists the specific resident codes that will trigger a RAP. The remaining columns list the individual RAP titles.

To identify a triggered RAP, match the resident's MDS item responses with the "Code" column. If there is a "match", follow horizontally to the right until a trigger is indicated by one of the key symbols. If, for example, there is a solid circle in the column, the RAP titled at the top of that column is "triggered". This means that further assessment using the RAP Guideline is required for that particular condition.

3. Note which RAPs are triggered by particular MDS items. If desired, circle or highlight the trigger indicator or the title of the column.

4. Continue down the left column of the Trigger Legend matching recorded MDS item responses with trigger definitions until all triggered RAPs have been identified.

5. When the Trigger Legend review is completed, document on the RAP Summary form which RAPs triggered by checking the boxes in the column titled "Check if Triggered".

EXAMPLES

When Mrs. D. returns to her room after eating breakfast, she cannot recall eating breakfast, and always asks the nurse when breakfast will be served. MDS item Short Term Memory, B2a, has been coded 1 (Memory Problem), and the Cognitive Loss/Dementia RAP is triggered for further assessment.

Mr. F. is independent in cognitive skills for daily decision-making. His transferring ability varies throughout each day. He receives no assistance at some times and heavy weight-bearing assistance of one person at other times. The MDS item Decision Making, B4, is coded 0 (Independent). The MDS item Transferring, G1bA, is coded 3 (Limited Assistance). The ADL-Rehabilitation RAP is triggered for further assessment, focusing on a possible rehabilitative intervention. Rationale for trigger: Mr. F. has good cognitive skills for learning new ways to function and realize his potential.

Mr. P. is receiving an antipsychotic medication two times per day. He has fallen within the last 30 days. The MDS item Antipsychotics, O4a, is coded 7 (Received 7 days a week). The MDS item Falls (in past 30 days), J4a, is checked. The Psychotropic Drug Use RAP is triggered for further assessment. (Note: Because J4a is checked, the Falls RAP will also be triggered.)

Mrs. T. is highly involved in activities of the facility. When structured activities are not scheduled, she keeps busy reading, crocheting and writing a journal. Mrs. T. awakens early in the morning and rarely takes a nap. MDS item Awake Mornings, N1a, is checked. MDS item Involved in Activities, N2, is coded 0 (most of time). Both of these MDS items are required to trigger the Activities RAP; these factors in combination suggest that the focus of the assessment should be on reviewing the current activities plan.

Mrs. C. is limited in bed mobility (MDS item G1aA), with a physical restraint used during part of the day. The presence of any of these items is sufficient to trigger the Pressure Ulcer RAP, focusing on issues of problem avoidance in the future. (Note: other RAPs triggered include ADLs and Physical Restraints.)

Different types of triggers can change the focus of the RAP review. There are four types of triggers:

1. **Potential Problems** - Those factors that suggest the presence of a problem that warrants additional assessment and consideration of a care plan intervention. These are usually "narrowly" defined as factors that warrant additional assessment. They include clinical factors commonly seen as indicative of possible underlying problems and consequently have generally been well understood by facility staff members. Examples include the

presence of a pressure ulcer or use of a trunk restraint, both of which indicate the need for further review to determine what type of intervention is appropriate or whether underlying behavioral symptoms can be minimized or eliminated by treatment of the underlying cause (e.g., agitated depression).

2. **Broad Screening Triggers** - These are factors that assist staff to identify hard to diagnose problems. Because some problems are often difficult to assess in the elderly nursing home population, certain triggers have been "broadly" defined and consequently may have a fair number of "false positives" (i.e., the resident may trigger a RAP which is not automatically representative of a problem for the resident). Examples include factors related to delirium or dehydration. At the same time, experience has shown that many residents who have these problems were not identified prior to having triggered for review. Thus careful consideration of these triggered conditions is warranted.

3. **Prevention of Problems** - Those factors that assist staff to identify residents at risk of developing particular problems. Examples include risk factors for falling or developing a pressure ulcer.

4. **Rehabilitation Potential** - Those factors that are aimed at identifying candidates with rehabilitation potential. Not all triggers identify deficits or problems. Some triggers indicate areas of resident strengths. In general, these factors suggest consideration of programs to improve a resident's functioning or minimize decline. For example, MDS item responses indicating "Resident believes he or she is capable of increased independence in at least some ADLs" (G8a) may focus the assessment and care plan on functional areas most important to the resident or on the area with the highest potential for improvement.

Facility staff who are assessing a resident whose condition "triggers" a RAP should know what item responses on the MDS triggered that RAP. This step is often missed, especially if someone other than the person(s) who completed the MDS reviews the Trigger Legend or the triggering is automated. Referring to the Triggers section of the RAP to identify relevant triggers can help to "steer" the assessment to factors particular to the individual resident. For example, if a staff member assigned to assess a resident who has fallen or is at risk for falls knows that the Falls RAP was triggered because the resident had been dizzy during the MDS assessment period (MDS item J1f - Dizziness was checked), the RAP review would include a focus on causal factors and interventions for dizziness. While reviewing the RAP, other factors may come to light regarding the resident's risk for falls, but knowing the trigger condition clarifies or possibly rules out certain avenues of approach to the resident's problem.

At the same time, there can also be a tendency to believe that the RAP review is limited to only those MDS items that triggered the RAP. Such a view is false and can lead to key causal factors being unnoticed and a less than appropriate plan of care being initiated. Many of the trigger conditions serve to initiate a more comprehensive review process including specific causal factors (as referenced in the Guidelines) that are to be considered relative to the resident's status.

4.5 Assessment of the Resident Whose Condition Triggered RAPs (RAP Process - Step 2)

"Reviewing" a triggered RAP means doing an in-depth assessment of a resident who has a particular clinical condition in terms of the potential need for care plan interventions. The RAP is used to organize or guide the assessment process so that information needed to fully understand the resident's condition is not overlooked.

The triggered RAPs are used to glean information that pertains to the resident's condition. While reviewing the RAP, facility staff consider what MDS items caused the RAP to trigger and what type of trigger it is (i.e., potential problem, broad screen, prevention of problem or rehabilitation potential). This focuses the review on information that will be helpful in deciding if a care plan intervention is necessary, and what type of intervention is appropriate.

The information in the RAP is used to supplement clinical judgment and stimulate creative thinking when attempting to understand or resolve difficult or confusing symptoms and their causes. The Guidelines are an aide, a tool, a starting point. It is the understanding and insight of members of the interdisciplinary team that will help integrate these factors into a meaningful resident assessment and care plan.

4.6 Decision-making and Documentation of the RAP Findings (RAP Process - Steps 3 and 4)

It is recommended that staff who have participated in the assessment and who have documented information about the resident's status for triggered RAPs be a part of the interdisciplinary team that develops the resident's care plan. The team, including the resident, family or resident representative, makes the final decision to proceed to address the "triggered" condition on the care plan.

In order to provide continuity of care for the resident and good communication to all persons involved in the resident's care, it is important that information from the assessment that led the team to their care planning decision be clearly documented.

It is not necessary to record all of the items referred to in the RAP Guidelines, listing all factors that do and do not apply. Rather, documentation should focus on key issues, which may include:

- Why will you address or not address specific conditions in the care plan?
- What is it about the conditions that may affect the resident's daily functioning?
- Why did you decide the resident is at risk, that improvement is possible, or that decline can be minimized?
- Why could the resident benefit from consultation with an expert in a particular area (e.g., gynecologist, psychologist, surgeon, speech pathologist)?

Or, for triggered conditions that do not warrant care planning:

- Why did you determine that the triggered condition is not a problem for the resident?

Written documentation of the RAP findings and decision-making process may appear anywhere in the resident's record. It can be written in discipline specific flowsheets, progress notes, in the care plan summary notes, in a RAP summary narrative, on a RAP questionnaire, etc.

No matter where the information is recorded, use the "Location and Date of RAP Assessment Documentation" column on the RAP Summary form to note where the RAP review and decision-making documentation can be found in the resident's record. Also indicate in the column "Care Plan Decision" if the triggered problem is addressed in the care plan.

Examples of Resident Assessment Documentation using RAP Guidelines as a Framework

The following examples illustrate different ways to document resident status information that the assessor(s) gleaned using RAP Guidelines. This documentation would be referenced by facility staff on the RAP Summary form under the "Location of Information" column, or it could be referenced in a RAP Summary note. Please note that these examples are not related to any particular resident or case example. Also, they are not related to one another. They merely depict samples of written notes.

EXAMPLE #1: This is an example of a note that substantiates the initiation of problem evaluation using RAP Guidelines.

PROBLEM: BEHAVIORAL SYMPTOMS

In the past week Ms. E. has resisted physical care, puts up a good struggle with the nurse assistants, hits them and swears at them whenever they try to help her. Prior to admission 4 weeks ago Ms. E. had a stroke that has affected her right side. She also has an aphasia. During the first few weeks Ms. E. was lethargic and passive. She accepted total care from staff. She was difficult to evaluate in many areas because of her communication difficulties. She has been receiving physical therapy for range of motion exercises without difficulty. These behavioral symptoms with nursing staff are new. When I observed her interactions with staff today it appears that if she is approached from the right she lashes out; from the left she is fine. On a positive note, we are seeing that Ms. E. is beginning to have some response to her environment and situation and requires further evaluation regarding a new approach to nursing care, ophthalmology evaluation to rule out visual field deficits, speech therapy referral. We will discuss Ms. E.'s care at nursing rounds tomorrow and develop a revised plan to address these issues.

EXAMPLE #2: This is an example of 1) documentation in the progress notes of the clinical record clarifying that a problem is present and has been discussed with the resident, and 2) another note that describes the beginning of a work-up to evaluate and treat causes of the problem.

8/21/95 PROBLEM: URINARY INCONTINENCE
Nursing note:

Mrs. D.'s clothing has been found wet during the night on 3 occasions in the past two weeks. Her nurse assistants have also found that she has been tucking washcloths in her underwear. I spoke with her this morning. She admitted that she has been having some urinary accidents for some time but was hiding them. She cried, saying, "I am so ashamed". I reassured her that although incontinence is not normal, it is common, and should be evaluated for possible treatments. I proceeded to review the type of step by step evaluation that could be done, some which could be done here at the home and, if necessary, she would see some specialists. Mrs. D. seemed relieved and asked me to call her daughter with the information. I spoke with Ms. D. who agreed with the evaluation. She said that she has been noticing a faint odor of urine when she visits, but her mother always denied any problems. Will contact physician.

G. Hope, RN

EXAMPLE #3: This is an example of a note in a clinical record that could be referenced on the RAP Summary form to substantiate a team's decision to proceed to care planning when a RAP is triggered.

8/30/95 PROBLEM: DELIRIUM
Physician Progress note:

Mr. F. has had new symptoms in the past week of altered perceptions (thinks someone keeps jumping through his window at night when the curtain moves and has hallucinations), restlessness (pacing) and agitation, and is more confused. A review of his medication sheet shows that his Digoxin dose was increased from 0.125 mg every other day to 0.25 mg. daily 2 weeks ago during an episode of congestive heart failure. His appetite has also decreased and he says food is making him sick. He is delusional in his thinking that his food is poisoned. Mr. F.'s exam is unremarkable for signs of an acute illness or other causes of delirium. His symptoms are consistent with probable digoxin toxicity. We will obtain a digoxin level in the morning. In the meantime, I have asked the nursing staff to hold the digoxin and encourage fluids until we reevaluate in the morning. I will temporarily put him on a low dose of Haldol 0.5 mg twice daily in order to reduce his delusions and distress. I will review his status daily with the goal of tapering him off the Haldol once his mental status returns to baseline.

Ben Todd, M.D.

8/30/95 PROBLEM: DELIRIUM
Nursing note:

Until the acute confusion subsides, Mr. F will receive close observation, monitoring of his intake with encouragement of fluids, cueing during ADLs to help him focus. He will be allowed to pace in the confines of the unit and restricted to the unit until his confusion resolves. J. Doe, RN

EXAMPLE #4: This case illustrates summary documentation using RAP Guidelines to assess the resident's progress related to a previously noted condition, as well as the success of the care plan over time.

PROBLEM: PRESSURE ULCER OVER RIGHT TROCHANTER

Three months ago, Mr. H. developed a Stage III pressure ulcer over his right trochanter when he fell asleep on the spirals of a notebook while reading in bed (pressure). Mr. H. had been receiving Ambien 10mg at bedtime for sleep because he had difficulty falling asleep with a roommate who snores loudly. He was friendly with the roommate and did not want to switch rooms when the opportunity was offered. Deep sleep most likely contributed to his not responding to the spiral by shifting his weight. Mr. H. has since agreed to move in with a quieter roommate and discontinue the Ambien. We have been treating the ulcer with surgical debridement as necessary and wet to dry saline dressings three times daily, and the ulcer has cleared up nicely to a dime-size area with clean granulation tissue present. Dr. K. discontinued wet to dry dressings and it is being managed with a transparent dressing. Mr. H. is back to his usual activities and is adherent to his repositioning program when in bed. We will continue the current care plan.

EXAMPLE #5: This case illustrates documentation, using RAP Guidelines, to assess the progress of a long-stay resident who has chronic Urinary Incontinence AND Pressure Ulcer risk.

PROBLEM: LONG-STANDING URINARY INCONTINENCE AND PRESSURE ULCER RISK

Mr. F. is a severely demented gentleman who suffers from immobility secondary to dementia and disuse. He has tight contractures of his elbows, hips, knees, and ankles making toileting difficult. Mr. F. is frail, primarily bed- and recliner chair-bound. He is totally dependent on staff for care in ADLs, including eating. He has long-standing incontinence that has been managed for the past year with an external catheter to protect his skin (He has a history of rashes). When transferred he is always placed on pressure relieving devices. He receives a turning and positioning regimen. This regimen has been working and he is free of rashes and skin breakdown. We and his family are in agreement about continuing the current palliative approach to urinary incontinence and preventive approach to ulcer formation.

EXAMPLE #6: This example illustrates that it is not necessary to use the titles of the RAPs to document resident assessment information using RAP Guidelines. <u>The most important goal of</u>

documentation is to describe events in a way that everyone can understand what is happening to the resident.

PROBLEM: SIDE EFFECTS FROM MELLARIL

Mrs. L. has been disimpacted of hard, pasty stool twice during the last 6 days. Bowel elimination records show that she has been having infrequent movements. Staff say that she strains at stool. Mrs. L. has a long history of schizophrenia. Her psychosis has been managed with various antipsychotics over the years. Most recently (last 6 weeks) we switched her from Haldol to Mellaril 50 mg. TID daily for its sedative effects as she was agitated, wandering, and delusional. The Mellaril has calmed her down to the point that she is able to sit in on some unit activities without leaving them. The dose was then reduced but when symptoms recurred we went back to 50mg. TID. Her blood pressure has been stable at 138/86 - 146/90 and she has had no falls. The constipation is most likely related to the Mellaril. However, as her emotional state is currently stable and she is functioning better we will maintain the current dose, add Colace 100 mg. bid, assure adequate fluid intake, and consult with dietary for suggestions.

EXAMPLE #7: This is an example of a note that illustrates the assessment of multiple problems that were triggered by the MDS. The rationale for combining the assessment into one note is that the resident's risks, problems, causes, and treatments are all interrelated. On a RAP Summary form the following note could be referenced for several triggered RAPs: Falls, Psychotropic Drug Use, Cognitive Loss, Mood State.

PROBLEM: FALLS

Mrs. T.'s severely depressed mood has improved with Trazodone and involvement in a twice weekly expressive therapy group. She has been more attentive to her surroundings and has begun to socialize like her old self. She remains disoriented to time and continues to need many reminders for most tasks (her baseline). She has rejoined her baking group that meets every other day. Her appetite has picked up and she eats most meals that are offered. We are now concerned about 2 falling episodes this past week. She usually walks alone but is very slow. On Monday night she seemed to falter in the dining room but grabbed onto some chairs to steady herself. On Tuesday she was walking in the corridor with her daughter, faltered, and then her daughter caught her before she fell. Mrs. T. insisted that she felt O.K. She denied feeling dizzy or unsteady and said she just tripped over a chair. Yesterday, she fell to the floor in the dining room while getting up from a chair. She sustained no injuries but she was posturally hypotensive (See vital sign sheet). She was seen by Dr. R. who cut back on her Trazodone dose. We will monitor postural vital signs twice daily, and supervise all transfers and walking, and observe for changes in mood. She has been referred to PT for gait evaluation.

EXAMPLE #8: The following example illustrates how to document a situation when the resident functions at a consistent level over a long period of time. The MDS assessment always triggers the same RAP for the same reason, but the resident has shown neither improvement nor decline in function. Note that a nursing diagnosis is used in the problem title rather than the triggered RAP title of ADL-Functional Rehabilitation Potential.

7/6/95 PROBLEM: IMPAIRED PHYSICAL MOBILITY

Mrs. X. has impaired mobility related to Parkinson's disease. She transfers and ambulates with a walker and receives non-weight bearing physical assistance of one person to get in and out of bed and for all walking. Occasionally she "freezes" and her medications have been adjusted with success. Mrs. X. requires coaxing from staff to take twice daily walks as she would prefer to stay in her room. However, she enjoys and has been doing well in tri-weekly strength training and stretching classes on the unit. We will continue current care plan of walking, titrating weights per protocol (See Strength Training Progress form) and individual progress note.

OR, THE NOTE COULD LOOK LIKE THE FOLLOWING:

7/6/95 PROBLEM: IMPAIRED TRANSFER AND AMBULATION

S. "I hate exercising even if it's good for me. It's a good thing I like you."

O. See MDS re: function. Occasionally Mrs. X. "freezes" and her Sinemet dose has been adjusted by Dr. B. with good results. Mrs. X. requires coaxing from staff to take twice daily walks around the unit. She would prefer to stay in her room. However, she seems to enjoy and has made progress in tri-weekly strength training and stretching classes on the unit.

A. Level of mobility is being maintained by walking and strength training programs.

P. Continue current plan, titrating weights as per strength training protocol (See Strength Training Progress form) and progress.

EXAMPLE #9: This note illustrates a case where the resident's MDS assessment has not changed, and although it keeps triggering the same RAP, staff discover new ways of approaching the problem by using the RAP Guidelines.

6/8/95 PROBLEM: IMPAIRED AMBULATION

Mr. H. is 25 lbs. overweight and has severe osteoarthritis of both knees. His MDS walking assessments have not changed. He uses a walker and continues to receive weight bearing assistance of two persons for all transfers. Once he is standing he walks with one-person, non-weight bearing physical assistance. He has been involved in a tri-weekly strength training and daily walking program. During the last 3 months Mr. H.'s endurance has improved. He can now walk 20 feet without stopping to rest. He has lost 13 lbs. on a weight reduction program and is motivated to lose more. Plan: refer to PT for aerobic activities, refer to orthopedic surgeon to see if Mr. H. is a candidate for knee replacement surgery.

4.7 Development or Revision of the Care Plan (RAP Process - Step 5)

Following the decision to address a "triggered" condition on the care plan, key staff or the interdisciplinary team should:

- Review the current care plan if the condition is already addressed and make changes, as needed, to reflect the new assessment; and
- Develop new care plan problems, goals and approaches as needed.

Staff may choose to combine related "triggered" conditions into a single care plan problem that will address the initial set of causal problems and related outcomes identified in the RAP review.

Chapter 5 will address the development of resident care plans in more detail.

4.8 Frequently Asked Questions on RAP Documentation

Q: "Is it necessary to complete a RAP review if a resident always triggers for the same RAP in the same way? For example, Mrs. Peterson always triggers for the Nutritional Status RAP because she often leaves 25% of her food uneaten at most meals. She is not a big eater, and prefers to snack throughout the day - not to mention the portions on the tray are quite large. Do we need to do the entire RAP each time?"

A: No, it is not necessary to always review and document RAP findings on subsequent assessments the way you would on the initial assessment. Triggers identify areas warranting further assessment. The RAP guides this assessment. In this example, further assessment may reveal a swallowing problem, chewing problem, delirium, activity endurance problem, or a healthy life time pattern. If Mrs. Peterson chooses to eat frequent snacks, and still is consuming a nutritionally adequate diet, then there is no reason to complete the RAP in its entirety at each full assessment. In this example, clearly document the initial nutritional assessment including: preferences, information that confirms her diet is sufficient, any supporting weights or any lab values that give insight into nutrition. If she continues to trigger this RAP for the same reasons, make a one line entry referring to the original nutritional assessment and indicate that the resident's status has not changed. **On subsequent assessments, it is always necessary to assess the resident to validate that his or her status has not changed as compared to the original RAP assessment and documentation.**

Q: "Is it required to write a summary note documenting all of the RAP information?"

A: The requirement is that you document information from the resident's assessment and staff's decision making about care. This should already be an easily accessible part of the medical record, in which case a summary note may be redundant. Ask yourself this question: "If I was a newly hired care giver for this resident, will I be able to find and understand the assessment and decision making process?" If the answer is yes, then you should feel secure that your documentation is complete. If you answer no, consider pulling together key information or "filling in the gaps" in a short note.

Q: "I often hear different stories about what is required for RAP documentation. These stories seem to vary by nursing home, surveyors, care givers, books, software and even the day of the week! Why is that, and how can we find out what is expected in our written documentation?"

A: While interpretations of HCFA's requirements have varied, the RAP process was developed to reflect good clinical practice and RAP documentation expectations have never changed: RAPs guide further assessment of residents who have or are at risk of developing problems (triggered areas). This assessment is supposed to lend further insight into the problems identified by the MDS. RAP "documentation" involves only what should already be taking place: clearly written assessments, decision making by staff knowledge about the resident's condition, and care plans developed based on a comprehensive assessment of a resident's needs, strengths, and preferences.

Where staff often go astray is in the basics. What does clear documentation and decision making mean? The RAP guides the assessment piece and documentation should follow. Decision making is a written account of the team's clinical thought processes about the resident assessment findings. This seemingly simple process has left many people baffled and searching for "user friendly" alternatives to RAP documentation. As a result an industry of workbooks, flow sheets, check lists and software has been created. In some cases, these products may help staff by providing structure that facilitates the clinical assessment and decision-making process; in other cases, such products have tended to create a larger paper trail and made the process more complicated than necessary. Each facility should establish a documentation process that "works" for them and incorporate additional tools only if they are deemed of clear benefit in facilitating documentation and clinical decision-making.

Q: "I don't see how we can possibly do the Urinary Incontinence RAP in 14 days after admission. And, it seems everyone has a different idea about when these RAPs are due. Some say 7 days after admission, 14 days, 21 days, who is right?"

A: Statutory requirements dictate that the RAI be completed within 14 days after admission. As an integral part of the RAI, RAPs must be completed within 14 days, which means that the initial RAP Guideline review must be conducted and documented by the end of that time. However, the RAPs may point out the need for a more extensive evaluation which cannot be completed entirely within the time period. A good example is the Urinary Incontinence RAP. It is generally difficult to perform a complete work-up in 14 days. Even getting initial tests ordered and scheduled can take several weeks. Rather what is intended by "14 days after admission" is when the initial RAP assessment process and documentation must be completed. Certainly you do not wait several weeks to initiate the assessment and make care planning decisions. These initial plans should be outlined in the care plan along with the plan for further assessment.

Q: "Is the person who signs the 'Signature of RN Coordinator for RAP Assessment Process on the RAP Summary form, the same person as the MDS RN Coordinator? What dates are entered in #2 and #4 on the RAP Summary form, and whose name is placed in the 'Signature of Person Completing Care Planning Decision'?

A: The "Signature of RN Coordinator for RAP Assessment Process" does not need to be the same RN as is on the MDS assessment. The date entered in VB2 on the RAP Summary form is the date the RN Coordinator of the RAP process (i.e., the person who oversaw completion of the RAPs), indicated the triggered RAPs and completed the Location and Date of RAP Assessment Documentation section. This must be completed no later than 14 days after admission. The (Signature of) Person Completing Care Planning Decision can be any person(s) who facilitates the care planning decision-making. It is an interdisciplinary process. The care plan must be done no later than 21 days after admission or 7 days after MDS and RAPs are completed. The care-planning information on the RAP Summary form would be completed at that time, with the date to enter in #4 the day that #3 is signed.

4.9 When is the Resident Assessment Instrument not Enough?

Federal requirements support a facility's ongoing responsibility to assess a resident. The Quality of Care regulation[3] requires that "each resident must receive and the facility must provide the necessary care and services to attain or maintain the highest practicable physical, mental, and psychosocial well-being, in accordance with the comprehensive assessment and plan of care". Services provided or arranged by the facility must also meet professional standards of quality. Compliance with these regulations requires that the facility monitor the resident's condition and respond with appropriate careplanning interventions.

The MDS is a screening instrument and does not include detailed descriptions of all factors necessary for careplanning and evaluation. When completing the MDS, the assessor simply indicates whether or not a factor is present. For certain clinical situations, if the MDS indicates the presence of a potential resident problem, need, or strength, the assessor may need to investigate and document the resident's condition in more detail. For example, if a resident is noted as having a contracture on the MDS, additional documentation in the record may include the number of contractures present, sites, and degree of restriction in each affected joint. RAPs also assist in gathering additional information for some clinical conditions.

In addition, completion of the MDS/RAPs does not necessarily fulfill a facility's obligation to perform a comprehensive assessment. Facilities are responsible for assessing areas that are relevant to individual residents regardless of whether or not the appropriate areas are included in the RAI. For example, the MDS includes a listing of those diagnoses that affect the resident's functioning or needs in the past 7 days. While the MDS may indicate the presence of medical

[3] 42 CFR 483.25--(F 309)

problems, such as unstable diabetes or orthostatic hypotension, there should be evidence of additional assessment of these factors if relevant to the development of the careplan for an individual resident. The need for a physical examination detailing findings in pertinent body subsystems is another example.

Some facilities have reacted to the Federal requirements for resident assessment by creating lengthy and cumbersome assessment tools, which are completed for each resident in addition to the State RAI. This is not a Federal requirement and often not a desirable use of facility staff resources. Additional assessment is necessary only for factors that are relevant for an individual resident. For example, an extensive cognitive status assessment is not necessary if no deficits were noted using the MDS. Likewise, using multiple assessment tools that basically measure the same thing is often a poor use of clinical resources. All members of the interdisciplinary team should be trained in assessment and capable of determining what is necessary and appropriate for a particular resident. Elaborate assessment systems should not necessarily replace the judgment of the team members.

Case Example - MDS, RAP and Care Planning

This case example is structured from the point of view of the nurse responsible for coordinating the RAI and care planning processes. It is organized in a series of stages, corresponding to how the care team acquired and used information in the MDS and RAPs.

In this case example:

- The processes of completing the MDS/RAP assessment [RAI] and developing an individualized care plan are illustrated.
- The goal is to show how MDS assessment information leads you to further assessment (by reviewing triggered RAPs) and to care planning.
- The RAP Summary forms are shown as part of this example to illustrate how this specific form can aid in coordinating and facilitating the flow of assessment data and decision-making.

This example does NOT:

- Represent a functionally complete MDS, RAP review and care planning process. Certain assessment areas and elements of care, although very appropriate, are not presented as part of this example.

1. THE ASSESSMENT PROCESS

We begin the MDS assessment process with examples of notes from the clinical record and conversations between caregivers displaying assessment points over the first few days of residency. These examples illustrate that MDS and RAP assessment information is being gathered from the point of admission, although the MDS form itself may be completed later.

Day 1 (Initial Admission of Mr. S. from the hospital August 24, 1995).

Following his admission, the following SOAP note was written on August 24, 1995.

S: "Come sit with me, Joanne. I am so thirsty. Get me some water" says Mr. S. talking to wife Marion. (Joanne is his sister who expired 12 years ago.) Wife stated that he never refers to her as his sister, but that since he was admitted to the hospital he has been more confused.

O: Mr. S. admitted from the hospital, s/p left hip replacement. Mr. S. has a five year history of Alzheimer's disease, and has been attending the Cognitive Impairment Clinic at the hospital for three years.

According to hospital discharge summary, Mr. S. was agitated in the ER, and was given Haldol IM several times during his stay in the hospital. His dehydration was treated successfully with IV fluids. He was "very confused, more so than what the wife previously indicated". Other new medications include ranitidine (Zantac), Morphine, Bactrim DS for a diagnosed urinary tract infection. He remained restrained throughout his stay.

Mr. S. is oriented only to self and responds to his name only. He refers to his wife as his sister (new for him). He is not aware that he is in a nursing home, or that he was in a hospital. He continuously picks at his bed clothes, and fidgets with the call light.

A: Acute confusion possibly related to hospitalization, medications, urinary tract infection, pain and isolation.

P: Monitor closely for safety. Do not use restraints. Begin 15 minute checks while awake. Encourage out of room activities. Resident continuing on Bactrim DS for 6 more days. Consult with physician about medication regimen. Ask daughter to bring in some of Mr. S.'s favorite articles to reorient him. Encourage frequent visits from family, explaining to them about Mr. S.'s change in cognitive status. Monitor closely for hip pain. Medicate with Tylenol for discomfort. Maintain pain flow sheet in the clinical record to assess effectiveness of pain regimen.

Day 2 (Note by physician on her visit with Mr. S.).

I saw Mr. S. today in the home where he was newly admitted. He has a five year history of Alzheimer's disease, complicated by an acute confusional state. His hospitalization for hip repair was complicated by a urinary tract infection, dehydration, and acute confusional state. Whether the dehydration, infection, or medications was the cause of the cognitive changes is uncertain at this time. Wife reports that he was having difficulty urinating prior to admission, but thought that it was normal, considering his history of an enlarged prostate. I discontinued morphine and started Tylenol, 650 mg every 6 hours, since admission. Also, I changed his

Haldol to p.o. and will slowly decrease the dosage. Continue with Bactrim DS until course completed. Discontinue Zantac. It is unclear why he was started on it and it may be contributing to his confusion. Monitor Intake and Output for next 7 days. I will do a further exam of Mr. S. on Monday.

Day 4 **(The following is an example of a dialogue between the nurse and the social worker about what was learned in admission examinations. It does not represent documentation but serves to illustrate the interdisciplinary assessment processes. Also included on this day are the follow-up nursing notes and a separate physical therapy note. Staff's awareness of the needs and treatments for the resident is expanding.)**

SOCIAL WORKER (SW):

"I spoke with Mr. S., his wife Marion and oldest daughter, Susan, the first two days of admission. Throughout the conversation, Mr. S. was unable to answer simple questions. He was easily sidetracked and would become consumed with smoothing out his bedclothes. Marion and Susan said that normally he can't answer simple questions about his immediate needs, but he can talk endlessly about woodworking and opera."

NURSE (N):

"Mr. S. is much clearer today. Although he didn't remember meeting me before, he responded to his name, and stated that he was not in his home, but in an old person's home. His wife was present and he called her by her proper name."

SW: "Mary [the nurse on evenings] told me that his cognition will probably continue to improve once his delirium clears. I have shared this with the family who seemed relieved."

N: "She is probably right. The UTI, dehydration, morphine, Zantac and Haldol probably contributed to his acute confusion, but because he has Alzheimer's disease, it makes it difficult to assess his baseline."

SW: "Well, his family described a gregarious man, who enjoyed attending the Alzheimer's Day Care Program at the community center. He was diagnosed with Alzheimer's Disease five years ago although the daughter stated that she felt that he was having problems several years before the actual diagnosis. His wife also told me that Mr. S. was having increasing difficulties with his ADLs. She would have to break tasks down into sub-tasks. He required lots of cueing for dressing especially."

N: "He had his admission physical exam yesterday. Under the circumstances, everything seems O.K. His enlarged prostate probably causes some urinary retention which would have put him at greater risk for the urinary tract infection, but his surgical incision line was clean. He appears well hydrated, and the nurse assistants from the day and evening shift indicate that he is taking in ample fluids. He continues to manipulate bed clothes, which according to his wife is a new activity, but it is tapering off. This could represent a resolution of his acute confusion. We will continue to monitor his intake and output, and cognition in light of his acute confusion. He is at risk for falling. He still has a few more days on his antibiotic for his UTI. The physical therapist will be seeing him today in fact. I'm going to write a brief note to document the areas we covered in these conversations."

NURSING NOTE

Discussed Mr. S.'s condition with Social Worker. Mr. S. seems to be "clearer today". He is oriented to person, able to identify wife by her correct name, and is aware that he is not in his home. He identifies his property that his wife brought in from home (picture and opera posters), and his fidgeting with the bedcloths has lessened. As his acute confusion improves we should see a returning to baseline. On exam Mr. S. appeared well hydrated, I/O adequate according to reports from nurse assistants. He appears in mild discomfort only when he ambulates, and is receiving Tylenol regularly. His dose of Haldol is being slowly tapered. He does not appear to have any negative effects from this. K. Phillips, R.N.

PHYSICAL THERAPY NOTE

On August 14, 1995, he sustained the fall and fractured his left hip. He underwent a successful replacement of the hip, and was cleared for light weight bearing status on 8/21/95. Because of his worsening cognition, and additional problems, he has not been ambulating except out of bed to the commode with nursing staff.

According to the daughter, who was involved with his care at home, his fall was an isolated event. Usually he ambulates around his home, Adult Day Care, and takes frequent walks without event. Orthostatic blood pressures and pulses from the end of his hospitalization and since admission here have been within normal limits, with orthostatic changes noted upon admission to the hospital.

His fall at home occurred at 2 am. The resident was very restless the entire day. He appeared to be having difficulty urinating. His wife was planning to take him into the doctor's office in the morning. Mr. S. got out of bed and was found wandering around the house. His wife tried to get him to return to bed, but he went into the bathroom, got into the shower - with his clothing on - and fell. Wife is not certain if he slipped or just fell.

Upon examination, he did not have orthostatic changes in his blood pressure or heart rate from a lying to upright position. He was able to get out of bed to a standing position with contact guard. Using his new walker, he was able to move to the hallways - safely. He did seem confused about the walker, but followed my commands appropriately.

This resident is ready to bear full weight. Staff should walk with him three times a day using contact guard and cueing for the walker. A sign that reads "Mr. S. remember your pusher" (his word for walker) was placed by his bed and by the inside of the door. According to notes from the Cognitive Impairment Clinic, he is able to read and follow simple written directions.

Assessment: Mr. S. is at risk for future falls due to his recent fracture and hip replacement, cognitive impairments, new required use of walker (which he may get to a point that he doesn't need), and residual acute confusion. Plan: Monitor closely, contact guarding with all ambulation. Ambulate in hallway at least three times a day. Slowly increase distance, over the next two weeks, from room to dining room. J. Smith, P.T.

Day 5 (Example of documentation of additional information gathered that would be relevant to comprehensive resident assessment using the MDS and RAPs)

NURSING NOTE

Resident incontinent of urine all three shifts since admission. His normal pattern at home was to toilet himself as needed, with additional reminders from his wife before leaving the house and at bed time. Resident with a past history of enlarged prostate and urinary retention. Resident is moving his bowels daily and passing moderate amounts of soft, formed stool. Digital exam is negative for feces in rectum. Mr. S. is receiving tapering doses of Haldol. We expect the incontinence to resolve with diminishing Haldol doses, full treatment of UTI, and resolution of delirium. The decision was made to document bowel and bladder activity, I/O of fluids, assess for bladder distention, discuss with wife regarding past patterns for bathroom cueing, and to continue to review medications: Haldol, Bactrim DS.

K. Phillips, R.N.

2. DRAWING INFORMATION TOGETHER

The above are examples of the types of activities and dialogue that occur as staff gather information and structure care during the first few days of a resident's stay in the home. Using this and other information, staff would next fill out the MDS. Each discipline would complete their assigned portion of the MDS, cross check the assessment across disciplines and shifts for accuracy, and then have it signed off by the RN.

A completed MDS for Mr. S. follows. Note that this completed MDS form includes information presented in the examples above, as well as other information not available to the reader. In reviewing Mr. S.'s MDS, note the information that it contains for use by staff in using the RAP Guidelines.

Numeric Identifier 17349

MINIMUM DATA SET (MDS) — *VERSION 2.0*

FOR NURSING HOME RESIDENT ASSESSMENT AND CARE SCREENING

BASIC ASSESSMENT TRACKING FORM

SECTION AA. IDENTIFICATION INFORMATION

1.	RESIDENT NAME©	— (a. First) — (b. Middle Initial) S. (c. Last) (d. Jr/Sr)
2.	GENDER©	1. Male 2. Female — 1
3.	BIRTHDATE©	02-16-1910 (Month, Day, Year)
4.	RACE/© ETHNICITY	1. American Indian/Alaskan Native 2. Asian/Pacific Islander 3. Black, not of Hispanic origin 4. Hispanic 5. White, not of Hispanic origin — 5
5.	SOCIAL SECURITY© AND MEDICARE NUMBERS© [C in 1st box if non med. no.]	a. Social Security Number: 046-53-3371 b. Medicare number (or comparable railroad insurance number): 010534499T
6.	FACILITY PROVIDER NO.©	a. State No.: 8041100 b. Federal No.: 700222
7.	MEDICAID NO. ["+" *if pending*, "N" *if not a Medicaid recipient*]©	0105344994
8.	REASONS FOR ASSESS-MENT	[Note—Other codes do not apply to this form] a. Primary reason for assessment — 1 1. Admission assessment (required by day 14) 2. Annual assessment 3. Significant change in status assessment 4. Significant correction of prior assessment 5. Quarterly review assessment 0. *NONE OF ABOVE* b. ***Special codes for use with supplemental assessment types in Case Mix demonstration states or other states where required*** *1. 5 day assessment* *2. 30 day assessment* *3. 60 day assessment* *4. Quarterly assessment using full MDS form* *5. Readmission/return assessment* *6. Other state required assessment*
9.	SIGNATURES OF PERSONS COMPLETING THESE ITEMS:	a. Signatures: Margaret Doyle — Title: RN — Date: 8/25/95 b. — Date:

GENERAL INSTRUCTIONS

Complete this information for submission with all full and quarterly assessments (Admission, Annual, Significant Change, State or Medicare required assessments, or Quarterly Reviews, etc.)

© = Key items for computerized resident tracking

☐ = When box blank, must enter number or letter [a.] = When letter in box, check if condition applies

Resident MR. S. Numeric Identifier 17349

MINIMUM DATA SET (MDS) — *VERSION 2.0*

FOR NURSING HOME RESIDENT ASSESSMENT AND CARE SCREENING

BACKGROUND (FACE SHEET) INFORMATION AT ADMISSION

SECTION AB. DEMOGRAPHIC INFORMATION

1.	DATE OF ENTRY	*Date the stay began. Note — Does not include readmission if record was closed at time of temporary discharge to hospital, etc. In such cases, use prior admission date* 08 – 24 – 1995 Month Day Year	
2.	ADMITTED FROM (AT ENTRY)	1. Private home/apt. with no home health services 2. Private home/apt. with home health services 3. Board and care/assisted living/group home 4. Nursing home 5. Acute care hospital 6. Psychiatric hospital, MR/DD facility 7. Rehabilitation hospital 8. Other	5
3.	LIVED ALONE (PRIOR TO ENTRY)	0. No 1. Yes 2. In other facility	0
4.	ZIP CODE OF PRIOR PRIMARY RESIDENCE	02491	
5.	RESIDENTIAL HISTORY 5 YEARS PRIOR TO ENTRY	(**Check all settings** *resident* **lived in** *during 5 years prior to date of entry given in item AB1 above)* Prior stay at this nursing home a. Stay in other nursing home b. Other residential facility—board and care home, assisted living, group home c. MH/psychiatric setting d. MR/DD setting e. *NONE OF ABOVE* f.	f. ✓
6.	LIFETIME OCCUPATION(S) [Put "/" between two occupations]	CARPENTER	
7.	EDUCATION (*Highest Level Completed*)	1. No schooling 2. 8th grade/less 3. 9-11 grades 4. High school 5. Technical or trade school 6. Some college 7. Bachelor's degree 8. Graduate degree	5
8.	LANGUAGE	(*Code for correct response*) a. Primary Language 0. English 1. Spanish 2. French 3. Other b. If other, specify	0
9.	MENTAL HEALTH HISTORY	Does resident's RECORD indicate any history of mental retardation, mental illness, or developmental disability problem? 0. No 1. Yes	0
10.	CONDITIONS RELATED TO MR/DD STATUS	(**Check all conditions** *that are related to MR/DD status that were manifested before age 22, and are likely to continue indefinitely*) Not applicable—no MR/DD (Skip to AB11) a. MR/DD with organic condition Down's syndrome b. Autism c. Epilepsy d. Other organic condition related to MR/DD e. MR/DD with no organic condition f.	a. ✓
11.	DATE BACKGROUND INFORMATION COMPLETED	08 – 25 – 1995 Month Day Year	

SECTION AC. CUSTOMARY ROUTINE

1. CUSTOMARY ROUTINE (*In year prior to DATE OF ENTRY to this nursing home, or year last in community if now being admitted from another nursing home*)

(**Check all that apply.** *If all information UNKNOWN, check last box only.*)

Item		Check
CYCLE OF DAILY EVENTS		
Stays up late at night (e.g., after 9 pm)	a.	✓
Naps regularly during day (at least 1 hour)	b.	
Goes out 1+ days a week	c.	✓
Stays busy with hobbies, reading, or fixed daily routine	d.	✓
Spends most of time alone or watching TV	e.	
Moves independently indoors (with appliances, if used)	f.	✓
Use of tobacco products at least daily	g.	
NONE OF ABOVE	h.	
EATING PATTERNS		
Distinct food preferences	i.	
Eats between meals all or most days	j.	✓
Use of alcoholic beverage(s) at least weekly	k.	
NONE OF ABOVE	l.	
ADL PATTERNS		
In bedclothes much of day	m.	
Wakens to toilet all or most nights	n.	✓
Has irregular bowel movement pattern	o.	
Showers for bathing	p.	✓
Bathing in PM	q.	✓
NONE OF ABOVE	r.	
INVOLVEMENT PATTERNS		
Daily contact with relatives/close friends	s.	✓
Usually attends church, temple, synagogue (etc.)	t.	
Finds strength in faith	u.	
Daily animal companion/presence	v.	
Involved in group activities	w.	✓
NONE OF ABOVE	x.	
UNKNOWN—Resident/family unable to provide information	y.	

END

SECTION AD. FACE SHEET SIGNATURES

SIGNATURES OF PERSONS COMPLETING FACE SHEET:

a. Signature of RN Assessment Coordinator — Margaret Doyle RN — Date 8/25/95

b. Signatures Title Sections Date

c. Date

d. Date

e. Date

f. Date

g. Date

☐ = When box blank, must enter number or letter [a.] = When letter in box, check if condition applies

MDS 2.0 10/18/94N

Resident MR. S. Numeric Identifier 17349

MINIMUM DATA SET (MDS) — *VERSION 2.0*
FOR NURSING HOME RESIDENT ASSESSMENT AND CARE SCREENING
FULL ASSESSMENT FORM
(Status in last 7 days, unless other time frame indicated)

SECTION A. IDENTIFICATION AND BACKGROUND INFORMATION

1.	RESIDENT NAME	— — S. a. (First) b. (Middle Initial) c. (Last) d. (Jr/Sr)	
2.	ROOM NUMBER	530A	
3.	ASSESSMENT REFERENCE DATE	a. *Last day of MDS observation period* 09 - 06 - 1995 Month Day Year	
		b. Original (0) or corrected copy of form (enter number of correction)	0
4a.	DATE OF REENTRY	**Date of reentry from most recent temporary discharge to a hospital in last 90 days (or since last assessment or admission if less than 90 days)** __ __ - __ __ - __ __ __ __ Month Day Year	
5.	MARITAL STATUS	1. Never married 2. Married 3. Widowed 4. Separated 5. Divorced	2
6.	MEDICAL RECORD NO.	2QT2BS8	
7.	CURRENT PAYMENT SOURCES FOR N.H. STAY	(*Billing Office to indicate; **check all that apply in last 30 days***) Medicaid per diem a. Medicare per diem b. Medicare ancillary part A c. Medicare ancillary part B d. CHAMPUS per diem e. VA per diem f. ✓ Self or family pays for full per diem g. Medicaid resident liability or Medicare co-payment h. Private insurance per diem (including co-payment) i. Other per diem j.	
8.	REASONS FOR ASSESSMENT [*Note—If this is a discharge or reentry assessment, only a limited subset of MDS items need be completed*]	a. Primary reason for assessment 1. Admission assessment (required by day 14) 2. Annual assessment 3. Significant change in status assessment 4. Significant correction of prior assessment 5. Quarterly review assessment 6. Discharged—return not anticipated 7. Discharged—return anticipated 8. Discharged prior to completing initial assessment 9. Reentry 0. *NONE OF ABOVE*	1
		b. ***Special codes for use with supplemental assessment types in Case Mix demonstration states or other states where required*** *1. 5 day assessment* *2. 30 day assessment* *3. 60 day assessment* *4. Quarterly assessment using full MDS form* *5. Readmission/return assessment* *6. Other state required assessment*	
9.	RESPONSIBILITY/ LEGAL GUARDIAN	(***Check all that apply***) Legal guardian a. Other legal oversight b. Durable power of attorney/health care c. ✓ Durable power attorney/financial d. ✓ Family member responsible e. ✓ Patient responsible for self f. *NONE OF ABOVE* g.	
10.	ADVANCED DIRECTIVES	(*For those items with supporting documentation in the medical record, **check all that apply***) Living will a. ✓ Do not resuscitate b. ✓ Do not hospitalize c. Organ donation d. Autopsy request e. Feeding restrictions f. Medication restrictions g. Other treatment restrictions h. *NONE OF ABOVE* i.	

SECTION B. COGNITIVE PATTERNS

1.	COMATOSE	(*Persistent vegetative state/no discernible consciousness*) 0. No 1. Yes **(If yes, skip to Section G)**	0
2.	MEMORY	(*Recall of what was learned or known*) a. Short-term memory OK—seems/appears to recall after 5 minutes 0. Memory OK 1. Memory problem	1
		b. Long-term memory OK—seems/appears to recall long past 0. Memory OK 1. Memory problem	1
3.	MEMORY/ RECALL ABILITY	(***Check all that resident was normally able to recall during last 7 days***) Current season a. ✓ Location of own room b. Staff names/faces c. That he/she is in a nursing home d. ✓ *NONE OF ABOVE* are recalled e.	
4.	COGNITIVE SKILLS FOR DAILY DECISION-MAKING	(*Made decisions regarding tasks of daily life*) 0. *INDEPENDENT*—decisions consistent/reasonable 1. *MODIFIED INDEPENDENCE*—some difficulty in new situations only 2. *MODERATELY IMPAIRED*—decisions poor; cues/supervision required 3. *SEVERELY IMPAIRED*—never/rarely made decisions	2
5.	INDICATORS OF DELIRIUM—PERIODIC DISORDERED THINKING/ AWARENESS	(*Code for behavior in the last 7 days.*) **[Note: *Accurate assessment requires conversations with staff and family who have direct knowledge of resident's behavior over this time*].** 0. Behavior not present 1. Behavior present, not of recent onset 2. Behavior present, over last 7 days appears different from resident's usual functioning (e.g., new onset or worsening)	
		a. EASILY DISTRACTED—(e.g., difficulty paying attention; gets sidetracked)	2
		b. PERIODS OF ALTERED PERCEPTION OR AWARENESS OF SURROUNDINGS—(e.g., moves lips or talks to someone not present; believes he/she is somewhere else; confuses night and day)	2
		c. EPISODES OF DISORGANIZED SPEECH—(e.g., speech is incoherent, nonsensical, irrelevant, or rambling from subject to subject; loses train of thought)	0
		d. PERIODS OF RESTLESSNESS—(e.g., fidgeting or picking at skin, clothing, napkins, etc; frequent position changes; repetitive physical movements or calling out)	2
		e. PERIODS OF LETHARGY—(e.g., sluggishness; staring into space; difficult to arouse; little body movement)	0
		f. MENTAL FUNCTION VARIES OVER THE COURSE OF THE DAY—(e.g., sometimes better, sometimes worse; behaviors sometimes present, sometimes not)	2
6.	CHANGE IN COGNITIVE STATUS	Resident's cognitive status, skills, or abilities have changed as compared to status of **90 days ago** (or since last assessment if less than 90 days) 0. No change 1. Improved 2. Deteriorated	2

SECTION C. COMMUNICATION/HEARING PATTERNS

1.	HEARING	(*With hearing appliance, if used*) 0. *HEARS ADEQUATELY*—normal talk, TV, phone 1. *MINIMAL DIFFICULTY* when not in quiet setting 2. *HEARS IN SPECIAL SITUATIONS ONLY*—speaker has to adjust tonal quality and speak distinctly 3. *HIGHLY IMPAIRED*/absence of useful hearing	0
2.	COMMUNICATION DEVICES/ TECHNIQUES	(***Check all that apply** during last 7 days*) Hearing aid, present and used a. Hearing aid, present and not used regularly b. ✓ Other receptive comm. techniques used (e.g., lip reading) c. *NONE OF ABOVE* d.	
3.	MODES OF EXPRESSION	(***Check all used** by resident to make needs known*) Speech a. ✓ Writing messages to express or clarify needs b. American sign language or Braille c. Signs/gestures/sounds d. ✓ Communication board e. Other f. *NONE OF ABOVE* g.	
4.	MAKING SELF UNDERSTOOD	(*Expressing information content—however able*) 0. *UNDERSTOOD* 1. *USUALLY UNDERSTOOD*—difficulty finding words or finishing thoughts 2. *SOMETIMES UNDERSTOOD*—ability is limited to making concrete requests 3. *RARELY/NEVER UNDERSTOOD*	2
5.	SPEECH CLARITY	(*Code for speech in the **last 7 days***) 0. *CLEAR SPEECH*—distinct, intelligible words 1. *UNCLEAR SPEECH*—slurred, mumbled words 2. *NO SPEECH*—absence of spoken words	0
6.	ABILITY TO UNDERSTAND OTHERS	(*Understanding verbal information content—however able*) 0. *UNDERSTANDS* 1. *USUALLY UNDERSTANDS*—may miss some part/intent of message 2. *SOMETIMES UNDERSTANDS*—responds adequately to simple, direct communication 3. *RARELY/NEVER UNDERSTANDS*	2
7.	CHANGE IN COMMUNICATION/ HEARING	Resident's ability to express, understand, or hear information has changed as compared to status of **90 days ago** (or since last assessment if less than 90 days) 0. No change 1. Improved 2. Deteriorated	2

[ ] = When box blank, must enter number or letter [a.] = When letter in box, check if condition applies

MDS 2.0 10/18/94N

Resident MR. S.

Numeric Identifier 17349

SECTION D. VISION PATTERNS

1.	VISION	(*Ability to see in adequate light and with glasses if used*) 0. *ADEQUATE*—sees fine detail, including regular print in newspapers/books 1. *IMPAIRED*—sees large print, but not regular print in newspapers/books 2. *MODERATELY IMPAIRED*—limited vision; not able to see newspaper headlines, but can identify objects 3. *HIGHLY IMPAIRED*—object identification in question, but eyes appear to follow objects 4. *SEVERELY IMPAIRED*—no vision or sees only light, colors, or shapes; eyes do not appear to follow objects	1
2.	VISUAL LIMITATIONS/ DIFFICULTIES	Side vision problems—decreased peripheral vision (e.g., leaves food on one side of tray, difficulty traveling, bumps into people and objects, misjudges placement of chair when seating self)	a.
		Experiences any of following: sees halos or rings around lights; sees flashes of light; sees "curtains" over eyes	b.
		NONE OF ABOVE	c. ✓
3.	VISUAL APPLIANCES	Glasses; contact lenses; magnifying glass 0. No 1. Yes	1

SECTION E. MOOD AND BEHAVIOR PATTERNS

1.	INDICATORS OF DEPRES-SION, ANXIETY, SAD MOOD	(***Code for indicators observed in last 30 days, irrespective of the assumed cause***) 0. Indicator not exhibited in last 30 days 1. Indicator of this type exhibited up to five days a week 2. Indicator of this type exhibited daily or almost daily (6, 7 days a week)	
		VERBAL EXPRESSIONS OF DISTRESS	
		a. Resident made negative statements—e.g., "*Nothing matters; Would rather be dead; What's the use; Regrets having lived so long; Let me die*"	0
		b. Repetitive questions—e.g., "*Where do I go; What do I do?*"	0
		c. Repetitive verbalizations—e.g., calling out for help, ("*God help me*")	0
		d. Persistent anger with self or others—e.g., easily annoyed, anger at placement in nursing home; anger at care received	0
		e. Self deprecation—e.g., "*I am nothing; I am of no use to anyone*"	0
		f. Expressions of what appear to be unrealistic fears—e.g., fear of being abandoned, left alone, being with others	0
		g. Recurrent statements that something terrible is about to happen—e.g., believes he or she is about to die, have a heart attack	1
		h. Repetitive health complaints—e.g., persistently seeks medical attention, obsessive concern with body functions	0
		i. Repetitive anxious complaints/concerns (non-health related) e.g., persistently seeks attention/ reassurance regarding schedules, meals, laundry, clothing, relationship issues	0
		SLEEP-CYCLE ISSUES	
		j. Unpleasant mood in morning	0
		k. Insomnia/change in usual sleep pattern	1
		SAD, APATHETIC, ANXIOUS APPEARANCE	
		l. Sad, pained, worried facial expressions—e.g., furrowed brows	2
		m. Crying, tearfulness	0
		n. Repetitive physical movements—e.g., pacing, hand wringing, restlessness, fidgeting, picking	2
		LOSS OF INTEREST	
		o. Withdrawal from activities of interest—e.g., no interest in long standing activities or being with family/friends	0
		p. Reduced social interaction	2
2.	MOOD PERSIS-TENCE	One or more indicators of depressed, sad or anxious mood **were not easily altered by attempts to "cheer up", console, or reassure the resident over last 7 days** 0. No mood indicators 1. Indicators present, easily altered 2. Indicators present, not easily altered	2
3.	CHANGE IN MOOD	Resident's mood status has changed as compared to status of **90 days ago** (or since last assessment if less then 90 days) 0. No change 1. Improved 2. Deteriorated	2

			(A)	(B)
4.	BEHAVIORAL SYMPTOMS	(A) ***Behavioral symptom frequency in last 7 days*** 0. Behavior not exhibited in last 7 days 1. Behavior of this type occurred 1 to 3 days in last 7 days 2. Behavior of this type occurred 4 to 6 days, but less than daily 3. Behavior of this type occurred daily (B) ***Behavioral symptom alterability in last 7 days*** 0. Behavior not present OR behavior was easily altered 1. Behavior was not easily altered		
		a. WANDERING (moved with no rational purpose, seemingly oblivious to needs or safety)	0	0
		b. VERBALLY ABUSIVE BEHAVIORAL SYMPTOMS (others were threatened, screamed at, cursed at)	0	0
		c. PHYSICALLY ABUSIVE BEHAVIORAL SYMPTOMS (others were hit, shoved, scratched, sexually abused)	0	0
		d. SOCIALLY INAPPROPRIATE/DISRUPTIVE BEHAVIORAL SYMPTOMS (made disruptive sounds, noisiness, screaming, self-abusive acts, sexual behavior or disrobing in public, smeared/threw food/feces, hoarding, rummaged through others' belongings)	0	0
		e. RESISTS CARE (resisted taking medications/ injections, ADL assistance, or eating)	0	0

5.	CHANGE IN BEHAVIORAL SYMPTOMS	Resident's behavior status has changed as compared to **status of 90 days ago** (or since last assessment if less than 90 days) 0. No change 1. Improved 2. Deteriorated	0

SECTION F. PSYCHOSOCIAL WELL-BEING

1.	SENSE OF INITIATIVE/ INVOLVE-MENT	At ease interacting with others	a.
		At ease doing planned or structured activities	b. ✓
		At ease doing self-initiated activities	c.
		Establishes own goals	d.
		Pursues involvement in life of facility (e.g., makes/keeps friends; involved in group activities; responds positively to new activities; assists at religious services)	e.
		Accepts invitations into most group activities	f. ✓
		NONE OF ABOVE	g.
2.	UNSETTLED RELATION-SHIPS	Covert/open conflict with or repeated criticism of staff	a.
		Unhappy with roommate	b.
		Unhappy with residents other than roommate	c.
		Openly expresses conflict/anger with family/friends	d.
		Absence of personal contact with family/friends	e.
		Recent loss of close family member/friend	f.
		Does not adjust easily to change in routines	g. ✓
		NONE OF ABOVE	h.
3.	PAST ROLES	Strong identification with past roles and life status	a.
		Expresses sadness/anger/empty feeling over lost roles/status	b.
		Resident perceives that daily routine (customary routine, activities) is very different from prior pattern in the community	c.
		NONE OF ABOVE	d. ✓

SECTION G. PHYSICAL FUNCTIONING AND STRUCTURAL PROBLEMS

1. (A) ADL SELF-PERFORMANCE—(***Code for resident's PERFORMANCE OVER ALL SHIFTS during last 7 days***—*Not including setup*)

0. *INDEPENDENT*—No help or oversight —OR— Help/oversight provided only 1 or 2 times during last 7 days
1. SUPERVISION—Oversight, encouragement or cueing provided 3 or more times during last7 days —OR— Supervision (3 or more times) plus physical assistance provided only 1 or 2 times during last 7 days
2. *LIMITED ASSISTANCE*—Resident highly involved in activity; received physical help in guided maneuvering of limbs or other nonweight bearing assistance 3 or more times —OR—More help provided only 1 or 2 times during last 7 days
3. *EXTENSIVE ASSISTANCE*—While resident performed part of activity, over last 7-day period, help of following type(s) provided 3 or more times:
   — Weight-bearing support
   — Full staff performance during part (but not all) of last 7 days
4. *TOTAL DEPENDENCE*—Full staff performance of activity during entire 7 days
8. *ACTIVITY DID NOT OCCUR* during entire 7 days

(B) ADL SUPPORT PROVIDED—(***Code for MOST SUPPORT PROVIDED OVER ALL SHIFTS during last 7 days; code regardless** of resident's self-performance classification*)

0. No setup or physical help from staff
1. Setup help only
2. One person physical assist
3. Two+ persons physical assist
8. ADL activity itself did not occur during entire 7 days

			(A) SELF-PERF	(B) SUPPORT
a.	BED MOBILITY	How resident moves to and from lying position, turns side to side, and positions body while in bed	2	2
b.	TRANSFER	How resident moves between surfaces—to/from: bed, chair, wheelchair, standing position (EXCLUDE to/from bath/toilet)	3	2
c.	WALK IN ROOM	How resident walks between locations in his/her room	2	2
d.	WALK IN CORRIDOR	How resident walks in corridor on unit	2	2
e.	LOCOMO-TION ON UNIT	How resident moves between locations in his/her room and adjacent corridor on same floor. If in wheelchair, self-sufficiency once in chair	2	2
f.	LOCOMO-TION OFF UNIT	How resident moves to and returns from off unit locations (e.g., areas set aside for dining, activities, or treatments). **If facility has only one floor,** how resident moves to and from distant areas on the floor. If in wheelchair, self-sufficiency once in chair	8	8
g.	DRESSING	How resident puts on, fastens, and takes off all items of **street clothing**, including donning/removing prosthesis	3	2
h.	EATING	How resident eats and drinks (regardless of skill). Includes intake of nourishment by other means (e.g., tube feeding, total parenteral nutrition)	1	1
i.	TOILET USE	How resident uses the toilet room (or commode, bedpan, urinal); transfer on/off toilet, cleanses, changes pad, manages ostomy or catheter, adjusts clothes	3	2
j.	PERSONAL HYGIENE	How resident maintains personal hygiene, including combing hair, brushing teeth, shaving, applying makeup, washing/drying face, hands, and perineum (EXCLUDE baths and showers)	3	2

Resident: Mr. S. Numeric Identifier: 17349

2.	BATHING	How resident takes full-body bath/shower, sponge bath, and transfers in/out of tub/shower (EXCLUDE washing of back and hair.) **Code for most dependent in self-performance and support.** (A) BATHING SELF-PERFORMANCE codes appear below 0. Independent—No help provided 1. Supervision—Oversight help only 2. Physical help limited to transfer only 3. Physical help in part of bathing activity 4. Total dependence 8. Activity itself did not occur during entire 7 days (*Bathing support codes are as defined in Item 1, code B above*)	(A) 4 (B) 2
3.	TEST FOR BALANCE (see training manual)	(*Code for ability during test in the last 7 days*) 0. Maintained position as required in test 1. Unsteady, but able to rebalance self without physical support 2. Partial physical support during test; or stands (sits) but does not follow directions for test 3. Not able to attempt test without physical help a. Balance while standing b. Balance while sitting—position, trunk control	a. 3 b. 2
4.	FUNCTIONAL LIMITATION IN RANGE OF MOTION (see training manual)	(*Code for limitations during last 7 days that interfered with daily functions or placed resident at risk of injury*) (A) *RANGE OF MOTION*: 0. No limitation; 1. Limitation on one side; 2. Limitation on both sides (B) *VOLUNTARY MOVEMENT*: 0. No loss; 1. Partial loss; 2. Full loss a. Neck — (A) 0 (B) 0 b. Arm—Including shoulder or elbow — (A) 0 (B) 0 c. Hand—Including wrist or fingers — (A) 0 (B) 0 d. Leg—Including hip or knee — (A) 1 (B) 1 e. Foot—Including ankle or toes — (A) 0 (B) 0 f. Other limitation or loss — (A) 0 (B) 0	
5.	MODES OF LOCOMOTION	(*Check all that apply during last 7 days*) Cane/walker/crutch a. ✓ Wheeled self b. Other person wheeled c. Wheelchair primary mode of locomotion d. *NONE OF ABOVE* e.	
6.	MODES OF TRANSFER	(*Check all that apply during last 7 days*) Bedfast all or most of time a. Bed rails used for bed mobility or transfer b. ✓ Lifted manually c. Lifted mechanically d. Transfer aid (e.g., slide board, trapeze, cane, walker, brace) e. ✓ *NONE OF ABOVE* f.	
7.	TASK SEGMENTATION	Some or all of ADL activities were broken into subtasks during **last 7 days** so that resident could perform them 0. No 1. Yes	1
8.	ADL FUNCTIONAL REHABILITATION POTENTIAL	Resident believes he/she is capable of increased independence in at least some ADLs a. Direct care staff believe resident is capable of increased independence in at least some ADLs b. ✓ Resident able to perform tasks/activity but is very slow c. ✓ Difference in ADL Self-Performance or ADL Support, comparing mornings to evenings d. ✓ *NONE OF ABOVE* e.	
9.	CHANGE IN ADL FUNCTION	Resident's ADL self-performance status has changed as compared to status of **90 days ago** (or since last assessment if less than 90 days) 0. No change 1. Improved 2. Deteriorated	2

SECTION H. CONTINENCE IN LAST 14 DAYS

1.	CONTINENCE SELF-CONTROL CATEGORIES (*Code for resident's PERFORMANCE OVER ALL SHIFTS*) 0. *CONTINENT*—Complete control [*includes use of indwelling urinary catheter or ostomy device that does not leak urine or stool*] 1. *USUALLY CONTINENT*—BLADDER, incontinent episodes once a week or less; BOWEL, less than weekly 2. *OCCASIONALLY INCONTINENT*—BLADDER, 2 or more times a week but not daily; BOWEL, once a week 3. *FREQUENTLY INCONTINENT*—BLADDER, tended to be incontinent daily, but some control present (e.g., on day shift); BOWEL, 2-3 times a week 4. *INCONTINENT*—Had inadequate control BLADDER, multiple daily episodes; BOWEL, all (or almost all) of the time		
a.	BOWEL CONTINENCE	Control of bowel movement, with appliance or bowel continence programs, if employed	0
b.	BLADDER CONTINENCE	Control of urinary bladder function (if dribbles, volume insufficient to soak through underpants), with appliances (e.g., foley) or continence programs, if employed	4
2.	BOWEL ELIMINATION PATTERN	Bowel elimination pattern regular—at least one movement every three days a. ✓ Constipation b. Diarrhea c. Fecal impaction d. *NONE OF ABOVE* e.	
3.	APPLIANCES AND PROGRAMS	Any scheduled toileting plan a. ✓ Bladder retraining program b. ✓ External (condom) catheter c. Indwelling catheter d. Intermittent catheter e. Did not use toilet room/commode/urinal f. Pads/briefs used g. Enemas/irrigation h. Ostomy present i. *NONE OF ABOVE* j.	
4.	CHANGE IN URINARY CONTINENCE	Resident's urinary continence has changed as compared to status of **90 days ago** (or since last assessment if less than 90 days) 0. No change 1. Improved 2. Deteriorated	2

SECTION I. DISEASE DIAGNOSES

Check only those diseases that have a relationship to current ADL status, cognitive status, mood and behavior status, medical treatments, nursing monitoring, or risk of death. (Do not list inactive diagnoses)

1.	DISEASES	(*If none apply, CHECK the NONE OF ABOVE box*) **ENDOCRINE/METABOLIC/ NUTRITIONAL** Diabetes mellitus a. Hyperthyroidism b. Hypothyroidism c. **HEART/CIRCULATION** Arteriosclerotic heart disease (ASHD) d. Cardiac dysrhythmias e. Congestive heart failure f. Deep vein thrombosis g. Hypertension h. Hypotension i. Peripheral vascular disease j. Other cardiovascular disease k. **MUSCULOSKELETAL** Arthritis l. Hip fracture m. ✓ Missing limb (e.g., amputation) n. Osteoporosis o. Pathological bone fracture p. **NEUROLOGICAL** Alzheimer's disease q. ✓ Aphasia r. Cerebral palsy s. Cerebrovascular accident (stroke) t. Dementia other than Alzheimer's disease u. Hemiplegia/Hemiparesis v. Multiple sclerosis w. Paraplegia x. Parkinson's disease y. Quadriplegia z. Seizure disorder aa. Transient ischemic attack (TIA) bb. Traumatic brain injury cc. **PSYCHIATRIC/MOOD** Anxiety disorder dd. Depression ee. Manic depression (bipolar disease) ff. Schizophrenia gg. **PULMONARY** Asthma hh. Emphysema/COPD ii. **SENSORY** Cataracts jj. Diabetic retinopathy kk. Glaucoma ll. Macular degeneration mm. **OTHER** Allergies nn. Anemia oo. Cancer pp. Renal failure qq. *NONE OF ABOVE* rr.
2.	INFECTIONS	(*If none apply, CHECK the NONE OF ABOVE box*) Antibiotic resistant infection (e.g., Methicillin resistant staph) a. Clostridium difficile (c. diff.) b. Conjunctivitis c. HIV infection d. Pneumonia e. Respiratory infection f. Septicemia g. Sexually transmitted diseases h. Tuberculosis i. Urinary tract infection in last 30 days j. ✓ Viral hepatitis k. Wound infection l. NONE OF ABOVE m.
3.	OTHER CURRENT OR MORE DETAILED DIAGNOSES AND ICD-9 CODES	a. acute confusion 291.0 b. c. d. e.

SECTION J. HEALTH CONDITIONS

1.	PROBLEM CONDITIONS	(*Check all problems present in last 7 days unless other time frame is indicated*) **INDICATORS OF FLUID STATUS** Weight gain or loss of 3 or more pounds within a 7 day period a. Inability to lie flat due to shortness of breath b. Dehydrated; output exceeds input c. Insufficient fluid; did NOT consume all/almost all liquids provided during last 3 days d. OTHER Delusions e. Dizziness/Vertigo f. Edema g. Fever h. Hallucinations i. Internal bleeding j. Recurrent lung aspirations in **last 90 days** k. Shortness of breath l. Syncope (fainting) m. Unsteady gait n. Vomiting o. *NONE OF ABOVE* p. ✓

Resident MR. S. Numeric Identifier 17349

2.	PAIN SYMPTOMS	(*Code the **highest level of pain** present in the **last 7 days***) a. **FREQUENCY** with which resident complains or shows evidence of pain 0. No pain (***skip to J4***) 1. Pain less than daily 2. Pain daily	2
		b. **INTENSITY** of pain 1. Mild pain 2. Moderate pain 3. Times when pain is horrible or excruciating	1
3.	PAIN SITE	(*If pain present, **check all sites** that apply in **last 7 days***)	
		Back pain	a.
		Bone pain	b.
		Chest pain while doing usual activities	c.
		Headache	d.
		Hip pain	e. ✓
		Incisional pain	f. ✓
		Joint pain (other than hip)	g.
		Soft tissue pain (e.g., lesion, muscle)	h.
		Stomach pain	i.
		Other	j.
4.	ACCIDENTS	(***Check all that apply***)	
		Fell in **past 30 days**	a. ✓
		Fell in **past 31-180 days**	b.
		Hip fracture in **last 180 days**	c. ✓
		Other fracture in **last 180 days**	d.
		NONE OF ABOVE	e.
5.	STABILITY OF CONDITIONS	Conditions/diseases make resident's cognitive, ADL, mood or behavior patterns unstable—(fluctuating, precarious, or deteriorating)	a. ✓
		Resident experiencing an acute episode or a flare-up of a recurrent or chronic problem	b.
		End-stage disease, 6 or fewer months to live	c.
		NONE OF ABOVE	d.

SECTION K. ORAL/NUTRITIONAL STATUS

1.	ORAL PROBLEMS	Chewing problem	a.
		Swallowing problem	b.
		Mouth pain	c.
		NONE OF ABOVE	d. ✓
2.	HEIGHT AND WEIGHT	*Record **(a.) height in inches** and **(b.) weight in pounds**. Base weight on most recent measure in **last 30 days**; measure weight consistently in accord with standard facility practice—e.g., in a.m. after voiding, before meal, with shoes off, and in nightclothes* a. HT (in.) 67 b. WT (lb.) 162	
3.	WEIGHT CHANGE	a. **Weight loss**—5 % or more in **last 30 days**; or 10 % or more in **last 180 days** 0. No 1. Yes	0
		b. **Weight gain**—5 % or more in **last 30 days**; or 10 % or more in **last 180 days** 0. No 1. Yes	0
4.	NUTRITIONAL PROBLEMS	Complains about the taste of many foods	a.
		Regular or repetitive complaints of hunger	b.
		Leaves 25% or more of food uneaten at most meals	c.
		NONE OF ABOVE	d. ✓
5.	NUTRITIONAL APPROACHES	(***Check all that apply in last 7 days***)	
		Parenteral/IV	a.
		Feeding tube	b.
		Mechanically altered diet	c.
		Syringe (oral feeding)	d.
		Therapeutic diet	e.
		Dietary supplement between meals	f. ✓
		Plate guard, stabilized built-up utensil, etc.	g.
		On a planned weight change program	h.
		NONE OF ABOVE	i.
6.	PARENTERAL OR ENTERAL INTAKE	(***Skip to Section L if neither 5a nor 5b is checked***) a. Code the proportion of **total calories** the resident received through parenteral or tube feedings in the **last 7 days** 0. None 1. 1% to 25% 2. 26% to 50% 3. 51% to 75% 4. 76% to 100%	
		b. Code the average **fluid intake** per day by IV or tube in **last 7 days** 0. None 1. 1 to 500 cc/day 2. 501 to 1000 cc/day 3. 1001 to 1500 cc/day 4. 1501 to 2000 cc/day 5. 2001 or more cc/day	

SECTION L. ORAL/DENTAL STATUS

1.	ORAL STATUS AND DISEASE PREVENTION	Debris (soft, easily movable substances) present in mouth prior to going to bed at night	a.
		Has dentures or removable bridge	b. ✓
		Some/all natural teeth lost—does not have or does not use dentures (or partial plates)	c.
		Broken, loose, or carious teeth	d.
		Inflamed gums (gingiva); swollen or bleeding gums; oral abscesses; ulcers or rashes	e.
		Daily cleaning of teeth/dentures or daily mouth care—by resident or staff	f. ✓
		NONE OF ABOVE	g.

SECTION M. SKIN CONDITION

			Number at Stage
1.	ULCERS (Due to any cause)	(*Record the number of ulcers at each ulcer stage—regardless of cause. If none present at a stage, record "0" (zero). Code all that apply during **last 7 days**. Code 9 = 9 or more.*) ***[Requires full body exam.]***	
		a. Stage 1. A persistent area of skin redness (without a break in the skin) that does not disappear when pressure is relieved.	0
		b. Stage 2. A partial thickness loss of skin layers that presents clinically as an abrasion, blister, or shallow crater.	0
		c. Stage 3. A full thickness of skin is lost, exposing the subcutaneous tissues - presents as a deep crater with or without undermining adjacent tissue.	0
		d. Stage 4. A full thickness of skin and subcutaneous tissue is lost, exposing muscle or bone.	0
2.	TYPE OF ULCER	(*For each type of ulcer, **code for the highest stage in the last 7 days** using scale in item M1—i.e., 0=none; stages 1, 2, 3, 4*)	
		a. Pressure ulcer—any lesion caused by pressure resulting in damage of underlying tissue	0
		b. Stasis ulcer—open lesion caused by poor circulation in the lower extremities	0
3.	HISTORY OF RESOLVED ULCERS	Resident had an ulcer that was resolved or cured in **LAST 90 DAYS** 0. No 1. Yes	0
4.	OTHER SKIN PROBLEMS OR LESIONS PRESENT	(***Check all that apply** during **last 7 days***)	
		Abrasions, bruises	a.
		Burns (second or third degree)	b.
		Open lesions other than ulcers, rashes, cuts (e.g., cancer lesions)	c.
		Rashes—e.g., intertrigo, eczema, drug rash, heat rash, herpes zoster	d.
		Skin desensitized to pain or pressure	e.
		Skin tears or cuts (other than surgery)	f.
		Surgical wounds	g. ✓
		NONE OF ABOVE	h.
5.	SKIN TREATMENTS	(***Check all that apply during last 7 days***)	
		Pressure relieving device(s) for chair	a. ✓
		Pressure relieving device(s) for bed	b. ✓
		Turning/repositioning program	c. ✓
		Nutrition or hydration intervention to manage skin problems	d.
		Ulcer care	e.
		Surgical wound care	f. ✓
		Application of dressings (with or without topical medications) other than to feet	g.
		Application of ointments/medications (other than to feet)	h.
		Other preventative or protective skin care (other than to feet)	i. ✓
		NONE OF ABOVE	j.
6.	FOOT PROBLEMS AND CARE	(***Check all that apply during last 7 days***)	
		Resident has one or more foot problems—e.g., corns, callouses, bunions, hammer toes, overlapping toes, pain, structural problems	a. ✓
		Infection of the foot—e.g., cellulitis, purulent drainage	b.
		Open lesions on the foot	c.
		Nails/calluses trimmed during **last 90 days**	d. ✓
		Received preventative or protective foot care (e.g., used special shoes, inserts, pads, toe separators)	e. ✓
		Application of dressings (with or without topical medications)	f.
		NONE OF ABOVE	g.

SECTION N. ACTIVITY PURSUIT PATTERNS

1.	TIME AWAKE	(***Check appropriate time periods over last 7 days***) Resident awake all or most of time (i.e., naps no more than one hour per time period) in the:	
		Morning	a.
		Afternoon	b. ✓
		Evening	c. ✓
		NONE OF ABOVE	d.
		(If resident is comatose, skip to Section O)	
2.	AVERAGE TIME INVOLVED IN ACTIVITIES	**(When awake and not receiving treatments or ADL care)** 0. Most—more than 2/3 of time 1. Some—from 1/3 to 2/3 of time 2. Little—less than 1/3 of time 3. None	2
3.	PREFERRED ACTIVITY SETTINGS	(***Check all settings** in which activities are preferred*)	
		Own room	a. ✓
		Day/activity room	b. ✓
		Inside NH/off unit	c.
		Outside facility	d.
		NONE OF ABOVE	e.
4.	GENERAL ACTIVITY PREFERENCES (adapted to resident's current abilities)	(***Check all PREFERENCES** whether or not activity is currently available to resident*)	
		Cards/other games	a.
		Crafts/arts	b. ✓
		Exercise/sports	c.
		Music	d. ✓
		Reading/writing	e.
		Spiritual/religious activities	f.
		Trips/shopping	g.
		Walking/wheeling outdoors	h. ✓
		Watching TV	i.
		Gardening or plants	j.
		Talking or conversing	k.
		Helping others	l.
		NONE OF ABOVE	m.

Resident MR. S. Numeric Identifier 17349

5.	PREFERS CHANGE IN DAILY ROUTINE	Code for resident preferences in daily routines 0. No change 1. Slight change 2. Major change	
		a. Type of activities in which resident is currently involved	0
		b. Extent of resident involvement in activities	0

SECTION O. MEDICATIONS

1.	NUMBER OF MEDICATIONS	(Record the number of different medications used in the last 7 days; enter "0" if none used)	03
2.	NEW MEDICATIONS	(Resident currently receiving medications that were initiated during the last 90 days) 0. No 1. Yes	1
3.	INJECTIONS	(Record the number of DAYS injections of any type received during the last 7 days; enter "0" if none used)	0
4.	DAYS RECEIVED THE FOLLOWING MEDICATION	(Record the number of DAYS during last 7 days; enter "0" if not used. Note—enter "1" for long-acting meds used less than weekly) a. Antipsychotic 7 b. Antianxiety 0 c. Antidepressant 0 d. Hypnotic 0 e. Diuretic 0	

SECTION P. SPECIAL TREATMENTS AND PROCEDURES

1.	SPECIAL TREATMENTS, PROCEDURES, AND PROGRAMS	a. SPECIAL CARE—Check treatments or programs received during the last 14 days	
		TREATMENTS	
		Chemotherapy	a.
		Dialysis	b.
		IV medication	c.
		Intake/output	d. ✓
		Monitoring acute medical condition	e. ✓
		Ostomy care	f.
		Oxygen therapy	g.
		Radiation	h.
		Suctioning	i.
		Tracheostomy care	j.
		Transfusions	k.
		Ventilator or respirator	l.
		PROGRAMS	
		Alcohol/drug treatment program	m.
		Alzheimer's/dementia special care unit	n.
		Hospice care	o.
		Pediatric unit	p.
		Respite care	q.
		Training in skills required to return to the community (e.g., taking medications, house work, shopping, transportation, ADLs)	r. ✓
		NONE OF ABOVE	s.

b. THERAPIES - Record the number of days and total minutes each of the following therapies was administered (for at least 15 minutes a day) in the last 7 calendar days (Enter 0 if none or less than 15 min. daily)
[Note—count only post admission therapies]
(A) = # of days administered for 15 minutes or more
(B) = total # of minutes provided in last 7 days

	DAYS (A)	MIN (B)
a. Speech - language pathology and audiology services	0	0
b. Occupational therapy	2	30
c. Physical therapy	4	60
d. Respiratory therapy	0	0
e. Psychological therapy (by any licensed mental health professional)	0	0

2.	INTERVENTION PROGRAMS FOR MOOD, BEHAVIOR, COGNITIVE LOSS	(Check all interventions or strategies used in last 7 days—no matter where received)	
		Special behavior symptom evaluation program	a. ✓
		Evaluation by a licensed mental health specialist in last 90 days	b. ✓
		Group therapy	c.
		Resident-specific deliberate changes in the environment to address mood/behavior patterns—e.g., providing bureau in which to rummage	d. ✓
		Reorientation—e.g., cueing	e. ✓
		NONE OF ABOVE	f.

3. NURSING REHABILITATION/RESTORATIVE CARE — Record the NUMBER OF DAYS each of the following rehabilitation or restorative techniques or practices was provided to the resident for more than or equal to 15 minutes per day in the last 7 days (Enter 0 if none or less than 15 min. daily.)

a. Range of motion (passive)	0	f. Walking	7
b. Range of motion (active)	7	g. Dressing or grooming	4
c. Splint or brace assistance	0	h. Eating or swallowing	0
TRAINING AND SKILL PRACTICE IN:		i. Amputation/prosthesis care	0
d. Bed mobility	3	j. Communication	0
e. Transfer	7	k. Other	0

4.	DEVICES AND RESTRAINTS	(Use the following codes for last 7 days:) 0. Not used 1. Used less than daily 2. Used daily	
		Bed rails	
		a. — Full bed rails on all open sides of bed	0
		b. — Other types of side rails used (e.g., half rail, one side)	2
		c. Trunk restraint	0
		d. Limb restraint	0
		e. Chair prevents rising	0
5.	HOSPITAL STAY(S)	Record number of times resident was admitted to hospital with an overnight stay in last 90 days (or since last assessment if less than 90 days). (Enter 0 if no hospital admissions)	01
6.	EMERGENCY ROOM (ER) VISIT(S)	Record number of times resident visited ER without an overnight stay in last 90 days (or since last assessment if less than 90 days). (Enter 0 if no ER visits)	00
7.	PHYSICIAN VISITS	In the LAST 14 DAYS (or since admission if less than 14 days in facility) how many days has the physician (or authorized assistant or practitioner) examined the resident? (Enter 0 if none)	02
8.	PHYSICIAN ORDERS	In the LAST 14 DAYS (or since admission if less than 14 days in facility) how many days has the physician (or authorized assistant or practitioner) changed the resident's orders? Do not include order renewals without change. (Enter 0 if none)	02
9.	ABNORMAL LAB VALUES	Has the resident had any abnormal lab values during the last 90 days (or since admission)? 0. No 1. Yes	1

SECTION Q. DISCHARGE POTENTIAL AND OVERALL STATUS

1.	DISCHARGE POTENTIAL	a. Resident expresses/indicates preference to return to the community 0. No 1. Yes	1
		b. Resident has a support person who is positive towards discharge 0. No 1. Yes	1
		c. Stay projected to be of a short duration— discharge projected within 90 days (do not include expected discharge due to death) 0. No 2. Within 31-90 days 1. Within 30 days 3. Discharge status uncertain	1
2.	OVERALL CHANGE IN CARE NEEDS	Resident's overall self sufficiency has changed significantly as compared to status of 90 days ago (or since last assessment if less than 90 days) 0. No change 1. Improved—receives fewer supports, needs less restrictive level of care 2. Deteriorated—receives more support	2

SECTION R. ASSESSMENT INFORMATION

1.	PARTICIPATION IN ASSESSMENT	a. Resident: 0. No 1. Yes	1
		b. Family: 0. No 1. Yes 2. No family	1
		c. Significant other: 0. No 1. Yes 2. None	0

2. SIGNATURES OF PERSONS COMPLETING THE ASSESSMENT:

Katie Phillips, R.N.

a. Signature of RN Assessment Coordinator (sign on above line)

b. Date RN Assessment Coordinator signed as complete: 09 (Month) – 04 (Day) – 1995 (Year)

	Other Signatures	Title	Sections	Date
c.	B. Godbout	RN	B,G,I,J,O,P	9/2/95
d.	P. Arbuthnof	LPN	D,H,L,M	9/2/95
e.	R. Ross	RD	K	9/3/95
f.	J. Amirani	ACSW	A,E,F,Q	9/4/95
g.	D. Wilcox	Activity Director	N	9/4/95
h.	D. Oatway	Speech Pathologist	C	9/4/95

3. FURTHER ASSESSMENT USING RAP GUIDELINES

The RAP review and assessment process provides a time for staff to think about and discuss key areas of concern related to the resident. There are many ways to structure this assessment process, e.g. who leads the discussion or assessment, who participates, and how the resident, family and physician are involved. But in each case, staff should:

- Discuss the triggered problems and any current treatment goals and related approaches to care.
- Identify the key causal factors (i.e., why the problem is present).
- Review the associated and confounding factors referenced in the RAP Guidelines (i.e., things that contribute to the problem or add to the complexity of the situation).
- Ensure that information regarding the resident's status and clinical decision-making is documented, and that the RAP Summary form identifies where this documentation can be found.
- Proceed to Care Planning.

The following RAP Summary form indicates which RAPs were triggered for Mr. S., where documentation can be found, and whether a care plan has been developed. Before turning to the RAP Summary form, you may wish to review the MDS to determine which RAPs should be triggered. Using Delirium as an example, the following are examples of how staff might proceed.

1. As shown here, the Delirium RAP was used throughout the initial assessment period. It was clear from admission that Mr. S. had acute confusion. Predictably the Delirium RAP was triggered. Staff documentation throughout the first weeks of residency capture the key elements of the Delirium RAP assessment. The location and date of this documentation is entered on the RAP Summary form. The decision to care plan is indicated. As key information is clearly documented in this example and readily accessible to all staff, there is no additional documentation required beyond the RAP Summary form and referenced notations and care plan.

2. In some cases, a staff person may want to write a summary of the RAP assessment. This could be for several reasons: e.g., while the assessment documentation is in the record it is incomplete, unclear, too scattered or not focused. It may also be useful to have the information summarized for quick reference by staff. If this is the case, the summary note for Delirium could look like this:

SECTION V. RESIDENT ASSESSMENT PROTOCOL SUMMARY

Numeric Identifier 17349

Resident's Name: Mr. S	Medical Record No.: 2QT2B28

1. Check if RAP is triggered.
2. For each triggered RAP, use the RAP guidelines to identify areas needing further assessment. Document relevant assessment information regarding the resident's status.
   - Describe:
     - — Nature of the condition (may include presence or lack of objective data and subjective complaints).
     - — Complications and risk factors that affect your decision to proceed to care planning.
     - — Factors that must be considered in developing individualized care plan interventions.
     - — Need for referrals/further evaluation by appropriate health professionals.
   - Documentation should support your decision-making regarding whether to proceed with a care plan for a triggered RAP and the type(s) of care plan interventions that are appropriate for a particular resident.
   - Documentation may appear anywhere in the clinical record (e.g., progress notes, consults, flowsheets, etc.).
3. Indicate under the Location of RAP Assessment Documentation column where information related to the RAP assessment can be found.
4. For each triggered RAP, indicate whether a new care plan, care plan revision, or continuation of current care plan is necessary to address the problem(s) identified in your assessment. The Care Planning Decision column must be completed within 7 days of completing the RAI (MDS and RAPs).

A. RAP PROBLEM AREA	(a) Check if triggered	Location and Date of RAP Assessment Documentation	(b) Care Planning Decision—check if addressed in care plan
1. DELIRIUM	✓	Nsg note: 8/24/95 MD note: 8/25/95, Nsg note: 8/28/95	✓
2. COGNITIVE LOSS	✓	MD note: 8/25/95, Nursing note: 8/28/95	✓
3. VISUAL FUNCTION			
4. COMMUNICATION	✓	Nursing note: 8/25/95	✓
5. ADL FUNCTIONAL/ REHABILITATION POTENTIAL	✓	OT note: 8/28/95, 9/1/95	✓
6. URINARY INCONTINENCE AND INDWELLING CATHETER	✓	MD note: 8/25/95; Nsg note: 8/24/95; 8/28/95	✓
7. PSYCHOSOCIAL WELL-BEING			
8. MOOD STATE	✓	Social service note: 8/24/95	✓
9. BEHAVIORAL SYMPTOMS			
10. ACTIVITIES	✓	RAP Summary note, 9/6/95	✓
11. FALLS	✓	Nursing note: 8/24/95, PT note: 8/28/95	✓
12. NUTRITIONAL STATUS			
13. FEEDING TUBES			
14. DEHYDRATION/FLUID MAINTENANCE	✓	I+O 8/24/95 - 9/2/95, Nsg note: 8/28/95, MD note: 8/25/95	✓
15. DENTAL CARE			
16. PRESSURE ULCERS	✓	RAP Summary note: 9/5/95	✓
17. PSYCHOTROPIC DRUG USE	✓	MD note: 8/25/95 med kardex	✓
18. PHYSICAL RESTRAINTS			

B. K. Phillips, RN
1. Signature of RN Coordinator for RAP Assessment Process

2. 09 – 06 – 1995 (Month – Day – Year)

S. Honemaker, RN
3. Signature of Person Completing Care Planning Decision

4. 09 – 13 – 1995 (Month – Day – Year)

Delirium: RAP Summary Example 1

Mr. S. admitted from hospital with diagnosis of acute confusion. Since admission his cognition has steadily cleared. Indicators of delirium, such as being easily distracted, having altered perception or awareness of surroundings, and restlessness have lessened, but are not completely gone. Mr. S. has a history of Alzheimer's Disease, family have been very helpful in describing his baseline mentation. The team believes that delirium is related to his UTI, relocation, Haldol, Morphine, Zantac, and dehydration. To this end, his Haldol is being tapered with the goal of elimination (he was not on this drug prior to hospitalization), Morphine and Zantac have been discontinued, UTI has been treated with Bactrim DS - a follow up U/A C+S will be sent upon completion, I/O is being monitored and fluids being encouraged, and the family has been helping us simulate a homelike environment with Mr. S.'s possessions and routine.

Another example could look like this:

Delirium: RAP Summary Example 2

Mr. S. triggered for delirium. RAP was used as a guideline for assessment by team. (See nursing notes: 8/24/95, 8/28/95, MD note 8/25). Possible causal factors: UTI, Medication, Dehydration, Relocation have been identified and treatment plans are indicated. Refer to Delirium care plan.

4. CARE PLAN SPECIFICATION

The following is an example care plan for Delirium. It contains general points, rather than specific prescriptions. It is meant to show general culmination of the assessment process in the plan of care.

Objective	Intervention	Evaluation
Mr. S. will remain safe and have no injuries in next 30 days	Keep night light on in room at night. Have family bring in familiar articles (bedspread, pictures). 15 minute checks while in room, encourage out of room activities. Involve in low stimulus activities. Keep pathways clear and free from clutter. Toilet q 2 hours while awake and q 4 hours during night. Offer frequent snacks including beverages.	Resident remained safe in last 30 days, with no evidence of injury.

Mr. S.'s cognitive function will return to baseline[4] in 30 days	Taper Haldol as ordered. Continue to review all medications with physician. Assess for adequate hydration by monitoring daily fluid intake. Review requested notes from Adult Day Care to gain further insight into baseline. Continue with Tylenol for pain, give PRN dose before Physical Therapy and if resident appears agitated or withdrawn.	Resident's cognitive functioning appears similar to baseline [4] according to: family, documentation from Adult Day Care and cognitive clinic at hospital. Resident received Tylenol as ordered, and did not appear to be in pain.
Mr. S. and family will be acclimated to the unit in 30 days as evidenced by recognizing his own room and participating in unit activities with minimal supervision	Primary team to meet with family to work on care plan and tour unit. Involve family in all aspects of care. Assess family's level of knowledge about Alzheimer's disease and acute confusion. Reorient Mr. S. to his room and surrounding unit. As acute confusion begins to clear, involve Mr. S. in more of unit activities.	Family met with primary care team and toured the unit. Mr. S. is able to recognize his room and attend unit activities with a staff prompt.
Resident will maintain adequate nutrition and hydration over next 30 days as evidenced by eating at least 3/4 of his meals and drinking 2 liters of fluid each day	See urinary incontinence care plan. Carefully assess fluid intake from meal trays. Offer supplemental fluids in between meals. Involve family in determining the best fluids, Mr. S likes chocolate milk and apple juice. Review monitored intake and output sheets from last 7 days. Continue if intake is not at least 2000 ml/day. Monitor skin turgor and mucous membranes.	Mr. S.'s intake was at least 2000. Resident received supplemental beverages in between meal. Skin turgor is intact and mucous membranes are moist.

[4] Assumes description of baseline is documented elsewhere in the clinical record.

CHAPTER 5: LINKING ASSESSMENT TO INDIVIDUALIZED CARE PLANS

Assessment (MDS/other) → Decision-making (RAPs/other) → Care Plan Development → Care Plan Implementation → Evaluation

5.1 Overview of the RAI and Care Planning

Throughout this manual the concept of linkages has been stressed. That is, good assessment forms the basis for a solid care plan, and the RAPs serve as the link between the MDS and care planning.

This chapter provides a discussion of how the care plan is driven not only by identified resident problems, but also by a resident's unique characteristics, strengths and needs. When the care plan is implemented in accordance with standards of good clinical practice, then the care plan becomes powerful, practical and represents the best approach to providing for the quality of care and quality of life needs of an individual resident.

The process of care planning is one of looking at a resident as a whole, building on the individual resident characteristics measured using standardized MDS items and definitions. The MDS was designed to allow the interdisciplinary team to observe and evaluate the resident's status with these detailed, consistently applied definitions. Once the separate items in the MDS have been reviewed, the RAP process provides guidance to the staff on how to use this information to assess triggered problems and ultimately to arrive at a holistic view of the person.

Once the resident has been assessed using triggered RAPs, the opportunity for development or modification of the care plan exists. The triggering of a RAP indicates the need for further review which is carried out utilizing the Guidelines that have been developed for each RAP. Staff use RAP Guidelines to determine whether a new care plan is needed or changes are needed in a resident's existing care plan. It is important to remember that even though a RAP may not have been "triggered" in the assessment process, the interdisciplinary team must address, in the care plan, a resident problem in that area if clinically warranted. **(See Chapter 4 for additional information on the use and documentation of RAPs.)**

The care-planning process in long term care facilities has been the subject of countless books, journal articles, conferences and discussions. Often this discussion has focused more on the structure or content of care plans than on the course of action needed to attain or maintain a resident's highest practicable level of well-being. It is not the intent of this chapter to specify a care plan structure or format. Rather the intent is to reinforce that the care plan is based on using fundamental information gathered by the MDS, further review and assessment "triggered" by the MDS, and distillation of all final assessment information, through the RAP Guidelines, into an appropriate blueprint for meeting the needs of the individual resident. An appropriate care plan results from analysis of the resident by the interdisciplinary team based on communication about the resident that is reliable, consistent and understood by all team members. This benefits the resident by ensuring that the entire interdisciplinary team and all "hands on" caregivers are following the same process based upon a common knowledge base.

Properly executed, the assessment and care planning processes flow together into a seamless circular process that:

- Looks at each resident as a "whole" human being with unique characteristics and strengths.
- Breaks the resident into distinct functional areas for the purpose of gaining knowledge about the resident's functional status (MDS).
- Re-groups the information gathered to identify possible problems the resident may have (Triggers).
- Provides additional assessment of potential problems by looking at possible causes and risks, and how these causes and risks can be addressed to provide for a resident's highest practicable level of well-being (RAP Guidelines).
- Develops and implements an interdisciplinary care plan based on the complete assessment information gathered by the RAI process, with necessary monitoring and follow-up.
- Re-evaluates the resident's status at prescribed intervals (i.e., quarterly, annually, or if a significant change in status occurs) using the RAI and then modifies the resident's care plan as appropriate and necessary.

Care planning is a process that has several steps that may occur at the same time or in sequence. The following list of care planning components may help the interdisciplinary team finalize the care plan after completing the comprehensive assessment:

1. The RAI process (i.e., MDS and RAPs) is completed as the basis for care plan decision-making. By regulation, this process may be completed solely by the RN Coordinator, but ideally the RAI is completed as a cohesive effort by the members of the interdisciplinary team that will develop the resident's care plan.

2. The team may find during their discussions that several problem conditions have a related cause but appear as one problem for the resident. They may also find that they stand alone and are unique. Goals and approaches for each problem condition may be overlapping, and consequently the interdisciplinary team may decide to address the problem conditions in combination on the care plan.

3. After using RAP Guidelines to assess the resident, staff may decide that a "triggered" condition does not affect the resident's functioning or well-being and therefore should not be addressed on the care plan.

4. The existence of a care planning issue (i.e., a resident problem, need or strength) should be documented as part of the RAP review documentation. Documentation may be done by individual staff members who have completed assessments using the RAP Guidelines or who participated in care planning, or as a joint note by members of the interdisciplinary team.

5. The resident, family or resident representative should be part of the team discussion or join the care planning process whenever they choose. The individual team members may have already discussed preliminary care plan ideas with the resident, family or resident representative in order to get suggestions, confirm agreement, or clarify reasons for developing specific goals and approaches.

6. In some cases a resident may refuse particular services or treatments that the interdisciplinary team believes may assist the resident to meet their highest practicable level of well-being. The resident's wishes should be documented in the clinical record.

7. When the interdisciplinary team has identified problems, conditions, limitations, maintenance levels or improvement possibilities, etc., they should be stated, to the extent possible, in functional or behavioral terms (e.g., how is the condition a problem for the resident; how does the condition limit or jeopardize the resident's ability to complete the tasks of daily life or affect the resident's well-being in some way).

EXAMPLES

- Mr. Smith cannot find his room independently.
- Mrs. Jones slaps at the faces of direct care staff while they are giving personal care.
- Mr. Brown is unable to walk more than 15 feet because of shortness of breath.

8. The interdisciplinary team agrees on intermediate goal(s) that will lead to an outcome objective.

9. The intermediate goal(s) should be measurable and have a time frame for completion or evaluation.

10. The parts of the goal statement should include:

    The **Subject** — the **Verb** — **Modifiers** — the **Time frame**.

EXAMPLE

Subject	Verb	Modifiers		Time frame
Mr. Jones	will walk	up and down 5 stairs	with the help of one nursing assistant	daily for the next 30 days.

11. Depending upon the conclusions of the assessment, types of goals may include improvement goals, prevention goals, palliative goals or maintenance goals.

12. Specific, individualized steps or approaches that staff will take to assist the resident to achieve the goal(s) will be identified. These approaches serve as instructions for resident care and provide for continuity of care by all staff. Short and concise instructions, which can be understood by all staff, should be written.

13. The final care plan should be discussed with the resident or the resident's representative.

14. The goals and their accompanying approaches are to be communicated to all direct care staff who were not directly involved in the development of the care plan.

15. The effectiveness of the care plan must be evaluated from its initiation and modified as necessary.

16. Changes to the care plan should occur as needed in accordance with professional standards of practice and documentation (e.g., signing and dating entries to the care plan). Communication about care plan changes should be ongoing among interdisciplinary team members.

5.2 The Care-Planning Process

In order to provide a backdrop for understanding care planning, how it is supported by the RAI process, and what is required by the regulations, this section has been organized around a **Question and Answer** format based on the interpretive guideline probes for the care planning requirements at 42 CFR 483.20. The appropriate **F Tags** have been added to the end of each question to guide the reader back to the regulation. The regulatory language and associated probes may be found in **Appendix P** of the State Operations Manual (SOM).

42 CFR 483.20 (d)(1)

Is the care plan oriented toward preventing avoidable declines in functioning or functional levels? - F 279

The care plan is a guide for all staff to ensure that decline is avoided, if possible. Not only is the resolution of clinical problems important (e.g., treatment of a pressure ulcer), so is the prevention of further decline. For example, for the resident with pressure ulcers, a program of bed mobility as well as efforts at improving the resident's mood to increase willingness to get out of bed, will improve chances for slowing decline. There must be a realistic, directed effort to provide quality care in addressing immediate concerns while, at the same time, attempting to ensure that functional decline does not occur. This is "proactive" involvement by the interdisciplinary team to make sure that declines in resident functioning are avoided if possible.

How does the care plan attempt to manage risk factors? - F 279

The RAPs are excellent identifiers of resident factors that may increase the chance of decline or for a problem to develop. Risk factors must not be overlooked when designing an effective care plan. Through the RAP review, the interdisciplinary team can identify certain resident characteristics that put the resident at risk for problems. For example, a resident may suddenly become at risk for falls when a change is made to certain medications. The team should identify this potential risk and identify the necessary precautions as part of the care plan (e.g. orthostatic blood pressure checks for a period of time).

Does the care plan build on resident strengths? - F 279

Care planning is usually thought of as a facility staff effort to solve or eliminate resident problems. While this view is often valid, it is also important for the interdisciplinary team to carefully look at the resident's strengths and use them to prevent decline or improve the resident's functional status. The RAI process not only identifies concerns but also pinpoints areas of resident vitality. These strengths or areas of vitality should be used in the care planning process to improve resident quality of care and quality of life through improved functional ability and self-esteem.

Does the care plan reflect standards of current professional practice? - F 279

It is important for all facility staff to be aware of and utilize current standards of professional practice. This can be accomplished through a routine, up-to-date in-house training program or through the use of qualified external training resources. New and more effective treatment modalities, resident activities, etc. are continually being identified which will benefit residents if built into their care plans.

Do treatment objectives have measurable outcomes? - F 279

Measurable outcomes require current knowledge about the resident to establish a baseline (e.g. how many times does a resident behavior or symptom occur in a certain time frame or how does a resident experience pain). Next, a target, goal or outcome is required (e.g., reduction of behaviors to a certain level or reduction of pain). Finally, some way of measuring if the care plan has moved the resident from the baseline to the target outcome is needed. Without measurable outcomes there is no way to truly identify that a care plan has been successful. The care plan is a dynamic document that needs to be continually evaluated and appropriately modified based on measurable outcomes. This continual evaluation takes into consideration resident change relative to the initial baseline—in other words, if the resident has declined, stayed the same, or improved at a lesser rate than expected, then a modification in the care plan may be necessary.

Has information regarding the resident's goals and wishes for treatment been obtained — especially if a resident wishes to refuse treatment? Has the resident been given sufficient information about his or her treatment so that an informed choice can be made? - F 279

Residents should, if possible, be involved in planning their treatment. This means that staff must talk to the resident about what goals the resident would like to achieve and whether they believe these goals can be achieved. Residents also have a right to refuse treatment. The interdisciplinary team should ensure that the resident has all of the necessary information about how a particular treatment will affect the care they receive and their general well-being so that the resident can make an informed choice about whether or not they wish to receive treatment.

If a resident refuses treatment, does the care plan reflect the facility's efforts to find alternative means to address the problem? - F 279

If a resident refuses treatment, the team should seek options with the help of the attending physician, resident and family. Often one method of treatment may not be acceptable to a resident, but another choice of treatment may. For example, a resident may refuse to take a prescribed anti-depressant medication for treatment of depression. Alternative courses of action could be explored with the resident that would use the expertise of mental health professionals. Consequently, rather than a care plan which indicates only that a resident refused treatment, the care plan would reflect other goals and methods of addressing the problem(s). Involve staff who have regular, first hand knowledge of the resident (e.g., nursing or activity assistants) in reviewing possible options. They can provide insights on why the resident may be refusing care and how to devise a better approach to the problem.

<u>42 CFR 483.20 (d)(2)</u>

Was interdisciplinary expertise utilized to develop a care plan to improve a resident's functional abilities? - F 280

It is of the utmost importance that the staff most knowledgeable about the resident, in coordination with staff having the most expertise in a given resident problem area, work with the resident and ~~their~~ family or other representative in the care planning process.

The medical model of care, while most common in the acute care setting, should not necessarily be the driving force in planning the resident's care unless the resident's medical condition is unstable and needs continuous clinical monitoring. The key is to identify those needs which affect the resident's day-to-day well-being. Such needs cover a broad range of areas and may vary among residents.

Although nursing staff are usually the "first responders" to resident problems and are responsible for the heaviest burden of documentation, each member of the interdisciplinary team brings a unique perspective and body of knowledge to the care planning process. As such, each members' contribution should be sought and valued.

In what ways do staff involve residents, families, and other resident representatives in care planning? - F 280

As emphasized in the Federal regulations as well as throughout this manual, the resident, resident's family or other resident representatives should be involved in the care planning process. The resident is the most appropriate individual to describe what is meaningful in his or her life. Family and friends may also contribute in a very meaningful way in describing what is important to a resident, especially for those residents who cannot speak for themselves. Although they may be knowledgeable about the resident and care practices, interdisciplinary team members do not know all of a resident's life history and experience which may affect his or her individual needs or dictate approaches.

It is important for the interdisciplinary team members to speak directly with the resident and the resident's family, friends and representatives during both the assessment and care planning process if an appropriate care plan is to be developed which will address all of the resident's individual quality of life and quality of care needs. If there is a legally designated proxy, staff should be aware of this fact and that individual should be given the opportunity to participate in the assessment and care planning process.

Is there evidence of assessment and care planning sufficient to meet the needs of newly admitted residents, prior to the completion of the first comprehensive assessment? - F 282

Some care planning needs to occur for immediate care of the resident after admission or after a significant change in status. Physician orders for immediate care (42 CFR 483.20 (a)/F 271) are the written orders facility staff need in order to provide essential care to the resident, consistent with the resident's physical and mental status at admission. These orders, at a minimum, should include dietary, medication (if necessary) and routine care instructions to maintain or improve the resident's functional abilities until facility staff can conduct a comprehensive resident assessment and develop an interdisciplinary care plan.

The interdisciplinary team may wish to conduct an initial RAP review for any identified problem or potential problem even before the MDS is completed. This review can be documented at the time, and a written update completed when the interdisciplinary team completes the RAI process and documents final care plan decisions.

For example, if a resident was re-admitted from the hospital with a physical restraint but the resident was not previously restrained, the interdisciplinary team should immediately assess the resident for the need for a restraint. Since the team would know that the Physical Restraint RAP would be triggered by the MDS, they would use the RAP to guide their assessment of the resident and make preliminary plans about how to handle the restraint issue. When the comprehensive assessment is completed, the interdisciplinary team would then make a final decision regarding the resident's current status and need for a restraint.

Similarly, if a resident is incontinent of urine at the first admission, or newly incontinent at re-admission, good practice would dictate that 14 days is too long to wait for completion of an initial assessment of the incontinence. Again, the Urinary Incontinence RAP can be used to guide the immediate care plan intervention. The documentation of the RAP review would then be updated following the completion of the comprehensive assessment.

Are direct care staff fully informed about the care, services and expected outcomes of the care they provide? Do direct care staff have general knowledge of the care and services provided by other staff and the relationship of those services to the resident's expected outcomes? - F 282

Direct care staff (e.g., nursing assistants, aides) must be directly involved in the care planning process. The importance of the communication between direct care staff and the interdisciplinary team cannot be overstated. Since direct care staff have the most frequent contact with residents, they may be the most knowledgeable about a resident's daily life, needs, problems and strengths.

Direct care staff who have not participated in the formal care plan decision-making process must be informed about how the care and services they provide is intended to improve, maintain or minimize decline in the resident's condition and well-being. Without knowing the reasons they are performing particular tasks, direct care staff may not understand the relationship between the care and services they provide for a resident and the expected outcomes for that resident. Similarly, for nursing staff to understand how the resident is responding to a plan of care, the input of direct care staff is crucial. In many ways, they are the best source of information on how the program has been implemented, how the resident has responded, and whether specific program variations might be useful.

What are some general care planning areas that could be considered in the Long Term Care setting? - F 280

The following are six general care planning areas that are useful in the long term care setting. This list is not prescriptive or all-inclusive. Ultimately the resident's status determines what should be addressed on the care plan.

<u>**Functional Status**</u>

Functional status limitations are identified using the MDS and triggers. All conditions determined to need care plan intervention, after using the RAPs to guide further assessment, must appear on the care plan. The conditions identified by the RAI should be clearly linked to the problems addressed on the care plan.

Rehabilitation/Restorative Nursing

A resident's potential for physical, occupational, speech, psychological and other types of rehabilitation needs to be assessed and care planned. The risk of immobility, for example, should be assessed, and restorative nursing interventions planned accordingly. Complications of immobility, such as damage to the muscular system as indicated by weakness, difficulty walking, posture problems, foot drop, contractures, edema, constipation, calcium depletion, depression, agitation, etc., should be assessed as appropriate. These assessments may include causes, particular risk factors, clinical impressions and the need for referrals.

Health Maintenance

Health maintenance includes monitoring of disease processes that are currently being treated. These would include both stable and unstable conditions that need monitoring such as a history of cardiac problems, hypertension, CHF, pain, dehydration, mental illness, etc. If a resident is taking medications for conditions, regular monitoring of edema, vital signs, blood glucose, etc., may be appropriate.

The interdisciplinary team may also decide whether or not to list problems on the care plan that no longer affect the resident, are controlled or need no monitoring. This will depend on the team's decision about how a given problem affects the resident's overall functioning or well-being.

Other areas of health maintenance may include terminal care, and special treatments such as peritoneal dialysis or ventilator support.

Discharge Potential

Discharge potential for each resident needs to be assessed at admission, annually, and as needed. The assessment for discharge potential should focus on what needs to happen before the resident can safely be discharged. If the resident has discharge potential or if discharge is actively being pursued, documentation should appear in the resident's plan of care.

Medications

On at least a yearly basis, a comprehensive assessment of drug therapy should be completed **(See 483.20 (b)(1)(2)(xiii))**. This assessment can be documented anywhere in the resident's record and should include dose, frequency, existing and most likely side effects, relevant lab results, parameter comparisons, and justifications for use. Pharmacists review the drug regimen and discuss irregularities with appropriate facilities staff using **Appendix N of the State Operations Manual** on a monthly basis.

It is the interdisciplinary team's decision whether medications need to be addressed in the care plan. For example, consideration might be given to recent changes in medications, the use of multiple medications, or medications which may put the resident in jeopardy for a decline in functional status. The care plan should alert the staff to medication side effects for which the resident is at particular risk. The interdisciplinary team may decide to identify a drug(s) as an approach to meeting a goal. The interdisciplinary team should determine if any medications that the resident is taking are listed in a triggered RAP. If so, use of the medication needs to be assessed as a potential contributing cause to the RAP concern.

Daily Care Needs

Some facilities put all resident daily care needs and standard practice approaches on the care plan. Daily care needs that are specific to the resident and are out of the ordinary must be addressed on the care plan. Facility staff must use their professional judgment when making these decisions.

APPENDIX A

STATE AGENCY CONTACTS RESPONSIBLE FOR ANSWERING RAI QUESTIONS

STATE AGENCY CONTACTS

Alabama
Ellen Mullins
Alabama Department of Public Health
Division Of Licensure and Certification
671 South Perry Street
Montgomery, AL 36104
(334) 240-3528

Alaska
Shellie Smith
Office of Health Facilities Cert. and Lic.
4730 Business Park Blvd, Ste. 18
Anchorage, AK 99503-7137
(907) 561-8081

Arizona
Ed Welsh
Office of Health Care Licensure
Department of Health Services
1647 E. Morten
Phoenix, AZ 85020
(602) 255-1177

Arkansas
Shirley Gamble, Director
Office of Long Term Care
P.O. Box 8050, Slot 400
Little Rock, AR 72203-8059
(501) 682-8486

California
Elissa Hinson
Department of Health Services, Licensure and Certification
1800 3rd Street, Suite 210
Sacramento, CA 95814
(916) 324-8627

Colorado
Diane Carter
Health Facilities Division
Colorado Department of Health
4300 Cherry Creek Drive South
Denver, CO 80222-1530
(303) 692-2833

Connecticut
Wendy Furniss, R.N.C., M.S.
Health Services Supervision, Certification
Hospital and Medical Care Division
Department of Public Health
150 Washington Street
Hartford, CT 06106
(203) 566-5758

Delaware
Jacquelyn Rohrbaugh
Office of Health Facilities Cert. and Lic.
3 Mill Road, Room 308
Wilmington, DE 19806
(302) 577-6666

District of Columbia
Judy McPherson
Service Facility Regulation Administration
Department of Consumer and Regulatory Affairs
614 H Street, NW
Tenth Floor
Washington, D.C. 20001
(202) 727-7200

Florida
Pat Hall
Office of Licensure and Certification
Department of Health and Rehabilitation Services
2727 Mahan Dr.
Tallahassee, FL 32308
(904) 487-3513

Georgia
Joyce Bridges
Office of Regulatory Services
Georgia Department of Human Resources
2 Peachtree St., NW 22nd Floor
Atlanta, Georgia 30303
(404) 656-5153

Hawaii
Karen Nishimura
Hospital and Medical Facilities Branch
Department of Health
P.O. Box 3378
Honolulu, HI 96801
(808) 586-4090

Idaho
Marie Ballard
Licensure and Certification
Department of Health and Welfare
P.O. Box 83720
Boise, ID 83720-0036
(208) 334-6626

Illinois
Donna Lounsberry R.N., Chief
Education and Training Section
State RAI Coordinator
Illinois Department of Public Health
Office of Health Care Regulation
525 W. Jefferson Street
Springfield, IL 62761
(217) 785-5132

Indiana
Lynn Carter, RAI Coordinator
Manager, Information Technology
Indiana State Department of Health
Long-Term Care
1330 West Michigan Street, P.O. Box 1964
Indianapolis, IN 46206-1964
(317) 383-6537

Iowa
Karen Mueller
Division of Health Facilities
Department of Inspections and Appeals
Lucas State Office Bldg., 3rd Floor
Des Moines, IA 50319
(515) 242-5991

Kansas
Patricia Maben
Director, Adult Care Home Program
Bureau of Adult and Child Care Facilities
Department of Health and Environment
Landon State Office Bldg., 10th Floor
900 Southwest Jackson
Topeka, KS 66612-1290
(913) 296-1246

Kentucky
Jenny Mitchell
Division Of Licensure and Regulation
Department of Human Resources
CHR Building, 4th Floor East
275 E. Main Street
Frankfort, KY 40601
(502) 564-2800

Louisiana
Barbara Anthony
Bureau of Health Standards
Office of Licensure and Certification
P.O. Box 3767
Baton Rouge, LA 70821
(504) 342-0138

Maine
Carole Kus
Case Mix Project
249 Western Ave.
State House--Station 11
Augusta, ME 04333
(207) 287-6482

Maryland
Fran Miller, Supervisor
Ed. and Training
Office of Licensure and Certification
Department of Health and Mental Hygiene
4th Floor Metro Executive Center
4201 Patterson Ave.
Baltimore, MD 21215
(410) 764-4970

Massachusetts
Mary Tess Crotty
Division of Health Care Quality
Department of Public Health
10 West Street, 5th Floor
Boston, MA 02111
(617) 727-5860 x395

Michigan
Cherie-Nan Jansen, RN, BSN, MPH
Staff Development Consultant
Program Development Section
Division of Licensing and Certification
3423 N. Martin Luther King Jr. Blvd.
P.O. Box 30195
Lansing, MI 48909
(517) 334-8470

Minnesota
Laurel Koster
Clinical Nurse Specialist, Licensing and Certification
Department of Health
393 N. Dunlap St.
P.O. Box 64900
St. Paul, MN 55164
(612) 643-2131

Mississippi
Sammy Rea
Department of Health, Division of Licensure and Certification
P.O. Box 1700
Jackson, MS 39215-1700
(601) 354-7300

Missouri
Betty Markway
Department of Social Services
Division of Aging
P.O. Box 1337
Jefferson City, MO 65102
(314)751-3082

Montana
Bobbie Sutherlin
Department of Public Health and Human Services
Health Facilities Program
PO Box 200901
Helena, MT 59620-0901
(406) 444-4749

Nebraska
Nancy Olson, Unit Manager,
Medical Services Division
Department of Social Services
301 Centennial Mall South, P.O. Box 95026
Lincoln, NE 68509-5026
(402) 471-9360

Nevada
Jennifer Dunaway
Bureau of Licensure and Certification
505 E. King Street, Room 202
Carson City, NV 89710
(702) 486-5061

New Hampshire
Carol Currier
Medicaid Agency
Office of Medical Services
6 Hazen Dr.
Concord, NH 03301-6521
(603) 271-4607

Judith Boska
Health Facilities Administration
Certification Coordinator
Office of Medical Services
6 Hazen Dr.
Concord, NH 03301-6521
(603) 271-4592

New Jersey
Anne Brodowski
Assistant Director
New Jersey State Health Department
CN 367
Trenton, NJ 08625-0367
(609) 588-7735

New Mexico
Matt Gervase
LTC Program Manager
525 Camino de los Marquez, Suite 2
P.O. Box 26110
Santa Fe, NM 87502-6110
(505) 827-4225

New York
Barbara Page, RNC, MA
Nursing Services Consultant
Bureau of LTC Services
1882 Corning Tower Building
Empire State Plaza
Albany, NY 12237-0732
(518) 474-2052

North Carolina
Cindy DePorter
Division of Facility Services
PO Box 29530
Raleigh, NC 27626-0530
(919) 733-7461

North Dakota
Darleen Bartz, Manager
Standards Development
North Dakota Department of Health
Division of Health Facilities
600 East Boulevard Ave.
Bismarck, ND 58505-0200
(701) 328-2352

Ohio
Nancy Whittenburg (Clinical Issues)
Asst. Chief, Bureau of HSQ
246 N. High Street
Columbus, OH 43215
(614) 752-9524

Sheila Lambowitz (Payment Issues)
Chief, Case Mix Section
Office of Medicaid
Bureau of Long Term Care Administration
30E. Broad Street, 33rd Floor
Columbus, OH 43266
(614) 466-1510

Oklahoma
Marietta Lynch
Licensing and Certification Division
Department of Health
P.O. Box 1299
Oklahoma City, OK 73117-1299
(405) 271-4085

Oregon
Linda Nickolisen
Albany Client Care Monitoring Unit
118 Second Avenue SE
Suite G.
Albany, Oregon 97321
(503) 967-2186

Pennsylvania
Marjorie K. Key
Room 528
Health and Welfare Building
Harrisburg, PA 17120
(717) 783-1927

Puerto Rico
Mirta Fernandez
Commonwealth of PR Department of Health
Assistant Secretariat for the Regulation and Accreditation of Health Facilities
Former Ruiz Soler Hospital
Bayamon, PR 00959
(809) 782-3395

Rhode Island
Gloria Roberto
Division of Facilities Regulation
Department of Health
3 Capitol Hill
Providence, RI 02908
(401) 277-2566

South Carolina
Sarah Granger
Bureau of Health Licensure and Certification
Department of Health and Environmental Control
2600 Bull St.
Columbia, SC 29201
(803) 737-7205

Janet D. Clayton
Department of Health and Human Services
P.O. Box 8206
1801 Main Street, 7th Floor
Columbis, SC 29202-8206
(803) 253-6182

South Dakota
Peggy E. Williams, Public Health Advisor
SD Department Of Health
445 E. Capitol
Pierre, SD 57501
(605) 773-3356

Carol Job, Case Mix Project Coordinator
SD Department of Social Services
700 Govenor's Drive
Pierre, SD 57501
(605) 773-3656

Texas
Shari Malloy
Utilization and Assessment Review
Texas Department of Human Services
P.O. Box 149030, Mail Code Y-919
Austin, TX 78714-9030
(512) 338-6493

Tennessee
Norma Miller
c/o Virginia Anderson
Health Care Facilities
Department of Health and Environment
283 Plus Park Blvd.
Nashville, TN 37217
(615) 367-6316

Utah
Carolyn Reese
Bureau of Facility Review
Patient Assessment Section
288 North 1460 West
P.O. Box 16990
Salt Lake City, UT 84116-0990
(801) 538-6599

Vermont
Laine Lucenti
Division of Licensure and Protection
Department of Rehabilitation and Aging
Ladd Hall
103 Main St.
Waterbury, VT 05671
(802) 241-2345

Virginia
Ann Adkins
Office of Health Facilities Regulation
3600 W. Broad Street
Richmond, VA 23230
(804) 367-2100

Washington
Marlene Black
Aging and Adult Services Admin.
Deparment of Social and Health Services
4413 Woodview Drive, SE, QG-16
Olympia, WA 98504
(360) 493-2573

West Virginia
Joan G. Armbruster, Coordinator
Nursing Home Services
Bureau for Medical Services
7012 MacCorkle Ave., SE
Charleston, West Virginia 25304
(304) 926-1712

Beverly Hissom
Office of Health Facility Licensure and Certification
Capitol Complex, Building 3
Charleston, West Virginia 25305
(304) 558-0050

Wisconsin
Billie March
Bureau of Quality Compliance
Department of Health and Social Services
1 West Wilson St., Room 150
Madison, WI 53701
(608) 266-7188

Wyoming
Marge Uelmen
Division of Preventive Medicine
Department of Health
First Bank Building, 8th Floor
2020 Carey Ave.
Cheyenne, WY 82002-0480
(307) 777-7121

REGIONAL OFFICE CONTACTS

Region I
Sharon Lounsbury
HCFA/DHSQ, Room 2275
JFK Federal Building
Boston, MA 02203-0003
(617) 565-1300

Region II
Margaret DiBari
HCFA/DHSQ
26 Federal Plaza, Room 3821
New York, NY 10278-0063
(212) 264-3496 x349

Region III
Gloria Speller
HCFA/DHSQ
P.O. Box 7760
Philadelphia, PA 19101-7760
(215) 596-4550

Region IV
Pat Bendert
HCFA/DHSQ
101 Marietta Tower, Ste. 601
Atlanta, GA 30323-2711
(404) 730-2723

Region V
Alice Fields (312) 353-2851 or,
Pauline Swalina (312) 353-2853 or,
Sally Wieling (312) 353-8853 at:
HCFA/DHSQ
105 W. Adams Street, 15th Floor
Chicago, IL 60603-6201

Region VI
Dan McElroy
HCFA/DHSQ
1200 Main Street, Ste. 1940
Dallas, TX 75202-4348
(214) 767-2077

Region VII
Mary Alice Futrell
HCFA/DHSQ
601 E. 12 Street, Room 242
New Federal Office Bldg.
Kansas City, MO 64106-2808
(816) 426-2011

Region VIII
Dottie Brinkmeyer
HCFA/DHSQ
Federal Office Bldg., Room 1185
1961 Stout St.
Denver, CO 80294-3538
(303) 844-4721 x435

Region IX
Mary Frances Colvin
HCFA/DHSQ
75 Hawthorne St., 4th Floor
San Francisco, CA 94105-3903
(415) 744-3693

Region X
Judy Ramberg
HCFA/DHSQ
Blanchard Plaza Bldg.
2201 Sixth Ave., Mail Stop RX-42
Seattle, WA 98121-2500
(206) 615-2321

APPENDIX B

MDS and QUARTERLY REVIEW FORMS FOR VERSION 2.0

Numeric Identifier________________

MINIMUM DATA SET (MDS) — *VERSION 2.0*

FOR NURSING HOME RESIDENT ASSESSMENT AND CARE SCREENING

BASIC ASSESSMENT TRACKING FORM

SECTION AA. IDENTIFICATION INFORMATION

1.	RESIDENT NAME⊙	a. (First) b. (Middle Initial) c. (Last) d. (Jr/Sr)
2.	GENDER⊙	1. Male 2. Female
3.	BIRTHDATE⊙	Month — Day — Year
4.	RACE/⊙ ETHNICITY	1. American Indian/Alaskan Native 2. Asian/Pacific Islander 3. Black, not of Hispanic origin 4. Hispanic 5. White, not of Hispanic origin
5.	SOCIAL SECURITY⊙ AND MEDICARE NUMBERS⊙ [C in 1st box if non med. no.]	a. Social Security Number b. Medicare number (or comparable railroad insurance number)
6.	FACILITY PROVIDER NO.⊙	a. State No. b. Federal No.
7.	MEDICAID NO. ["+" *if pending*, "N" *if not a Medicaid recipient*]⊙	
8.	REASONS FOR ASSESS-MENT	[Note—Other codes do not apply to this form] a. Primary reason for assessment 1. Admission assessment (required by day 14) 2. Annual assessment 3. Significant change in status assessment 4. Significant correction of prior assessment 5. Quarterly review assessment 0. *NONE OF ABOVE* *b. Special codes for use with supplemental assessment types in Case Mix demonstration states or other states where required* *1. 5 day assessment* *2. 30 day assessment* *3. 60 day assessment* *4. Quarterly assessment using full MDS form* *5. Readmission/return assessment* *6. Other state required assessment*
9.	SIGNATURES OF PERSONS COMPLETING THESE ITEMS:	

a. Signatures	Title	Date
b.		Date

GENERAL INSTRUCTIONS

Complete this information for submission with all full and quarterly assessments (Admission, Annual, Significant Change, State or Medicare required assessments, or Quarterly Reviews, etc.)

⊙ = Key items for computerized resident tracking

☐ = When box blank, must enter number or letter [a.] = When letter in box, check if condition applies

Resident ______________________ Numeric Identifier ______________________

MINIMUM DATA SET (MDS) — *VERSION 2.0*

FOR NURSING HOME RESIDENT ASSESSMENT AND CARE SCREENING

BACKGROUND (FACE SHEET) INFORMATION AT ADMISSION

SECTION AB. DEMOGRAPHIC INFORMATION

1.	DATE OF ENTRY	*Date the stay began. Note — Does not include readmission if record was closed at time of temporary discharge to hospital, etc. In such cases, use prior admission date* [ ][ ] — [ ][ ] — [ ][ ][ ][ ] Month Day Year
2.	ADMITTED FROM (AT ENTRY)	1. Private home/apt. with no home health services 2. Private home/apt. with home health services 3. Board and care/assisted living/group home 4. Nursing home 5. Acute care hospital 6. Psychiatric hospital, MR/DD facility 7. Rehabilitation hospital 8. Other
3.	LIVED ALONE (PRIOR TO ENTRY)	0. No 1. Yes 2. In other facility
4.	ZIP CODE OF PRIOR PRIMARY RESIDENCE	[ ][ ][ ][ ][ ]
5.	RESIDENTIAL HISTORY 5 YEARS PRIOR TO ENTRY	(***Check all settings** resident **lived in** during 5 years prior to date of entry given in item AB1 above)* Prior stay at this nursing home — a. Stay in other nursing home — b. Other residential facility—board and care home, assisted living, group home — c. MH/psychiatric setting — d. MR/DD setting — e. *NONE OF ABOVE* — f.
6.	LIFETIME OCCUPATION(S) [Put "/" between two occupations]	
7.	EDUCATION (*Highest Level Completed*)	1. No schooling 2. 8th grade/less 3. 9-11 grades 4. High school 5. Technical or trade school 6. Some college 7. Bachelor's degree 8. Graduate degree
8.	LANGUAGE	*(Code for correct response)* **a.** Primary Language 0. English 1. Spanish 2. French 3. Other **b. If other, specify**
9.	MENTAL HEALTH HISTORY	Does resident's RECORD indicate any history of mental retardation, mental illness, or developmental disability problem? 0. No 1. Yes
10.	CONDITIONS RELATED TO MR/DD STATUS	(***Check all conditions** that are related to MR/DD status that were manifested before age 22, and are likely to continue indefinitely)* Not applicable—no MR/DD (Skip to AB11) — a. MR/DD with organic condition Down's syndrome — b. Autism — c. Epilepsy — d. Other organic condition related to MR/DD — e. MR/DD with no organic condition — f.
11.	DATE BACKGROUND INFORMATION COMPLETED	[ ][ ] — [ ][ ] — [ ][ ][ ][ ] Month Day Year

SECTION AC. CUSTOMARY ROUTINE

1\. CUSTOMARY ROUTINE (*In year prior to DATE OF ENTRY to this nursing home, or year last in community if now being admitted from another nursing home*)

(***Check all that apply.** If all information UNKNOWN, check last box only.*)

CYCLE OF DAILY EVENTS	
Stays up late at night (e.g., after 9 pm)	a.
Naps regularly during day (at least 1 hour)	b.
Goes out 1+ days a week	c.
Stays busy with hobbies, reading, or fixed daily routine	d.
Spends most of time alone or watching TV	e.
Moves independently indoors (with appliances, if used)	f.
Use of tobacco products at least daily	g.
NONE OF ABOVE	h.
EATING PATTERNS	
Distinct food preferences	i.
Eats between meals all or most days	j.
Use of alcoholic beverage(s) at least weekly	k.
NONE OF ABOVE	l.
ADL PATTERNS	
In bedclothes much of day	m.
Wakens to toilet all or most nights	n.
Has irregular bowel movement pattern	o.
Showers for bathing	p.
Bathing in PM	q.
NONE OF ABOVE	r.
INVOLVEMENT PATTERNS	
Daily contact with relatives/close friends	s.
Usually attends church, temple, synagogue (etc.)	t.
Finds strength in faith	u.
Daily animal companion/presence	v.
Involved in group activities	w.
NONE OF ABOVE	x.
UNKNOWN—Resident/family unable to provide information	y.

END

SECTION AD. FACE SHEET SIGNATURES

SIGNATURES OF PERSONS COMPLETING FACE SHEET:

a. Signature of RN Assessment Coordinator			Date
b. Signatures	Title	Sections	Date
c.			Date
d.			Date
e.			Date
f.			Date
g.			Date

[ ] = When box blank, must enter number or letter [a.] = When letter in box, check if condition applies

MINIMUM DATA SET (MDS) — *VERSION 2.0*
FOR NURSING HOME RESIDENT ASSESSMENT AND CARE SCREENING
FULL ASSESSMENT FORM
(Status in last 7 days, unless other time frame indicated)

SECTION A. IDENTIFICATION AND BACKGROUND INFORMATION

1.	RESIDENT NAME	a. (First) b. (Middle Initial) c. (Last) d. (Jr/Sr)
2.	ROOM NUMBER	☐☐☐☐☐
3.	ASSESSMENT REFERENCE DATE	a. *Last day of MDS observation period* ☐☐—☐☐—☐☐☐☐ Month Day Year b. Original (0) or corrected copy of form (enter number of correction)
4a.	DATE OF REENTRY	**Date of reentry from most recent temporary discharge to a hospital in last 90 days (or since last assessment or admission if less than 90 days)** ☐☐—☐☐—☐☐☐☐ Month Day Year
5.	MARITAL STATUS	1. Never married 2. Married 3. Widowed 4. Separated 5. Divorced
6.	MEDICAL RECORD NO.	☐☐☐☐☐☐☐☐☐☐☐☐
7.	CURRENT PAYMENT SOURCES FOR N.H. STAY	(*Billing Office to indicate;* ***check all that apply in last 30 days***) Medicaid per diem a. Medicare per diem b. Medicare ancillary part A c. Medicare ancillary part B d. CHAMPUS per diem e. VA per diem f. Self or family pays for full per diem g. Medicaid resident liability or Medicare co-payment h. Private insurance per diem (including co-payment) i. Other per diem j.
8.	REASONS FOR ASSESSMENT (*Note—If this is a discharge or reentry assessment, only a limited subset of MDS items need be completed*)	a. Primary reason for assessment 1. Admission assessment (required by day 14) 2. Annual assessment 3. Significant change in status assessment 4. Significant correction of prior assessment 5. Quarterly review assessment 6. Discharged—return not anticipated 7. Discharged—return anticipated 8. Discharged prior to completing initial assessment 9. Reentry 0. *NONE OF ABOVE* b. ***Special codes for use with supplemental assessment types in Case Mix demonstration states or other states where required*** *1. 5 day assessment* *2. 30 day assessment* *3. 60 day assessment* *4. Quarterly assessment using full MDS form* *5. Readmission/return assessment* *6. Other state required assessment*
9.	RESPONSIBILITY/ LEGAL GUARDIAN	(***Check all that apply***) Legal guardian a. Other legal oversight b. Durable power of attorney/health care c. Durable power attorney/financial d. Family member responsible e. Patient responsible for self f. *NONE OF ABOVE* g.
10.	ADVANCED DIRECTIVES	(*For those items with supporting* ***documentation*** *in the medical record,* ***check all that apply***) Living will a. Do not resuscitate b. Do not hospitalize c. Organ donation d. Autopsy request e. Feeding restrictions f. Medication restrictions g. Other treatment restrictions h. *NONE OF ABOVE* i.

SECTION B. COGNITIVE PATTERNS

1.	COMATOSE	(*Persistent vegetative state/no discernible consciousness*) 0. No 1. Yes **(If yes, skip to Section G)**
2.	MEMORY	(*Recall of what was learned or known*) a. Short-term memory OK—seems/appears to recall after 5 minutes 0. Memory OK 1. Memory problem b. Long-term memory OK—seems/appears to recall long past 0. Memory OK 1. Memory problem
3.	MEMORY/ RECALL ABILITY	(***Check all that resident was normally able to recall during last 7 days***) Current season a. Location of own room b. Staff names/faces c. That he/she is in a nursing home d. *NONE OF ABOVE* are recalled e.
4.	COGNITIVE SKILLS FOR DAILY DECISION-MAKING	(*Made decisions regarding tasks of daily life*) 0. *INDEPENDENT*—decisions consistent/reasonable 1. *MODIFIED INDEPENDENCE*—some difficulty in new situations only 2. *MODERATELY IMPAIRED*—decisions poor; cues/supervision required 3. *SEVERELY IMPAIRED*—never/rarely made decisions
5.	INDICATORS OF DELIRIUM—PERIODIC DISORDERED THINKING/ AWARENESS	(*Code for behavior in the last 7 days.*) [***Note: Accurate assessment requires conversations with staff and family who have direct knowledge of resident's behavior over this time***]. 0. Behavior not present 1. Behavior present, not of recent onset 2. Behavior present, over last 7 days appears different from resident's usual functioning (e.g., new onset or worsening) a. EASILY DISTRACTED—(e.g., difficulty paying attention; gets sidetracked) b. PERIODS OF ALTERED PERCEPTION OR AWARENESS OF SURROUNDINGS—(e.g., moves lips or talks to someone not present; believes he/she is somewhere else; confuses night and day) c. EPISODES OF DISORGANIZED SPEECH—(e.g., speech is incoherent, nonsensical, irrelevant, or rambling from subject to subject; loses train of thought) d. PERIODS OF RESTLESSNESS—(e.g., fidgeting or picking at skin, clothing, napkins, etc; frequent position changes; repetitive physical movements or calling out) e. PERIODS OF LETHARGY—(e.g., sluggishness; staring into space; difficult to arouse; little body movement) f. MENTAL FUNCTION VARIES OVER THE COURSE OF THE DAY—(e.g., sometimes better, sometimes worse; behaviors sometimes present, sometimes not)
6.	CHANGE IN COGNITIVE STATUS	Resident's cognitive status, skills, or abilities have changed as compared to status of **90 days ago** (or since last assessment if less than 90 days) 0. No change 1. Improved 2. Deteriorated

SECTION C. COMMUNICATION/HEARING PATTERNS

1.	HEARING	(*With hearing appliance, if used*) 0. *HEARS ADEQUATELY*—normal talk, TV, phone 1. *MINIMAL DIFFICULTY* when not in quiet setting 2. *HEARS IN SPECIAL SITUATIONS ONLY*—speaker has to adjust tonal quality and speak distinctly 3. *HIGHLY IMPAIRED*/absence of useful hearing
2.	COMMUNICATION DEVICES/ TECHNIQUES	(***Check all that apply*** *during last 7 days*) Hearing aid, present and used a. Hearing aid, present and not used regularly b. Other receptive comm. techniques used (e.g., lip reading) c. *NONE OF ABOVE* d.
3.	MODES OF EXPRESSION	(***Check all used*** *by resident to make needs known*) Speech a. Writing messages to express or clarify needs b. American sign language or Braille c. Signs/gestures/sounds d. Communication board e. Other f. *NONE OF ABOVE* g.
4.	MAKING SELF UNDERSTOOD	(*Expressing information content—however able*) 0. *UNDERSTOOD* 1. *USUALLY UNDERSTOOD*—difficulty finding words or finishing thoughts 2. *SOMETIMES UNDERSTOOD*—ability is limited to making concrete requests 3. *RARELY/NEVER UNDERSTOOD*
5.	SPEECH CLARITY	(*Code for speech in the last 7 days*) 0. *CLEAR SPEECH*—distinct, intelligible words 1. *UNCLEAR SPEECH*—slurred, mumbled words 2. *NO SPEECH*—absence of spoken words
6.	ABILITY TO UNDERSTAND OTHERS	(*Understanding verbal information content—however able*) 0. *UNDERSTANDS* 1. *USUALLY UNDERSTANDS*—may miss some part/intent of message 2. *SOMETIMES UNDERSTANDS*—responds adequately to simple, direct communication 3. *RARELY/NEVER UNDERSTANDS*
7.	CHANGE IN COMMUNICATION/ HEARING	Resident's ability to express, understand, or hear information has changed as compared to status of **90 days ago** (or since last assessment if less than 90 days) 0. No change 1. Improved 2. Deteriorated

☐ = When box blank, must enter number or letter

a. = When letter in box, check if condition applies

SECTION D. VISION PATTERNS

1.	VISION	(*Ability to see in adequate light and with glasses if used*) 0. *ADEQUATE*—sees fine detail, including regular print in newspapers/books 1. *IMPAIRED*—sees large print, but not regular print in newspapers/books 2. *MODERATELY IMPAIRED*—limited vision; not able to see newspaper headlines, but can identify objects 3. *HIGHLY IMPAIRED*—object identification in question, but eyes appear to follow objects 4. *SEVERELY IMPAIRED*—no vision or sees only light, colors, or shapes; eyes do not appear to follow objects	
2.	VISUAL LIMITATIONS/ DIFFICULTIES	Side vision problems—decreased peripheral vision (e.g., leaves food on one side of tray, difficulty traveling, bumps into people and objects, misjudges placement of chair when seating self)	a.
		Experiences any of following: sees halos or rings around lights; sees flashes of light; sees "curtains" over eyes	b.
		NONE OF ABOVE	c.
3.	VISUAL APPLIANCES	Glasses; contact lenses; magnifying glass 0. No 1. Yes	

SECTION E. MOOD AND BEHAVIOR PATTERNS

1.	INDICATORS OF DEPRES-SION, ANXIETY, SAD MOOD	(***Code for indicators observed in last 30 days, irrespective of the assumed cause***) 0. Indicator not exhibited in last 30 days 1. Indicator of this type exhibited up to five days a week 2. Indicator of this type exhibited daily or almost daily (6, 7 days a week)	
		VERBAL EXPRESSIONS OF DISTRESS	
		a. Resident made negative statements—e.g., "*Nothing matters; Would rather be dead; What's the use; Regrets having lived so long; Let me die*"	
		b. Repetitive questions—e.g., "*Where do I go; What do I do?*"	
		c. Repetitive verbalizations—e.g., calling out for help, ("*God help me*")	
		d. Persistent anger with self or others—e.g., easily annoyed, anger at placement in nursing home; anger at care received	
		e. Self deprecation—e.g., "*I am nothing; I am of no use to anyone*"	
		f. Expressions of what appear to be unrealistic fears—e.g., fear of being abandoned, left alone, being with others	
		g. Recurrent statements that something terrible is about to happen—e.g., believes he or she is about to die, have a heart attack	
		h. Repetitive health complaints—e.g., persistently seeks medical attention, obsessive concern with body functions	
		i. Repetitive anxious complaints/concerns (non-health related) e.g., persistently seeks attention/ reassurance regarding schedules, meals, laundry, clothing, relationship issues	
		SLEEP-CYCLE ISSUES	
		j. Unpleasant mood in morning	
		k. Insomnia/change in usual sleep pattern	
		SAD, APATHETIC, ANXIOUS APPEARANCE	
		l. Sad, pained, worried facial expressions—e.g., furrowed brows	
		m. Crying, tearfulness	
		n. Repetitive physical movements—e.g., pacing, hand wringing, restlessness, fidgeting, picking	
		LOSS OF INTEREST	
		o. Withdrawal from activities of interest—e.g., no interest in long standing activities or being with family/friends	
		p. Reduced social interaction	
2.	MOOD PERSIS-TENCE	**One or more indicators of depressed, sad or anxious mood were not easily altered by attempts to "cheer up", console, or reassure the resident over last 7 days** 0. No mood indicators 1. Indicators present, easily altered 2. Indicators present, not easily altered	
3.	CHANGE IN MOOD	Resident's mood status has changed as compared to status of **90 days ago** (or since last assessment if less then 90 days) 0. No change 1. Improved 2. Deteriorated	

			(A)	(B)
4.	BEHAVIORAL SYMPTOMS	(A) ***Behavioral symptom frequency in last 7 days*** 0. Behavior not exhibited in last 7 days 1. Behavior of this type occurred 1 to 3 days in last 7 days 2. Behavior of this type occurred 4 to 6 days, but less than daily 3. Behavior of this type occurred daily (B) ***Behavioral symptom alterability in last 7 days*** 0. Behavior not present OR behavior was easily altered 1. Behavior was not easily altered		
		a. WANDERING (moved with no rational purpose, seemingly oblivious to needs or safety)		
		b. VERBALLY ABUSIVE BEHAVIORAL SYMPTOMS (others were threatened, screamed at, cursed at)		
		c. PHYSICALLY ABUSIVE BEHAVIORAL SYMPTOMS (others were hit, shoved, scratched, sexually abused)		
		d. SOCIALLY INAPPROPRIATE/DISRUPTIVE BEHAVIORAL SYMPTOMS (made disruptive sounds, noisiness, screaming, self-abusive acts, sexual behavior or disrobing in public, smeared/threw food/feces, hoarding, rummaged through others' belongings)		
		e. RESISTS CARE (resisted taking medications/ injections, ADL assistance, or eating)		

5.	CHANGE IN BEHAVIORAL SYMPTOMS	Resident's behavior status has changed as compared to **status of 90 days ago** (or since last assessment if less than 90 days) 0. No change 1. Improved 2. Deteriorated	

SECTION F. PSYCHOSOCIAL WELL-BEING

1.	SENSE OF INITIATIVE/ INVOLVE-MENT	At ease interacting with others	a.
		At ease doing planned or structured activities	b.
		At ease doing self-initiated activities	c.
		Establishes own goals	d.
		Pursues involvement in life of facility (e.g., makes/keeps friends; involved in group activities; responds positively to new activities; assists at religious services)	e.
		Accepts invitations into most group activities	f.
		NONE OF ABOVE	g.
2.	UNSETTLED RELATION-SHIPS	Covert/open conflict with or repeated criticism of staff	a.
		Unhappy with roommate	b.
		Unhappy with residents other than roommate	c.
		Openly expresses conflict/anger with family/friends	d.
		Absence of personal contact with family/friends	e.
		Recent loss of close family member/friend	f.
		Does not adjust easily to change in routines	g.
		NONE OF ABOVE	h.
3.	PAST ROLES	Strong identification with past roles and life status	a.
		Expresses sadness/anger/empty feeling over lost roles/status	b.
		Resident perceives that daily routine (customary routine, activities) is very different from prior pattern in the community	c.
		NONE OF ABOVE	d.

SECTION G. PHYSICAL FUNCTIONING AND STRUCTURAL PROBLEMS

			(A) SELF-PERF	(B) SUPPORT
1.	(A) ADL SELF-PERFORMANCE—(*Code for resident's **PERFORMANCE OVER ALL SHIFTS during last 7 days**—Not including setup*) 0. *INDEPENDENT*—No help or oversight —OR— Help/oversight provided only 1 or 2 times during last 7 days 1. SUPERVISION—Oversight, encouragement or cueing provided 3 or more times during last7 days —OR— Supervision (3 or more times) plus physical assistance provided only 1 or 2 times during last 7 days 2. *LIMITED ASSISTANCE*—Resident highly involved in activity; received physical help in guided maneuvering of limbs or other nonweight bearing assistance 3 or more times —OR—More help provided only 1 or 2 times during last 7 days 3. *EXTENSIVE ASSISTANCE*—While resident performed part of activity, over last 7-day period, help of following type(s) provided 3 or more times: — Weight-bearing support — Full staff performance during part (but not all) of last 7 days 4. *TOTAL DEPENDENCE*—Full staff performance of activity during entire 7 days 8. *ACTIVITY DID NOT OCCUR* during entire 7 days (B) ADL SUPPORT PROVIDED—(***Code for MOST SUPPORT PROVIDED OVER ALL SHIFTS during last 7 days; code regardless** of resident's self-performance classification*) 0. No setup or physical help from staff 1. Setup help only 2. One person physical assist 3. Two+ persons physical assist 8. ADL activity itself did not occur during entire 7 days			
a.	BED MOBILITY	How resident moves to and from lying position, turns side to side, and positions body while in bed		
b.	TRANSFER	How resident moves between surfaces—to/from: bed, chair, wheelchair, standing position (EXCLUDE to/from bath/toilet)		
c.	WALK IN ROOM	How resident walks between locations in his/her room		
d.	WALK IN CORRIDOR	How resident walks in corridor on unit		
e.	LOCOMO-TION ON UNIT	How resident moves between locations in his/her room and adjacent corridor on same floor. If in wheelchair, self-sufficiency once in chair		
f.	LOCOMO-TION OFF UNIT	How resident moves to and returns from off unit locations (e.g., areas set aside for dining, activities, or treatments). **If facility has only one floor**, how resident moves to and from distant areas on the floor. If in wheelchair, self-sufficiency once in chair		
g.	DRESSING	How resident puts on, fastens, and takes off all items of **street clothing**, including donning/removing prosthesis		
h.	EATING	How resident eats and drinks (regardless of skill). Includes intake of nourishment by other means (e.g., tube feeding, total parenteral nutrition)		
i.	TOILET USE	How resident uses the toilet room (or commode, bedpan, urinal); transfer on/off toilet, cleanses, changes pad, manages ostomy or catheter, adjusts clothes		
j.	PERSONAL HYGIENE	How resident maintains personal hygiene, including combing hair, brushing teeth, shaving, applying makeup, washing/drying face, hands, and perineum (EXCLUDE baths and showers)		

Resident ____________

Numeric Identifier ____________

2.	BATHING	How resident takes full-body bath/shower, sponge bath, and transfers in/out of tub/shower (EXCLUDE washing of back and hair.) *Code for most dependent in self-performance and support.* (A) BATHING SELF-PERFORMANCE codes appear below 0. Independent—No help provided 1. Supervision—Oversight help only 2. Physical help limited to transfer only 3. Physical help in part of bathing activity 4. Total dependence 8. Activity itself did not occur during entire 7 days *(Bathing support codes are as defined in Item 1, code B above)*	(A) (B)
3.	TEST FOR BALANCE (see training manual)	*(Code for ability during test in the last 7 days)* 0. Maintained position as required in test 1. Unsteady, but able to rebalance self without physical support 2. Partial physical support during test; or stands (sits) but does not follow directions for test 3. Not able to attempt test without physical help a. Balance while standing b. Balance while sitting—position, trunk control	
4.	FUNCTIONAL LIMITATION IN RANGE OF MOTION (see training manual)	*(Code for limitations during* **last 7 days** *that interfered with daily functions or placed resident at risk of injury)* (A) *RANGE OF MOTION*: 0. No limitation; 1. Limitation on one side; 2. Limitation on both sides (B) *VOLUNTARY MOVEMENT*: 0. No loss; 1. Partial loss; 2. Full loss a. Neck b. Arm—Including shoulder or elbow c. Hand—Including wrist or fingers d. Leg—Including hip or knee e. Foot—Including ankle or toes f. Other limitation or loss	(A) (B)
5.	MODES OF LOCOMOTION	*(Check all that apply during last 7 days)* Cane/walker/crutch a. Wheeled self b. Other person wheeled c. Wheelchair primary mode of locomotion d. *NONE OF ABOVE* e.	
6.	MODES OF TRANSFER	*(Check all that apply during last 7 days)* Bedfast all or most of time a. Bed rails used for bed mobility or transfer b. Lifted manually c. Lifted mechanically d. Transfer aid (e.g., slide board, trapeze, cane, walker, brace) e. *NONE OF ABOVE* f.	
7.	TASK SEGMENTATION	Some or all of ADL activities were broken into subtasks during last 7 days so that resident could perform them 0. No 1. Yes	
8.	ADL FUNCTIONAL REHABILITATION POTENTIAL	Resident believes he/she is capable of increased independence in at least some ADLs a. Direct care staff believe resident is capable of increased independence in at least some ADLs b. Resident able to perform tasks/activity but is very slow c. Difference in ADL Self-Performance or ADL Support, comparing mornings to evenings d. *NONE OF ABOVE* e.	
9.	CHANGE IN ADL FUNCTION	Resident's ADL self-performance status has changed as compared to status of **90 days ago** (or since last assessment if less than 90 days) 0. No change 1. Improved 2. Deteriorated	

SECTION H. CONTINENCE IN LAST 14 DAYS

1.	CONTINENCE SELF-CONTROL CATEGORIES ***(Code for resident's PERFORMANCE OVER ALL SHIFTS)*** 0. *CONTINENT*—Complete control *[includes use of indwelling urinary catheter or ostomy device that does not leak urine or stool]* 1. *USUALLY CONTINENT*—BLADDER, incontinent episodes once a week or less; BOWEL, less than weekly 2. *OCCASIONALLY INCONTINENT*—BLADDER, 2 or more times a week but not daily; BOWEL, once a week 3. *FREQUENTLY INCONTINENT*—BLADDER, tended to be incontinent daily, but some control present (e.g., on day shift); BOWEL, 2-3 times a week 4. *INCONTINENT*—Had inadequate control BLADDER, multiple daily episodes; BOWEL, all (or almost all) of the time		
a.	BOWEL CONTINENCE	Control of bowel movement, with appliance or bowel continence programs, if employed	
b.	BLADDER CONTINENCE	Control of urinary bladder function (if dribbles, volume insufficient to soak through underpants), with appliances (e.g., foley) or continence programs, if employed	
2.	BOWEL ELIMINATION PATTERN	Bowel elimination pattern regular—at least one movement every three days a. Constipation b. Diarrhea c. Fecal impaction d. *NONE OF ABOVE* e.	

3.	APPLIANCES AND PROGRAMS	Any scheduled toileting plan a. Bladder retraining program b. External (condom) catheter c. Indwelling catheter d. Intermittent catheter e. Did not use toilet room/commode/urinal f. Pads/briefs used g. Enemas/irrigation h. Ostomy present i. *NONE OF ABOVE* j.	
4.	CHANGE IN URINARY CONTINENCE	Resident's urinary continence has changed as compared to status of **90 days ago** (or since last assessment if less than 90 days) 0. No change 1. Improved 2. Deteriorated	

SECTION I. DISEASE DIAGNOSES

Check only those diseases that have a relationship to current ADL status, cognitive status, mood and behavior status, medical treatments, nursing monitoring, or risk of death. (Do not list inactive diagnoses)

1.	DISEASES	*(If none apply, CHECK the NONE OF ABOVE box)* **ENDOCRINE/METABOLIC/NUTRITIONAL** Diabetes mellitus a. Hyperthyroidism b. Hypothyroidism c. **HEART/CIRCULATION** Arteriosclerotic heart disease (ASHD) d. Cardiac dysrhythmias e. Congestive heart failure f. Deep vein thrombosis g. Hypertension h. Hypotension i. Peripheral vascular disease j. Other cardiovascular disease k. **MUSCULOSKELETAL** Arthritis l. Hip fracture m. Missing limb (e.g., amputation) n. Osteoporosis o. Pathological bone fracture p. **NEUROLOGICAL** Alzheimer's disease q. Aphasia r. Cerebral palsy s. Cerebrovascular accident (stroke) t. Dementia other than Alzheimer's disease u.	Hemiplegia/Hemiparesis v. Multiple sclerosis w. Paraplegia x. Parkinson's disease y. Quadriplegia z. Seizure disorder aa. Transient ischemic attack (TIA) bb. Traumatic brain injury cc. **PSYCHIATRIC/MOOD** Anxiety disorder dd. Depression ee. Manic depression (bipolar disease) ff. Schizophrenia gg. **PULMONARY** Asthma hh. Emphysema/COPD ii. **SENSORY** Cataracts jj. Diabetic retinopathy kk. Glaucoma ll. Macular degeneration mm. **OTHER** Allergies nn. Anemia oo. Cancer pp. Renal failure qq. *NONE OF ABOVE* rr.
2.	INFECTIONS	*(If none apply, CHECK the NONE OF ABOVE box)* Antibiotic resistant infection (e.g., Methicillin resistant staph) a. Clostridium difficile (c. diff.) b. Conjunctivitis c. HIV infection d. Pneumonia e. Respiratory infection f.	Septicemia g. Sexually transmitted diseases h. Tuberculosis i. Urinary tract infection in last 30 days j. Viral hepatitis k. Wound infection l. NONE OF ABOVE m.
3.	OTHER CURRENT OR MORE DETAILED DIAGNOSES AND ICD-9 CODES	a. ____ | | | | .| | b. ____ | | | | .| | c. ____ | | | | .| | d. ____ | | | | .| | e. ____ | | | | .| |	

SECTION J. HEALTH CONDITIONS

1.	PROBLEM CONDITIONS	*(Check all problems present in* **last 7 days** *unless other time frame is indicated)* **INDICATORS OF FLUID STATUS** Weight gain or loss of 3 or more pounds within a 7 day period a. Inability to lie flat due to shortness of breath b. Dehydrated; output exceeds input c. Insufficient fluid; did NOT consume all/almost all liquids provided during **last 3 days** d. **OTHER** Delusions e.	Dizziness/Vertigo f. Edema g. Fever h. Hallucinations i. Internal bleeding j. Recurrent lung aspirations in **last 90 days** k. Shortness of breath l. Syncope (fainting) m. Unsteady gait n. Vomiting o. *NONE OF ABOVE* p.

Resident ____________ Numeric Identifier ____________

2.	PAIN SYMPTOMS	(*Code the **highest level of pain** present in the **last 7 days***) a. **FREQUENCY** with which resident complains or shows evidence of pain 0. No pain (***skip to J4***) 1. Pain less than daily 2. Pain daily b. **INTENSITY** of pain 1. Mild pain 2. Moderate pain 3. Times when pain is horrible or excruciating	
3.	PAIN SITE	(*If pain present, **check all sites** that apply in **last 7 days***) Back pain — a. Bone pain — b. Chest pain while doing usual activities — c. Headache — d. Hip pain — e. Incisional pain — f. Joint pain (other than hip) — g. Soft tissue pain (e.g., lesion, muscle) — h. Stomach pain — i. Other — j.	
4.	ACCIDENTS	(***Check all that apply***) Fell in **past 30 days** — a. Fell in **past 31-180 days** — b. Hip fracture in **last 180 days** — c. Other fracture in **last 180 days** — d. *NONE OF ABOVE* — e.	
5.	STABILITY OF CONDITIONS	Conditions/diseases make resident's cognitive, ADL, mood or behavior patterns unstable—(fluctuating, precarious, or deteriorating) — a. Resident experiencing an acute episode or a flare-up of a recurrent or chronic-problem — b. End-stage disease, 6 or fewer months to live — c. *NONE OF ABOVE* — d.	

SECTION K. ORAL/NUTRITIONAL STATUS

1.	ORAL PROBLEMS	Chewing problem — a. Swallowing problem — b. Mouth pain — c. *NONE OF ABOVE* — d.	
2.	HEIGHT AND WEIGHT	*Record **(a.) height in inches** and **(b.) weight in pounds**. Base weight on most recent measure in **last 30 days**; measure weight consistently in accord with standard facility practice—e.g., in a.m. after voiding, before meal, with shoes off, and in nightclothes* a. HT (in.) b. WT (lb.)	
3.	WEIGHT CHANGE	**a. Weight loss**—5 % or more in **last 30 days**; or 10 % or more in **last 180 days** 0. No 1. Yes **b. Weight gain**—5 % or more in **last 30 days**; or 10 % or more in **last 180 days** 0. No 1. Yes	
4.	NUTRITIONAL PROBLEMS	Complains about the taste of many foods — a. Regular or repetitive complaints of hunger — b. Leaves 25% or more of food uneaten at most meals — c. *NONE OF ABOVE* — d.	
5.	NUTRITIONAL APPROACHES	(***Check all that apply in last 7 days***) Parenteral/IV — a. Feeding tube — b. Mechanically altered diet — c. Syringe (oral feeding) — d. Therapeutic diet — e. Dietary supplement between meals — f. Plate guard, stabilized built-up utensil, etc. — g. On a planned weight change program — h. *NONE OF ABOVE* — i.	
6.	PARENTERAL OR ENTERAL INTAKE	(***Skip to Section L if neither 5a nor 5b is checked***) a. Code the proportion of **total calories** the resident received through parenteral or tube feedings in the **last 7 days** 0. None 1. 1% to 25% 2. 26% to 50% 3. 51% to 75% 4. 76% to 100% b. Code the average **fluid intake** per day by IV or tube in **last 7 days** 0. None 1. 1 to 500 cc/day 2. 501 to 1000 cc/day 3. 1001 to 1500 cc/day 4. 1501 to 2000 cc/day 5. 2001 or more cc/day	

SECTION L. ORAL/DENTAL STATUS

1.	ORAL STATUS AND DISEASE PREVENTION	Debris (soft, easily movable substances) present in mouth prior to going to bed at night — a. Has dentures or removable bridge — b. Some/all natural teeth lost—does not have or does not use dentures (or partial plates) — c. Broken, loose, or carious teeth — d. Inflamed gums (gingiva); swollen or bleeding gums; oral abcesses; ulcers or rashes — e. Daily cleaning of teeth/dentures or daily mouth care—by resident or staff — f. *NONE OF ABOVE* — g.	

SECTION M. SKIN CONDITION

			Number at Stage
1.	ULCERS (Due to any cause)	(*Record the number of ulcers at each ulcer stage—regardless of cause. If none present at a stage, record "0" (zero). Code all that apply during **last 7 days**. Code 9 = 9 or more.) **[Requires full body exam.]*** a. Stage 1. A persistent area of skin redness (without a break in the skin) that does not disappear when pressure is relieved. b. Stage 2. A partial thickness loss of skin layers that presents clinically as an abrasion, blister, or shallow crater. c. Stage 3. A full thickness of skin is lost, exposing the subcutaneous tissues - presents as a deep crater with or without undermining adjacent tissue. d. Stage 4. A full thickness of skin and subcutaneous tissue is lost, exposing muscle or bone.	
2.	TYPE OF ULCER	(*For each type of ulcer, **code for the highest stage in the last 7 days** using scale in item M1—i.e., 0=none; stages 1, 2, 3, 4*) a. Pressure ulcer—any lesion caused by pressure resulting in damage of underlying tissue b. Stasis ulcer—open lesion caused by poor circulation in the lower extremities	
3.	HISTORY OF RESOLVED ULCERS	Resident had an ulcer that was resolved or cured **in LAST 90 DAYS** 0. No 1. Yes	
4.	OTHER SKIN PROBLEMS OR LESIONS PRESENT	(***Check all that apply** during **last 7 days***) Abrasions, bruises — a. Burns (second or third degree) — b. Open lesions other than ulcers, rashes, cuts (e.g., cancer lesions) — c. Rashes—e.g., intertrigo, eczema, drug rash, heat rash, herpes zoster — d. Skin desensitized to pain or pressure — e. Skin tears or cuts (other than surgery) — f. Surgical wounds — g. *NONE OF ABOVE* — h.	
5.	SKIN TREATMENTS	(***Check all that apply** during **last 7 days***) Pressure relieving device(s) for chair — a. Pressure relieving device(s) for bed — b. Turning/repositioning program — c. Nutrition or hydration intervention to manage skin problems — d. Ulcer care — e. Surgical wound care — f. Application of dressings (with or without topical medications) other than to feet — g. Application of ointments/medications (other than to feet) — h. Other preventative or protective skin care (other than to feet) — i. *NONE OF ABOVE* — j.	
6.	FOOT PROBLEMS AND CARE	(***Check all that apply** during **last 7 days***) Resident has one or more foot problems—e.g., corns, callouses, bunions, hammer toes, overlapping toes, pain, structural problems — a. Infection of the foot—e.g., cellulitis, purulent drainage — b. Open lesions on the foot — c. Nails/calluses trimmed during **last 90 days** — d. Received preventative or protective foot care (e.g., used special shoes, inserts, pads, toe separators) — e. Application of dressings (with or without topical medications) — f. *NONE OF ABOVE* — g.	

SECTION N. ACTIVITY PURSUIT PATTERNS

1.	TIME AWAKE	(***Check appropriate time periods over last 7 days***) Resident awake all or most of time (i.e., naps no more than one hour per time period) in the: Morning — a. Afternoon — b. Evening — c. *NONE OF ABOVE* — d.	
	(If resident is comatose, skip to Section O)		
2.	AVERAGE TIME INVOLVED IN ACTIVITIES	**(When awake and not receiving treatments or ADL care)** 0. Most—more than 2/3 of time 1. Some—from 1/3 to 2/3 of time 2. Little—less than 1/3 of time 3. None	
3.	PREFERRED ACTIVITY SETTINGS	(***Check all settings** in which activities are preferred*) Own room — a. Day/activity room — b. Inside NH/off unit — c. Outside facility — d. *NONE OF ABOVE* — e.	
4.	GENERAL ACTIVITY PREFERENCES (adapted to resident's current abilities)	(***Check all PREFERENCES** whether or not activity is currently available to resident*) Cards/other games — a. Crafts/arts — b. Exercise/sports — c. Music — d. Reading/writing — e. Spiritual/religious activities — f. Trips/shopping — g. Walking/wheeling outdoors — h. Watching TV — i. Gardening or plants — j. Talking or conversing — k. Helping others — l. *NONE OF ABOVE* — m.	

Resident ____________________ Numeric Identifier ____________________

5.	PREFERS CHANGE IN DAILY ROUTINE	*Code for resident preferences in daily routines* 0. No change 1. Slight change 2. Major change
		a. Type of activities in which resident is currently involved
		b. Extent of resident involvement in activities

SECTION O. MEDICATIONS

1.	NUMBER OF MEDICATIONS	***(Record the number of different** medications used in the last 7 days; enter "0" if none used)*
2.	NEW MEDICATIONS	*(Resident currently receiving medications that were initiated during the **last 90 days**)* 0. No 1. Yes
3.	INJECTIONS	***(Record the number of DAYS** injections of any type received during the **last 7 days**; enter "0" if none used)*
4.	DAYS RECEIVED THE FOLLOWING MEDICATION	***(Record the number of DAYS** during last 7 days; enter "0" if not used. Note—enter "1" for long-acting meds used less than weekly)*
		a. Antipsychotic; b. Antianxiety; c. Antidepressant; d. Hypnotic; e. Diuretic

SECTION P. SPECIAL TREATMENTS AND PROCEDURES

1.	SPECIAL TREATMENTS, PROCEDURES, AND PROGRAMS	a. **SPECIAL CARE—Check** *treatments or programs received during the **last 14 days***
		TREATMENTS: Chemotherapy a.; Dialysis b.; IV medication c.; Intake/output d.; Monitoring acute medical condition e.; Ostomy care f.; Oxygen therapy g.; Radiation h.; Suctioning i.; Tracheostomy care j.; Transfusions k.; Ventilator or respirator l.
		PROGRAMS: Alcohol/drug treatment program m.; Alzheimer's/dementia special care unit n.; Hospice care o.; Pediatric unit p.; Respite care q.; Training in skills required to return to the community (e.g., taking medications, house work, shopping, transportation, ADLs) r.; *NONE OF ABOVE* s.
		b. **THERAPIES** - *Record the number of days and total minutes each of the following therapies was administered (for at least 15 minutes a day) in the **last 7 calendar days** (Enter 0 if none or less than 15 min. daily)* **[Note—count only post admission therapies]**
		(A) = # of days administered for **15 minutes or more** — DAYS (A); **(B) = total # of minutes** provided in last 7 days — MIN (B)
		a. Speech - language pathology and audiology services
		b. Occupational therapy
		c. Physical therapy
		d. Respiratory therapy
		e. Psychological therapy (by any licensed mental health professional)
2.	INTERVENTION PROGRAMS FOR MOOD, BEHAVIOR, COGNITIVE LOSS	**(Check all interventions or strategies used in last 7 days**—no matter where received)
		Special behavior symptom evaluation program a.
		Evaluation by a licensed mental health specialist in **last 90 days** b.
		Group therapy c.
		Resident-specific deliberate changes in the environment to address mood/behavior patterns—e.g., providing bureau in which to rummage d.
		Reorientation—e.g., cueing e.
		NONE OF ABOVE f.
3.	NURSING REHABILITATION/ RESTORATIVE CARE	*Record the NUMBER OF DAYS each of the following rehabilitation or restorative techniques or practices was **provided to the resident for more than or equal to 15 minutes per day in the last 7 days** (Enter 0 if none or less than 15 min. daily.)*
		a. Range of motion (passive); b. Range of motion (active); c. Splint or brace assistance
		TRAINING AND SKILL PRACTICE IN: d. Bed mobility; e. Transfer; f. Walking; g. Dressing or grooming; h. Eating or swallowing; i. Amputation/prosthesis care; j. Communication; k. Other

4.	DEVICES AND RESTRAINTS	*(Use the following codes for **last 7 days**:)* 0. Not used 1. Used less than daily 2. Used daily
		Bed rails
		a. — Full bed rails on all open sides of bed
		b. — Other types of side rails used (e.g., half rail, one side)
		c. Trunk restraint
		d. Limb restraint
		e. Chair prevents rising
5.	HOSPITAL STAY(S)	Record number of times resident was admitted to hospital with an overnight stay **in last 90 days** (or since last assessment if less than 90 days). *(Enter 0 if no hospital admissions)*
6.	EMERGENCY ROOM (ER) VISIT(S)	Record number of times resident visited ER without an overnight stay **in last 90 days** (or since last assessment if less than 90 days). *(Enter 0 if no ER visits)*
7.	PHYSICIAN VISITS	In the **LAST 14 DAYS** (or since admission if less than 14 days in facility) how many days has the physician (or authorized assistant or practitioner) examined the resident? *(Enter 0 if none)*
8.	PHYSICIAN ORDERS	In the **LAST 14 DAYS** (or since admission if less than 14 days in facility) how many days has the physician (or authorized assistant or practitioner) changed the resident's orders? *Do not include order renewals without change. (Enter 0 if none)*
9.	ABNORMAL LAB VALUES	Has the resident had any abnormal lab values during the **last 90 days** (or since admission)? 0. No 1. Yes

SECTION Q. DISCHARGE POTENTIAL AND OVERALL STATUS

1.	DISCHARGE POTENTIAL	a. Resident expresses/indicates preference to return to the community — 0. No 1. Yes
		b. Resident has a support person who is positive towards discharge — 0. No 1. Yes
		c. Stay projected to be of a short duration— discharge projected **within 90 days** (do not include expected discharge due to death) 0. No 1. Within 30 days 2. Within 31-90 days 3. Discharge status uncertain
2.	OVERALL CHANGE IN CARE NEEDS	Resident's overall self sufficiency has changed significantly as compared to status of **90 days ago** (or since last assessment if less than 90 days) 0. No change 1. Improved—receives fewer supports, needs less restrictive level of care 2. Deteriorated—receives more support

SECTION R. ASSESSMENT INFORMATION

1.	PARTICIPATION IN ASSESSMENT	a. Resident:	0. No	1. Yes	
		b. Family:	0. No	1. Yes	2. No family
		c. Significant other:	0. No	1. Yes	2. None

2. SIGNATURES OF PERSONS COMPLETING THE ASSESSMENT:

a. Signature of RN Assessment Coordinator (sign on above line)

b. Date RN Assessment Coordinator signed as complete: Month — Day — Year

c. Other Signatures	Title	Sections	Date
d.			Date
e.			Date
f.			Date
g.			Date
h.			Date

Resident ______ Numeric Identifier ______

SECTION T. SUPPLEMENT—CASE MIX DEMO

1.	SPECIAL TREAT-MENTS AND PROCE-DURES	**a. RECREATION THERAPY**—*Enter number of days and total minutes of recreation therapy administered* (***for at least 15 minutes a day***) *in the* ***last 7 days*** (*Enter 0 if none*) DAYS (A) MIN (B) (A) = **# of days** administered for 15 minutes or more (B) = **total # of minutes** provided in last 7 days
		Skip unless this is a Medicare 5 day or initial admission assessment. **b. ORDERED THERAPIES**—*Has physician ordered any of following therapies to begin in FIRST 14 days of stay—physical therapy, occupational therapy, or speech pathology service?* 0. No 1. Yes ***If not ordered, skip to item 2*** **c.** Through day 15, provide an estimate of the number of days when at least 1 therapy service can be expected to have been delivered. **d.** Through day 15, provide an estimate of the number of therapy minutes (across the therapies) that can be expected to be delivered?
2.	WALKING WHEN MOST SELF SUFFICIENT	***Complete item 2 if ADL self-performance score for TRANSFER (G.1.b.A) is 0,1,2, or 3 AND at least one of the following are present:*** • Resident received physical therapy involving gait training (P.1.b.c) • Physical therapy was ordered for the resident involving gait training (T.2.b) • Resident received nursing rehabilitation for walking (P.3.f) • Physical therapy involving walking has been discontinued within the past 180 days ***Skip to item 3 if resident did not walk in last 7 days*** ***(FOR FOLLOWING FIVE ITEMS, BASE CODING ON THE EPISODE WHEN THE RESIDENT WALKED THE FARTHEST WITHOUT SITTING DOWN. INCLUDE WALKING DURING REHABILITATION SESSIONS.)***
		a. Furthest distance walked without sitting down during this episode. 0. 150+ feet 1. 51-149 feet 2. 26-50 feet 3. 10-25 feet 4. Less than 10 feet **b. Time walked** without sitting down during this episode. 0. 1-2 minutes 1. 3-4 minutes 2. 5-10 minutes 3. 11-15 minutes 4. 16-30 minutes 5. 31+ minutes **c. Self-Performance in walking** during this episode. 0. *INDEPENDENT*—No help or oversight 1. *SUPERVISION*—Oversight, encouragement or cueing provided 2. *LIMITED ASSISTANCE*—Resident highly involved in walking; received physical help in guided maneuvering of limbs or other nonweight bearing assistance 3. *EXTENSIVE ASSISTANCE*—Resident received weight bearing assistance while walking **d. Walking support provided** associated with this episode (code regardless of resident's self-performance classification). 0. No setup or physical help from staff 1. Setup help only 2. One person physical assist 3. Two+ persons physical assist **e. Parallel bars** used by resident in association with this episode. 0. No 1. Yes
3.	CASE MIX GROUP	**Medicare** State

SECTION U. MEDICATIONS—CASE MIX DEMO

List all medications that the resident **received** during the last 7 days. Include scheduled medications that are used regularly, but less than weekly .

1. **Medication Name and Dose Ordered.** Record the name of the medication and dose ordered.
2. **Route of Administration (RA).** Code the Route of Administration using the following list:

   1=by mouth (PO)
   2=sub lingual (SL)
   3=intramuscular (IM)
   4=intravenous (IV)
   5=subcutaneous (SQ)
   6=rectal (R)
   7=topical
   8=inhalation
   9=enteral tube
   10=other

3. **Frequency.** Code the number of times per day, week, or month the medication is administered using the following list:

PR=(PRN) as necessary
1H=(QH) every hour
2H=(Q2H) every two hours
3H=(Q3H) every three hours
4H=(Q4H) every four hours
6H=(Q6H) every six hours
8H=(Q8H) every eight hours
1D=(QD or HS) once daily
2D=(BID) two times daily (includes every 12 hrs)
3D=(TID) three times daily
4D=(QID) four times daily
5D=five times daily
1W=(Q week) once each wk
2W=two times every week
3W=three times every week
QO=every other day
4W=4 times each week
5W=five times each week
6W=six times each week
1M=(Q month) once every month
2M=twice every month
C=continuous
O=other

4. **Amount Administered (AA).** Record the number of tablets, capsules, suppositories, or liquid (any route) **per dose** administered to the resident. Code 999 for topicals, eye drops, inhalants and oral medications that need to be dissolved in water..

5. **PRN-number of days (PRN-n).** If the frequency code for the medication is "PR", record the number of times during the last 7 days each PRN medication was given. Code STAT medications as PRNs given once.

6. **NDC Codes.** Enter the National Drug Code for each medication given. Be sure to enter the correct NDC code for the drug name, strength , and form. The NDC code must match the drug dispensed by the pharmacy.

1. Medication Name and Dose Ordered	2. RA	3. Freq	4. AA	5. PRN-n	6. NDC Codes

MDS QUARTERLY ASSESSMENT FORM

Numeric Identifier ______________________

A1.	RESIDENT NAME	a. (First) b. (Middle Initial) c. (Last) d. (Jr/Sr)
A2.	ROOM NUMBER	
A3.	ASSESSMENT REFERENCE DATE	a. Last day of MDS observation period Month — Day — Year b. Original (0) or corrected copy of form (enter number of correction)
A4a	DATE OF REENTRY	**Date of reentry from most recent temporary discharge to a hospital in last 90 days (or since last assessment or admission if less than 90 days)** Month — Day — Year
A6.	MEDICAL RECORD NO.	
B1.	COMATOSE	(*Persistent vegetative state/no discernible consciousness*) 0. No 1. Yes (***Skip to Section G***)
B2.	MEMORY	(*Recall of what was learned or known*) a. Short-term memory OK—seems/appears to recall after 5 minutes 0. Memory OK 1. Memory problem b. Long-term memory OK—seems/appears to recall long past 0. Memory OK 1. Memory problem
B4.	COGNITIVE SKILLS FOR DAILY DECISION-MAKING	(*Made decisions regarding tasks of daily life*) 0. *INDEPENDENT*—decisions consistent/reasonable 1. *MODIFIED INDEPENDENCE*—some difficulty in new situations only 2. *MODERATELY IMPAIRED*—decisions poor; cues/supervision required 3. *SEVERELY IMPAIRED*—never/rarely made decisions
B5.	INDICATORS OF DELIRIUM—PERIODIC DISORDERED THINKING/AWARENESS	(*Code for behavior in the **last 7 days**.*) [***Note: Accurate assessment requires conversations with staff and family who have direct knowledge of resident's behavior over this time***]. 0. Behavior not present 1. Behavior present, not of recent onset 2. Behavior present, over last 7 days appears different from resident's usual functioning (e.g., new onset or worsening) a. EASILY DISTRACTED—(e.g., difficulty paying attention; gets sidetracked) b. PERIODS OF ALTERED PERCEPTION OR AWARENESS OF SURROUNDINGS—(e.g., moves lips or talks to someone not present; believes he/she is somewhere else; confuses night and day) c. EPISODES OF DISORGANIZED SPEECH—(e.g., speech is incoherent, nonsensical, irrelevant, or rambling from subject to subject; loses train of thought) d. PERIODS OF RESTLESSNESS—(e.g., fidgeting or picking at skin, clothing, napkins, etc; frequent position changes; repetitive physical movements or calling out) e. PERIODS OF LETHARGY—(e.g., sluggishness; staring into space; difficult to arouse; little body movement) f. MENTAL FUNCTION VARIES OVER THE COURSE OF THE DAY—(e.g., sometimes better, sometimes worse; behaviors sometimes present, sometimes not)
C4.	MAKING SELF UNDERSTOOD	(*Expressing information content—however able*) 0. *UNDERSTOOD* 1. *USUALLY UNDERSTOOD*—difficulty finding words or finishing thoughts 2. *SOMETIMES UNDERSTOOD*—ability is limited to making concrete requests 3. *RARELY/NEVER UNDERSTOOD*
C6.	ABILITY TO UNDERSTAND OTHERS	(*Understanding verbal information content—however able*) 0. *UNDERSTANDS* 1. *USUALLY UNDERSTANDS*—may miss some part/intent of message 2. *SOMETIMES UNDERSTANDS*—responds adequately to simple, direct communication 3. *RARELY/NEVER UNDERSTANDS*
E1.	INDICATORS OF DEPRESSION, ANXIETY, SAD MOOD	(***Code for indicators observed in last 30 days, irrespective of the assumed cause***) 0. Indicator not exhibited in last 30 days 1. Indicator of this type exhibited up to five days a week 2. Indicator of this type exhibited daily or almost daily (6, 7 days a week) **VERBAL EXPRESSIONS OF DISTRESS** a. Resident made negative statements—e.g., "*Nothing matters; Would rather be dead; What's the use; Regrets having lived so long; Let me die*" b. Repetitive questions—e.g., "*Where do I go; What do I do?*" c. Repetitive verbalizations—e.g., calling out for help, ("*God help me*") d. Persistent anger with self or others—e.g., easily annoyed, anger at placement in nursing home; anger at care received e. Self deprecation—e.g., "*I am nothing; I am of no use to anyone*"
E1.	INDICATORS OF DEPRESSION, ANXIETY, SAD MOOD (cont.)	**VERBAL EXPRESSIONS OF DISTRESS** f. Expressions of what appear to be unrealistic fears—e.g., fear of being abandoned, left alone, being with others g. Recurrent statements that something terrible is about to happen—e.g., believes he or she is about to die, have a heart attack h. Repetitive health complaints—e.g., persistently seeks medical attention, obsessive concern with body functions i. Repetitive anxious complaints/concerns (non-health related) e.g., persistently seeks attention/reassurance regarding schedules, meals, laundry, clothing, relationship issues **SLEEP-CYCLE ISSUES** j. Unpleasant mood in morning k. Insomnia/change in usual sleep pattern **SAD, APATHETIC, ANXIOUS APPEARANCE** l. Sad, pained, worried facial expressions—e.g., furrowed brows m. Crying, tearfulness n. Repetitive physical movements—e.g., pacing, hand wringing, restlessness, fidgeting, picking **LOSS OF INTEREST** o. Withdrawal from activities of interest—e.g., no interest in long standing activities or being with family/friends p. Reduced social interaction
E2.	MOOD PERSISTENCE	**One or more indicators of depressed, sad or anxious mood were not easily altered by attempts to "cheer up", console, or reassure the resident over last 7 days** 0. No mood indicators 1. Indicators present, easily altered 2. Indicators present, not easily altered
E4.	BEHAVIORAL SYMPTOMS	(A) ***Behavioral symptom frequency in last 7 days*** 0. Behavior not exhibited in last 7 days 1. Behavior of this type occurred 1 to 3 days in last 7 days 2. Behavior of this type occurred 4 to 6 days, but less than daily 3. Behavior of this type occurred daily (B) ***Behavioral symptom alterability in last 7 days*** 0. Behavior not present OR behavior was easily altered 1. Behavior was not easily altered (A) (B) a. WANDERING (moved with no rational purpose, seemingly oblivious to needs or safety) b. VERBALLY ABUSIVE BEHAVIORAL SYMPTOMS (others were threatened, screamed at, cursed at) c. PHYSICALLY ABUSIVE BEHAVIORAL SYMPTOMS (others were hit, shoved, scratched, sexually abused) d. SOCIALLY INAPPROPRIATE/DISRUPTIVE BEHAVIORAL SYMPTOMS (made disruptive sounds, noisiness, screaming, self-abusive acts, sexual behavior or disrobing in public, smeared/threw food/feces, hoarding, rummaged through others' belongings) e. RESISTS CARE (resisted taking medications/ injections, ADL assistance, or eating)

G1. (A) ADL SELF-PERFORMANCE—(***Code for resident's PERFORMANCE OVER ALL SHIFTS during last 7 days—Not including setup***)

0. *INDEPENDENT*—No help or oversight —OR— Help/oversight provided only 1 or 2 times during last 7 days
1. SUPERVISION—Oversight, encouragement or cueing provided 3 or more times during last7 days —OR— Supervision (3 or more times) plus physical assistance provided only 1 or 2 times during last 7 days
2. *LIMITED ASSISTANCE*—Resident highly involved in activity; received physical help in guided maneuvering of limbs or other nonweight bearing assistance 3 or more times —OR—More help provided only 1 or 2 times during last 7 days
3. *EXTENSIVE ASSISTANCE*—While resident performed part of activity, over last 7-day period, help of following type(s) provided 3 or more times:
   — Weight-bearing support
   — Full staff performance during part (but not all) of last 7 days
4. *TOTAL DEPENDENCE*—Full staff performance of activity during entire 7 days
8. *ACTIVITY DID NOT OCCUR* during entire 7 days

			(A)
a.	BED MOBILITY	How resident moves to and from lying position, turns side to side, and positions body while in bed	
b.	TRANSFER	How resident moves between surfaces—to/from: bed, chair, wheelchair, standing position (EXCLUDE to/from bath/toilet)	
c.	WALK IN ROOM	How resident walks between locations in his/her room.	
d.	WALK IN CORRIDOR	How resident walks in corridor on unit.	
e.	LOCOMOTION ON UNIT	How resident moves between locations in his/her room and adjacent corridor on same floor. If in wheelchair, self-sufficiency once in chair	
f.	LOCOMOTION OFF UNIT	How resident moves to and returns from off unit locations (e.g., areas set aside for dining, activities, or treatments). If facility has only one floor, how resident moves to and from distant areas on the floor. If in wheelchair, self-sufficiency once in chair	
g.	DRESSING	How resident puts on, fastens, and takes off all items of street clothing, including donning/removing prosthesis	
h.	EATING	How resident eats and drinks (regardless of skill). Includes intake of nourishment by other means (e.g., tube feeding, total parenteral nutrition).	

Resident ______________________ Numeric Identifier ______________________

i.	TOILET USE	How resident uses the toilet room (or commode, bedpan, urinal); transfer on/off toilet, cleanses, changes pad, manages ostomy or catheter, adjusts clothes	
j.	PERSONAL HYGIENE	How resident maintains personal hygiene, including combing hair, brushing teeth, shaving, applying makeup, washing/drying face, hands, and perineum (EXCLUDE baths and showers)	
G2.	BATHING	How resident takes full-body bath/shower, sponge bath, and transfers in/out of tub/shower (EXCLUDE washing of back and hair.) ***Code for most dependent in self-performance.*** (A) BATHING SELF PERFORMANCE codes appear below 0. Independent—No help provided 1. Supervision—Oversight help only 2. Physical help limited to transfer only 3. Physical help in part of bathing activity 4. Total dependence 8. Activity itself did not occur during entire 7 days	(A)
G4.	FUNCTIONAL LIMITATION IN RANGE OF MOTION	(*Code for limitations during **last 7 days** that interfered with daily functions or placed residents at risk of injury*) (A) *RANGE OF MOTION*: 0. No limitation; 1. Limitation on one side; 2. Limitation on both sides (B) *VOLUNTARY MOVEMENT*: 0. No loss; 1. Partial loss; 2. Full loss a. Neck b. Arm—Including shoulder or elbow c. Hand—Including wrist or fingers d. Leg—Including hip or knee e. Foot—Including ankle or toes f. Other limitation or loss	(A) (B)
G6.	MODES OF TRANSFER	(***Check all that apply** during **last 7 days***) Bedfast all or most of time — a. Bed rails used for bed mobility or transfer — b. *NONE OF ABOVE* — f.	
H1.	CONTINENCE SELF-CONTROL CATEGORIES (***Code for resident's PERFORMANCE OVER ALL SHIFTS***)	0. *CONTINENT*—Complete control *[includes use of indwelling urinary catheter or ostomy device that does not leak urine or stool]* 1. *USUALLY CONTINENT*—BLADDER, incontinent episodes once a week or less; BOWEL, less than weekly 2. *OCCASIONALLY INCONTINENT*—BLADDER, 2 or more times a week but not daily; BOWEL, once a week 3. *FREQUENTLY INCONTINENT*—BLADDER, tended to be incontinent daily, but some control present (e.g., on day shift); BOWEL, 2-3 times a week 4. *INCONTINENT*—Had inadequate control BLADDER, multiple daily episodes; BOWEL, all (or almost all) of the time	
a.	BOWEL CONTINENCE	Control of bowel movement, with appliance or bowel continence programs, if employed	
b.	BLADDER CONTINENCE	Control of urinary bladder function (if dribbles, volume insufficient to soak through underpants), with appliances (e.g., foley) or continence programs, if employed	
H2.	BOWEL ELIMINATION PATTERN	Fecal impaction — d. *NONE OF ABOVE* — e.	
H3.	APPLIANCES AND PROGRAMS	Any scheduled toileting plan — a. Bladder retraining program — b. External (condom) catheter — c. Indwelling catheter — d. Ostomy present — i. *NONE OF ABOVE* — j.	
I2.	INFECTIONS	Urinary tract infection in **last 30 days** — j. *NONE OF ABOVE* — m.	
I3.	OTHER CURRENT DIAGNOSES AND ICD-9 CODES	(*Include **only those diseases diagnosed in the last 90 days that have a relationship** to current ADL status, cognitive status, moodr or behavior status, medical treatments, nursing monitoring, or risk of death*) a. ______ | | | |•| | b. ______ | | | |•| |	
J1.	PROBLEM CONDITIONS	(***Check all problems present** in **last 7 days***) Dehydrated; output exceeds input — c. Hallucinations — i. *NONE OF ABOVE* — p.	
J2.	PAIN SYMPTOMS	(*Code the **highest level of pain** present in the **last 7 days***) a. **FREQUENCY** with which resident complains or shows evidence of pain 0. No pain (***skip to J4***) 1. Pain less than daily 2. Pain daily b. **INTENSITY** of pain 1. Mild pain 2. Moderate pain 3. Times when pain is horrible or excrutiating	
J4.	ACCIDENTS	(***Check all that apply***) Fell in **past 30 days** — a. Fell in **past 31-180 days** — b. Hip fracture in **last 180 days** — c. Other fracture in **last 180 days** — d. *NONE OF ABOVE* — e.	

J5.	STABILITY OF CONDITIONS	Conditions/diseases make resident's cognitive, ADL, mood or behavior status unstable—(fluctuating, precarious, or deteriorating) — a. Resident experiencing an acute episode or a flare-up of a recurrent or chronic problem — b. End-stage disease, 6 or fewer months to live — c. *NONE OF ABOVE* — d.	
K3.	WEIGHT CHANGE	a. **Weight loss**—5 % or more in **last 30 days**; or 10 % or more in **last 180 days** 0. No 1. Yes b. **Weight gain**—5 % or more in **last 30 days**; or 10 % or more in **last 180 days** 0. No 1. Yes	
K5.	NUTRITIONAL APPROACHES	Feeding tube — b. On a planned weight change program — h. *NONE OF ABOVE* — l.	
M1.	ULCERS (Due to any cause)	(*Record the number of ulcers at each ulcer stage—regardless of cause. If none present at a stage, record "0" (zero). Code all that apply during **last 7 days**. Code 9 = 9 or more.) **[Requires full body exam.]*** a. Stage 1. A persistent area of skin redness (without a break in the skin) that does not disappear when pressure is relieved. b. Stage 2. A partial thickness loss of skin layers that presents clinically as an abrasion, blister, or shallow crater. c. Stage 3. A full thickness of skin is lost, exposing the subcutaneous tissues - presents as a deep crater with or without undermining adjacent tissue. d. Stage 4. A full thickness of skin and subcutaneous tissue is lost, exposing muscle or bone.	Number at Stage
M2.	TYPE OF ULCER	(*For each type of ulcer, **code for the highest stage in the last 7 days** using scale in item M1—i.e., 0=none; stages 1, 2, 3, 4*) a. Pressure ulcer—any lesion caused by pressure resulting in damage of underlying tissue b. Stasis ulcer—open lesion caused by poor circulation in the lower extremities	
N1.	TIME AWAKE	(***Check appropriate time periods over last 7 days***) Resident awake all or most of time (i.e., naps no more than one hour per time period) in the: Morning — a. Afternoon — b. Evening — c. *NONE OF ABOVE* — d.	
(If resident is comatose, skip to Section O)			
N2.	AVERAGE TIME INVOLVED IN ACTIVITIES	**(When awake and not receiving treatments or ADL care)** 0. Most—more than 2/3 of time 1. Some—from 1/3 to 2/3 of time 2. Little—less than 1/3 of time 3. None	
O1.	NUMBER OF MEDICATIONS	(***Record the number of different medications used in the last 7 days; enter "0" if none used***)	
O4.	DAYS RECEIVED THE FOLLOWING MEDICATION	(***Record the number of DAYS** during **last 7 days**; enter "0" if not used. Note—enter "1" for long-acting meds used less than weekly*) a. Antipsychotic b. Antianxiety c. Antidepressant d. Hypnotic e. Diuretic	
P4.	DEVICES AND RESTRAINTS	*Use the following codes for **last 7 days**:* 0. Not used 1. Used less than daily 2. Used daily Bed rails a. — Full bed rails on all open sides of bed b. — Other types of side rails used (e.g., half rail, one side) c. Trunk restraint d. Limb restraint e. Chair prevents rising	
Q2.	OVERALL CHANGE IN CARE NEEDS	Resident's overall level of self sufficiency has changed significantly as compared to status of **90 days ago** (or since last assessment if less than 90 days) 0. No change 1. Improved—receives fewer supports, needs less restrictive level of care 2. Deteriorated—receives more support	

R2. SIGNATURES OF PERSONS COMPLETING THE ASSESSMENT:

____

a. Signature of RN Assessment Coordinator (sign on above line)

b. Date RN Assessment Coordinator signed as complete [ ][ ] — [ ][ ] — [ ][ ][ ][ ]
Month Day Year

c. Other Signatures	Title	Sections	Date
d.			Date
e.			Date
f.			Date
g.			Date

MDS QUARTERLY ASSESSMENT FORM
(OPTIONAL VERSION FOR RUG III)

Numeric Identifier ____________

A1. RESIDENT NAME — a. (First) b. (Middle Initial) c. (Last) d. (Jr/Sr)

A2. ROOM NUMBER

A3. ASSESSMENT REFERENCE DATE
a. Last day of MDS observation period
Month — Day — Year
b. Original (0) or corrected copy of form (enter number of correction)

A4. DATE OF READMISSION
Date of readmission from most recent temporary discharge due to hospitalization in last 90 days (or since last assessment or admission if less than 90 days)
Month — Day — Year

A6. MEDICAL RECORD NO.

B1. COMATOSE (*Persistent vegetative state/no discernible consciousness*)
0. No 1. Yes (*Skip to Section G*)

B2. MEMORY (*Recall of what was learned or known*)
a. Short-term memory OK—seems/appears to recall after 5 minutes
0. Memory OK 1. Memory problem
b. Long-term memory OK—seems/appears to recall long past
0. Memory OK 1. Memory problem

B3. MEMORY/RECALL ABILITY (***Check all** that resident was **normally able to recall during last 7 days***)
Current season a.
Location of own room b.
Staff names/faces c.
That he/she is in a nursing home d.
NONE OF ABOVE are recalled e.

B4. COGNITIVE SKILLS FOR DAILY DECISION-MAKING (*Made decisions regarding tasks of daily life*)
0. *INDEPENDENT*—decisions consistent/reasonable
1. *MODIFIED INDEPENDENCE*—some difficulty in new situations only
2. *MODERATELY IMPAIRED*—decisions poor; cues/supervision required
3. *SEVERELY IMPAIRED*—never/rarely made decisions

B5. INDICATORS OF DELIRIUM—PERIODIC DISORDERED THINKING/AWARENESS (*Code for behavior in the last 7 days.*) [***Note: Accurate assessment requires conversations with staff and family who have direct knowledge of resident's behavior over this time***].
0. Behavior not present
1. Behavior present, not of recent onset
2. Behavior present, over last 7 days appears different from resident's usual functioning (e.g., new onset or worsening)

a. EASILY DISTRACTED—(e.g., difficulty paying attention; gets sidetracked)
b. PERIODS OF ALTERED PERCEPTION OR AWARENESS OF SURROUNDINGS—(e.g., moves lips or talks to someone not present; believes he/she is somewhere else; confuses night and day)
c. EPISODES OF DISORGANIZED SPEECH—(e.g., speech is incoherent, nonsensical, irrelevant, or rambling from subject to subject; loses train of thought)
d. PERIODS OF RESTLESSNESS—(e.g., fidgeting or picking at skin, clothing, napkins, etc; frequent position changes; repetitive physical movements or calling out)
e. PERIODS OF LETHARGY—(e.g., sluggishness; staring into space; difficult to arouse; little body movement)
f. MENTAL FUNCTION VARIES OVER THE COURSE OF THE DAY—(e.g., sometimes better, sometimes worse; behaviors sometimes present, sometimes not)

C4. MAKING SELF UNDERSTOOD (*Expressing information content—however able*)
0. *UNDERSTOOD*
1. *USUALLY UNDERSTOOD*—difficulty finding words or finishing thoughts
2. *SOMETIMES UNDERSTOOD*—ability is limited to making concrete requests
3. *RARELY/NEVER UNDERSTOOD*

C6. ABILITY TO UNDERSTAND OTHERS (*Understanding verbal information content—however able*)
0. *UNDERSTANDS*
1. *USUALLY UNDERSTANDS*—may miss some part/intent of message
2. *SOMETIMES UNDERSTANDS*—responds adequately to simple, direct communication
3. *RARELY/NEVER UNDERSTANDS*

E1. INDICATORS OF DEPRESSION, ANXIETY, SAD MOOD (***Code for indicators observed in last 30 days, irrespective of the assumed cause***)
0. Indicator not exhibited in last 30 days
1. Indicator of this type exhibited up to five days a week
2. Indicator of this type exhibited daily or almost daily (6, 7 days a week)

E1. INDICATORS OF DEPRESSION, ANXIETY, SAD MOOD (continued)

VERBAL EXPRESSIONS OF DISTRESS
a. Resident made negative statements—e.g., "*Nothing matters; Would rather be dead; What's the use; Regrets having lived so long; Let me die*"
b. Repetitive questions—e.g., "*Where do I go; What do I do?*"
c. Repetitive verbalizations—e.g., calling out for help, ("*God help me*")
d. Persistent anger with self or others—e.g., easily annoyed, anger at placement in nursing home; anger at care received
e. Self deprecation—e.g., "*I am nothing; I am of no use to anyone*"
f. Expressions of what appear to be unrealistic fears—e.g., fear of being abandoned, left alone, being with others
g. Recurrent statements that something terrible is about to happen—e.g., believes he or she is about to die, have a heart attack
h. Repetitive health complaints—e.g., persistently seeks medical attention, obsessive concern with body functions
i. Repetitive anxious complaints/concerns (non-health related) e.g., persistently seeks attention/reassurance regarding schedules, meals, laundry, clothing, relationship issues

SLEEP-CYCLE ISSUES
j. Unpleasant mood in morning
k. Insomnia/change in usual sleep pattern

SAD, APATHETIC, ANXIOUS APPEARANCE
l. Sad, pained, worried facial expressions—e.g., furrowed brows
m. Crying, tearfulness
n. Repetitive physical movements—e.g., pacing, hand wringing, restlessness, fidgeting, picking

LOSS OF INTEREST
o. Withdrawal from activities of interest—e.g., no interest in long standing activities or being with family/friends
p. Reduced social interaction

E2. MOOD PERSISTENCE **One or more indicators** of depressed, sad or anxious mood **were not easily altered by attempts to "cheer up", console, or reassure the resident over last 7 days**
0. No mood indicators 1. Indicators present, easily altered 2. Indicators present, not easily altered

E4. BEHAVIORAL SYMPTOMS
(A) ***Behavioral symptom frequency in last 7 days***
0. Behavior not exhibited in last 7 days
1. Behavior of this type occurred 1 to 3 days in last 7 days
2. Behavior of this type occurred 4 to 6 days, but less than daily
3. Behavior of this type occurred daily

(B) ***Behavioral symptom alterability in last 7 days***
0. Behavior not present OR behavior was easily altered
1. Behavior was not easily altered

	(A)	(B)
a. WANDERING (moved with no rational purpose, seemingly oblivious to needs or safety)		
b. VERBALLY ABUSIVE BEHAVIORAL SYMPTOMS (others were threatened, screamed at, cursed at)		
c. PHYSICALLY ABUSIVE BEHAVIORAL SYMPTOMS (others were hit, shoved, scratched, sexually abused)		
d. SOCIALLY INAPPROPRIATE/DISRUPTIVE BEHAVIORAL SYMPTOMS (made disruptive sounds, noisiness, screaming, self-abusive acts, sexual behavior or disrobing in public, smeared/threw food/feces, hoarding, rummaged through others' belongings)		
e. RESISTS CARE (resisted taking medications/ injections, ADL assistance, or eating)		

G1. (A) ADL SELF-PERFORMANCE—(***Code for resident's PERFORMANCE OVER ALL SHIFTS during last 7 days**—Not including setup*)
0. *INDEPENDENT*—No help or oversight —OR— Help/oversight provided only 1 or 2 times during last 7 days
1. SUPERVISION—Oversight, encouragement or cueing provided 3 or more times during last7 days —OR— Supervision (3 or more times) plus physical assistance provided only 1 or 2 times during last 7 days
2. *LIMITED ASSISTANCE*—Resident highly involved in activity; received physical help in guided maneuvering of limbs or other nonweight bearing assistance 3 or more times —OR—More help provided only 1 or 2 times during last 7 days
3. *EXTENSIVE ASSISTANCE*—While resident performed part of activity, over last 7-day period, help of following type(s) provided 3 or more times:
— Weight-bearing support
— Full staff performance during part (but not all) of last 7 days
4. *TOTAL DEPENDENCE*—Full staff performance of activity during entire 7 days
8. *ACTIVITY DID NOT OCCUR* during entire 7 days

(B) ADL SUPPORT PROVIDED—(***Code for MOST SUPPORT PROVIDED OVER ALL SHIFTS during last 7 days; code regardless** of resident's self-performance classification*)
0. No setup or physical help from staff
1. Setup help only
2. One person physical assist
3. Two+ persons physical assist
8. ADL activity itself did not occur during entire 7 days

			(A) SELF-PERF	(B) SUPPORT
a.	BED MOBILITY	How resident moves to and from lying position, turns side to side, and positions body while in bed		
b.	TRANSFER	How resident moves between surfaces—to/from: bed, chair, wheelchair, standing position (EXCLUDE to/from bath/toilet)		

Resident______________________ Numeric Identifier______________________

G1.			(A)	(B)
c.	WALK IN ROOM	How resident walks between locations in his/her room		
d.	WALK IN CORRIDOR	How resident walks in corridor on unit		
e.	LOCOMOTION ON UNIT	How resident moves between locations in his/her room and adjacent corridor on same floor. If in wheelchair, self-sufficiency once in chair		
f.	LOCOMOTION OFF UNIT	How resident moves to and returns from off unit locations (e.g., areas set aside for dining, activities, or treatments). **If facility has only one floor**, how resident moves to and from distant areas on the floor. If in wheelchair, self-sufficiency once in chair		
g.	DRESSING	How resident puts on, fastens, and takes off all items of **street clothing**, including donning/removing prosthesis		
h.	EATING	How resident eats and drinks (regardless of skill). Includes intake of nourishment by other means (e.g., tube feeding, total parenteral nutrition)		
i.	TOILET USE	How resident uses the toilet room (or commode, bedpan, urinal); transfer on/off toilet, cleanses, changes pad, manages ostomy or catheter, adjusts clothes		
j.	PERSONAL HYGIENE	How resident maintains personal hygiene, including combing hair, brushing teeth, shaving, applying makeup, washing/drying face, hands, and perineum (EXCLUDE baths and showers)		

G2. BATHING — How resident takes full-body bath/shower, sponge bath, and transfers in/out of tub/shower (EXCLUDE washing of back and hair.) ***Code for most dependent** in self-performance.*

(A) BATHING SELF PERFORMANCE codes appear below — (A) ___

0. Independent—No help provided
1. Supervision—Oversight help only
2. Physical help limited to transfer only
3. Physical help in part of bathing activity
4. Total dependence
8. Activity itself did not occur during entire 7 days

G3. TEST FOR BALANCE (see training manual) — *(Code for ability during test in the **last 7 days**)*

0. Maintained position as required in test
1. Unsteady, but able to rebalance self without physical support
2. Partial physical support during test; or stands (sits) but does not follow directions for test
3. Not able to attempt test without physical help

a. Balance while standing ___

b. Balance while sitting—position, trunk control ___

G4. FUNCTIONAL LIMITATION IN RANGE OF MOTION — *(Code for limitations during **last 7 days** that interfered with daily functions or placed residents at risk of injury)*

(A) *RANGE OF MOTION*	(B) *VOLUNTARY MOVEMENT*
0. No limitation	0. No loss
1. Limitation on one side	1. Partial loss
2. Limitation on both sides	2. Full loss

	(A)	(B)
a. Neck		
b. Arm—Including shoulder or elbow		
c. Hand—Including wrist or fingers		
d. Leg—Including hip or knee		
e. Foot—Including ankle or toes		
f. Other limitation or loss		

G6. MODES OF TRANSFER — ***(Check all that apply** during **last 7 days**)*

Bedfast all or most of time	a.	*NONE OF ABOVE*	f.
Bed rails used for bed mobility or transfer	b.		

G7. TASK SEGMENTATION — Some or all of ADL activities were broken into subtasks during last 7 days so that resident could perform them
0. No 1. Yes

H1. CONTINENCE SELF-CONTROL CATEGORIES
(Code for resident's PERFORMANCE OVER ALL SHIFTS)

0. *CONTINENT*—Complete control *[includes use of indwelling urinary catheter or ostomy device that does not leak urine or stool]*
1. *USUALLY CONTINENT*—BLADDER, incontinent episodes once a week or less; BOWEL, less than weekly
2. *OCCASIONALLY INCONTINENT*—BLADDER, 2 or more times a week but not daily; BOWEL, once a week
3. *FREQUENTLY INCONTINENT*—BLADDER, tended to be incontinent daily, but some control present (e.g., on day shift); BOWEL, 2-3 times a week
4. *INCONTINENT*—Had inadequate control BLADDER, multiple daily episodes; BOWEL, all (or almost all) of the time

a.	BOWEL CONTINENCE	Control of bowel movement, with appliance or bowel continence programs, if employed	
b.	BLADDER CONTINENCE	Control of urinary bladder function (if dribbles, volume insufficient to soak through underpants), with appliances (e.g., foley) or continence programs, if employed	

H2. BOWEL ELIMINATION PATTERN

Diarrhea	c.	*NONE OF ABOVE*	e.
Fecal impaction	d.		

H3. APPLIANCES AND PROGRAMS

Any scheduled toileting plan	a.	Indwelling catheter	d.
Bladder retraining program	b.	Ostomy present	i.
External (condom) catheter	c.	*NONE OF ABOVE*	j.

Check only those diseases that have a relationship to current ADL status, cognitive status, mood and behavior status, medical treatments, nursing monitoring, or risk of death. (Do not list inactive diagnoses)

I1. DISEASES — *(If none apply, CHECK the NONE OF ABOVE box)*

MUSCULOSKELETAL		Hemiplegia/Hemiparesis	v.
Hip fracture	m.	Multiple sclerosis	w.
NEUROLOGICAL		**PSYCHIATRIC/MOOD**	
Aphasia	r.	Depression	ee.
Cerebral palsy	s.	Manic depressive (bipolar disease)	ff.
Cerebrovascular accident (stroke)	t.	**OTHER**	
Quadriplegia	z.	*NONE OF ABOVE*	rr.

I2. INFECTIONS — *(If none apply, CHECK the NONE OF ABOVE box)*

Antibiotic resistant infection (e.g., Methicillin resistant staph)	a.	Septicemia	g.
		Sexually transmitted diseases	h.
Clostridium difficile (c. diff.)	b.	Tuberculosis	i.
Conjunctivitis	c.	Urinary tract infection in last 30 days	j.
HIV infection	d.	Viral hepatitis	k.
Pneumonia	e.	Wound infection	l.
Respiratory infection	f.	NONE OF ABOVE	m.

I3. OTHER CURRENT DIAGNOSES AND ICD-9 CODES — *(Include **only those diseases diagnosed in the last 90 days that have a relationship** to current ADL status, cognitive status, mood or behavior status, medical treatments, nursing monitoring, or risk of death)*

a. ______________________ | | | | . | |

b. ______________________ | | | | | |

J1. PROBLEM CONDITIONS — ***(Check all problems present in last 7 days** unless other time frame is indicated)*

INDICATORS OF FLUID STATUS		**OTHER**	
		Delusions	e.
Weight gain or loss of 3 or more pounds within a 7 day period	a.	Edema	g.
		Fever	h.
		Hallucinations	i.
Inability to lie flat due to shortness of breath	b.	Internal bleeding	j.
Dehydrated; output exceeds input	c.	Recurrent lung aspirations in **last 90 days**	k.
		Shortness of breath	l.
Insufficient fluid; did NOT consume all/almost all liquids provided during **last 3 days**	d.	Unsteady gait	n.
		Vomiting	o.
		NONE OF ABOVE	p.

J2. PAIN SYMPTOMS — *(Code the highest level of pain present in the **last 7 days**)*

a. **FREQUENCY** with which resident complains or shows evidence of pain	b. **INTENSITY** of pain
0. No pain (***skip to J4***)	1. Mild pain
1. Pain less than daily	2. Moderate pain
2. Pain daily	3. Times when pain is horrible or excruciating

J4. ACCIDENTS — ***(Check all that apply)***

Fell in **past 30 days**	a.	Hip fracture in **last 180 days**	c.
Fell in **past 31-180 days**	b.	*NONE OF ABOVE*	e.

J5. STABILITY OF CONDITIONS

Conditions/diseases make resident's cognitive, ADL, mood or behavior status unstable—(fluctuating, precarious, or deteriorating)	a.
Resident experiencing an acute episode or a flare-up of a recurrent or chronic problem	b.
End-stage disease, 6 or fewer months to live	c.
NONE OF ABOVE	d.

K1. ORAL PROBLEMS

Chewing problem	a.
Swallowing problem	b.
NONE OF ABOVE	d.

K2. HEIGHT AND WEIGHT — *Record **(a.) height in inches** and **(b.) weight in pounds**. Base weight on most recent measure in **last 30 days**; measure weight consistently in accord with standard facility practice—e.g., in a.m. after voiding, before meal, with shoes off, and in nightclothes*

a. HT (in.) ___ b. WT (lb.) ___

K2. HEIGHT AND WEIGHT — *Record **(a.) height in inches** and **(b.) weight in pounds**. Base weight on most recent measure in **last 30 days**; measure weight consistently in accord with standard facility practice—e.g., in a.m. after voiding, before meal, with shoes off, and in nightclothes*

a. HT (in.) ___ b. WT (lb.) ___

K3. WEIGHT CHANGE — **a. Weight loss**—5 % or more in **last 30 days**; or 10 % or more in **last 180 days**
0. No 1. Yes

Resident________ Numeric Identifier________

K3.	WEIGHT CHANGE	b. Weight gain—5 % or more in last 30 days; or 10 % or more in last 180 days 0. No 1. Yes
K5.	NUTRITIONAL APPROACHES	(*Check all that apply in last 7 days*) Parenteral/IV a. Feeding tube b. On a planned weight change program h. *NONE OF ABOVE* i.
M1.	ULCERS (Due to any cause)	(*Record the number of ulcers at each ulcer stage—regardless of cause. If none present at a stage, record "0" (zero). Code all that apply during last 7 days. Code 9 = 9 or more.) [Requires full body exam.]* Number at Stage a. Stage 1. A persistent area of skin redness (without a break in the skin) that does not disappear when pressure is relieved. b. Stage 2. A partial thickness loss of skin layers that presents clinically as an abrasion, blister, or shallow crater. c. Stage 3. A full thickness of skin is lost, exposing the subcutaneous tissues - presents as a deep crater with or without undermining adjacent tissue. d. Stage 4. A full thickness of skin and subcutaneous tissue is lost, exposing muscle or bone.
M2.	TYPE OF ULCER	(*For each type of ulcer, code for the highest stage in the last 7 days using scale in item M1—i.e., 0=none; stages 1, 2, 3, 4*) a. Pressure ulcer—any lesion caused by pressure resulting in damage of underlying tissue b. Stasis ulcer—open lesion caused by poor circulation in the lower extremities
M4.	OTHER SKIN PROBLEMS OR LESIONS PRESENT	(*Check all that apply during last 7 days*) Abrasions, bruises a. Burns (second or third degree) b. Open lesions other than ulcers, rashes, cuts (e.g., cancer lesions) c. Rashes—e.g., intertrigo, eczema, drug rash, heat rash, herpes zoster d. Skin desensitized to pain or pressure e. Skin tears or cuts (other than surgery) f. Surgical wounds g. *NONE OF ABOVE* h.
M5.	SKIN TREATMENTS	(*Check all that apply during last 7 days*) Pressure relieving device(s) for chair a. Pressure relieving device(s) for bed b. Turning/repositioning program c. Nutrition or hydration intervention to manage skin problems d. Ulcer care e. Surgical wound care f. Application of dressings (with or without topical medications) other than to feet g. Application of ointments/medications (other than to feet) h. Other preventative or protective skin care (other than to feet) i. *NONE OF ABOVE* j.
M6.	FOOT PROBLEMS AND CARE	(*Check all that apply during last 7 days*) Resident has one or more foot problems—e.g., corns, callouses, bunions, hammer toes, overlapping toes, pain, structural problems a. Infection of the foot—e.g., cellulitis, purulent drainage b. Open lesions on the foot c. Nails/calluses trimmed during last 90 days d. Received preventative or protective foot care (e.g., used special shoes, inserts, pads, toe separators) e. Application of dressings (with or without topical medications) f. *NONE OF ABOVE* g.
N1.	TIME AWAKE	(*Check appropriate time periods over last 7 days*) Resident awake all or most of time (i.e., naps no more than one hour per time period) in the: Morning a. Afternoon b. Evening c. *NONE OF ABOVE* d.

(If resident is comatose, skip to Section O)

N2.	AVERAGE TIME INVOLVED IN ACTIVITIES	(When awake and not receiving treatments or ADL care) 0. Most—more than 2/3 of time 1. Some—from 1/3 to 2/3 of time 2. Little—less than 1/3 of time 3. None
O1.	NUMBER OF MEDICATIONS	(*Record the number of different medications used in the last 7 days; enter "0" if none used*)
O3.	INJECTIONS	(*Record the number of DAYS injections of any type received during the last 7 days; enter "0" if none used*)
O4.	DAYS RECEIVED THE FOLLOWING MEDICATION	(*Record the number of DAYS during last 7 days; enter "0" if not used. Note—enter "1" for long-acting meds used less than weekly*) a. Antipsychotic b. Antianxiety c. Antidepressant d. Hypnotic e. Diuretic

P1.	SPECIAL TREATMENTS, PROCEDURES, AND PROGRAMS	a. SPECIAL CARE—*Check treatments or programs received during the last 14 days* **TREATMENTS** Chemotherapy a. Dialysis b. IV medication c. Intake/output d. Monitoring acute medical condition e. Ostomy care f. Oxygen therapy g. Radiation h. Suctioning i. Tracheostomy care j. Transfusions k. Ventilator or respirator l. **PROGRAMS** Alcohol/drug treatment program m. Alzheimer's/dementia special care unit n. Hospice care o. Pediatric unit p. Respite care q. Training in skills required to return to the community (e.g., taking medications, house work, shopping, transportation, ADLs) r. *NONE OF ABOVE* s. b. THERAPIES - *Record the number of days and total minutes each of the following therapies was administered (for at least 15 minutes a day) in the last 7 calendar days (Enter 0 if none or less than 15 min. daily)* **[Note—count only post admission therapies]** (A) = # of days administered for 15 minutes or more — DAYS (A) (B) = total # of minutes provided in last 7 days — MIN (B) a. Speech - language pathology and audiology services b. Occupational therapy c. Physical therapy d. Respiratory therapy e. Psychological therapy (by any licensed mental health professional)
P3.	NURSING REHABILITATION/ RESTORATIVE CARE	*Record the NUMBER OF DAYS each of the following rehabilitation or restorative techniques or practices was provided to the resident for more than or equal to 15 minutes per day in the last 7 days (Enter 0 if none or less than 15 min. daily.)* a. Range of motion (passive) b. Range of motion (active) c. Splint or brace assistance TRAINING AND SKILL PRACTICE IN: d. Bed mobility e. Transfer f. Walking g. Dressing or grooming h. Eating or swallowing i. Amputation/prosthesis care j. Communication k. Other
P4.	DEVICES AND RESTRAINTS	*Use the following codes for last 7 days:* 0. Not used 1. Used less than daily 2. Used daily Bed rails a. — Full bed rails on all open sides of bed b. — Other types of side rails used (e.g., half rail, one side) c. Trunk restraint d. Limb restraint e. Chair prevents rising
P7.	PHYSICIAN VISITS	In the LAST 14 DAYS (or since admission if less than 14 days in facility) how many days has the physician (or authorized assistant or practitioner) examined the resident? (*Enter 0 if none*)
P8.	PHYSICIAN ORDERS	In the LAST 14 DAYS (or since admission if less than 14 days in facility) how many days has the physician (or authorized assistant or practitioner) changed the resident's orders? *Do not include order renewals without change. (Enter 0 if none)*
Q2.	OVERALL CHANGE IN CARE NEEDS	Resident's overall level of self sufficiency has changed significantly as compared to status of 90 days ago (or since last assessment if less than 90 days) 0. No change 1. Improved—receives fewer supports, needs less restrictive level of care 2. Deteriorated—receives more support

R2. SIGNATURES OF PERSONS COMPLETING THE ASSESSMENT:

a. Signature of RN Assessment Coordinator (sign on above line)

b. Date RN Assessment Coordinator signed as complete ☐☐ — ☐☐ — ☐☐☐☐
Month Day Year

	Title	Sections	Date
c. Other Signatures			Date
d.			Date
e.			Date
f.			Date
g.			Date
h.			Date

Numeric Identifier_______________

MINIMUM DATA SET (MDS) — *VERSION 2.0*

FOR NURSING HOME RESIDENT ASSESSMENT AND CARE SCREENING

DISCHARGE TRACKING FORM [*do not use for temporary visits home*]

SECTION AA. IDENTIFICATION INFORMATION

1.	RESIDENT NAME⊙	a. (First) b. (Middle Initial) c. (Last) d. (Jr/Sr)
2.	GENDER⊙	1. Male 2. Female
3.	BIRTHDATE⊙	Month — Day — Year
4.	RACE/ ETHNICITY⊙	1. American Indian/Alaskan Native 2. Asian/Pacific Islander 3. Black, not of Hispanic origin 4. Hispanic 5. White, not of Hispanic origin
5.	SOCIAL SECURITY⊙ AND MEDICARE NUMBERS⊙ [C in 1st box if non med. no.]	a. Social Security Number b. Medicare number (or comparable railroad insurance number)
6.	FACILITY PROVIDER NO.⊙	a. State No. b. Federal No.
7.	MEDICAID NO. [*"+" if pending, "N" if not a Medicaid recipient*]⊙	
8.	REASONS FOR ASSESS-MENT	[Note—Other codes do not apply to this form] a. Primary reason for assessment 6. Discharged—return not anticipated 7. Discharged—return anticipated 8. Discharged prior to completing initial assessment

9. SIGNATURES OF STAFF COMPLETING FORM

a. Signatures	Title	Sections	Date
b.			Date
c.			Date

SECTION AB. DEMOGRAPHIC INFORMATION

[*Complete only for stays less than 14 days*] (AA8a=8)

1.	DATE OF ENTRY	*Date the stay began. Note — Does not include readmission if record was closed at time of temporary discharge to hospital, etc. In such cases, use prior admission date* Month — Day — Year
2.	ADMITTED FROM (AT ENTRY)	1. Private home/apt. with no home health services 2. Private home/apt. with home health services 3. Board and care/assisted living/group home 4. Nursing home 5. Acute care hospital 6. Psychiatric hospital, MR/DD facility 7. Rehabilitation hospital 8. Other

SECTION A. IDENTIFICATION AND BACKGROUND INFORMATION

6.	MEDICAL RECORD NO.	

SECTION R. ASSESSMENT/DISCHARGE INFORMATION

3.	DISCHARGE STATUS	***Skip if not discharged*** *a. Code for resident disposition upon discharge* 1. Private home/apartment with no home health services 2. Private home/apartment with home health services 3. Board and care/assisted living 4. Another nursing facility 5. Acute care hospital 6. Psychiatric hospital, MR/DD facility 7. Rehabilitation hospital 8. Deceased 9. Other b. *Optional State Code*
4.	DISCHARGE DATE	*Date of death or discharge* Month — Day — Year

⊙ = Key items for computerized resident tracking

[ ] = When box blank, must enter number or letter [a.] = When letter in box, check if condition applies

Numeric Identifier_______________

MINIMUM DATA SET (MDS) — *VERSION 2.0*

FOR NURSING HOME RESIDENT ASSESSMENT AND CARE SCREENING

REENTRY TRACKING FORM

SECTION AA. IDENTIFICATION INFORMATION

1.	RESIDENT NAME⊙	a. (First) b. (Middle Initial) c. (Last) d. (Jr/Sr)
2.	GENDER⊙	1. Male 2. Female
3.	BIRTHDATE⊙	Month — Day — Year
4.	RACE/ ETHNICITY⊙	1. American Indian/Alaskan Native 2. Asian/Pacific Islander 3. Black, not of Hispanic origin 4. Hispanic 5. White, not of Hispanic origin
5.	SOCIAL SECURITY⊙ AND MEDICARE NUMBERS⊙ [C in 1st box if non med. no.]	a. Social Security Number b. Medicare number (or comparable railroad insurance number)
6.	FACILITY PROVIDER NO.⊙	a. State No. b. Federal No.
7.	MEDICAID NO. ["+" *if pending*, "N" *if not a Medicaid recipient*]⊙	
8.	REASONS FOR ASSESS-MENT	[Note—Other codes do not apply to this form] a. Primary reason for assessment 9. Reentry
9.	SIGNATURES OF PERSONS COMPLETING FORM	

a. Signatures	Title	Sections	Date
b.			Date
c.			Date

SECTION A. IDENTIFICATION AND BACKGROUND INFORMATION

4a.	DATE OF REENTRY	**Date of reentry** Month — Day — Year
4b.	ADMITTED FROM (AT REENTRY)	1. Private home/apt. with no home health services 2. Private home/apt. with home health services 3. Board and care/assisted living/group home 4. Nursing home 5. Acute care hospital 6. Psychiatric hospital, MR/DD facility 7. Rehabilitation hospital 8. Other
6.	MEDICAL RECORD NO.	

⊙ = Key items for computerized resident tracking

[ ] = When box blank, must enter number or letter [a.] = When letter in box, check if condition applies

APPENDIX C

Resident Assessment Protocols

SECTION V. RESIDENT ASSESSMENT PROTOCOL SUMMARY

Numeric Identifier ____________

Resident's Name:	Medical Record No.:

1. Check if RAP is triggered.
2. For each triggered RAP, use the RAP guidelines to identify areas needing further assessment. Document relevant assessment information regarding the resident's status.
   - Describe:
     — Nature of the condition (may include presence or lack of objective data and subjective complaints).
     — Complications and risk factors that affect your decision to proceed to care planning.
     — Factors that must be considered in developing individualized care plan interventions.
     — Need for referrals/further evaluation by appropriate health professionals.
   - Documentation should support your decision-making regarding whether to proceed with a care plan for a triggered RAP and the type(s) of care plan interventions that are appropriate for a particular resident.
   - Documentation may appear anywhere in the clinical record (e.g., progress notes, consults, flowsheets, etc.).
3. Indicate under the Location of RAP Assessment Documentation column where information related to the RAP assessment can be found.
4. For each triggered RAP, indicate whether a new care plan, care plan revision, or continuation of current care plan is necessary to address the problem(s) identified in your assessment. The Care Planning Decision column must be completed within 7 days of completing the RAI (MDS and RAPs).

A. RAP PROBLEM AREA	(a) Check if triggered	Location and Date of RAP Assessment Documentation	(b) Care Planning Decision—check if addressed in care plan
1. DELIRIUM	☐		☐
2. COGNITIVE LOSS	☐		☐
3. VISUAL FUNCTION	☐		☐
4. COMMUNICATION	☐		☐
5. ADL FUNCTIONAL/ REHABILITATION POTENTIAL	☐		☐
6. URINARY INCONTINENCE AND INDWELLING CATHETER	☐		☐
7. PSYCHOSOCIAL WELL-BEING	☐		☐
8. MOOD STATE	☐		☐
9. BEHAVIORAL SYMPTOMS	☐		☐
10. ACTIVITIES	☐		☐
11. FALLS	☐		☐
12. NUTRITIONAL STATUS	☐		☐
13. FEEDING TUBES	☐		☐
14. DEHYDRATION/FLUID MAINTENANCE	☐		☐
15. DENTAL CARE	☐		☐
16. PRESSURE ULCERS	☐		☐
17. PSYCHOTROPIC DRUG USE	☐		☐
18. PHYSICAL RESTRAINTS	☐		☐

B. ____

1. Signature of RN Coordinator for RAP Assessment Process

2. ☐☐–☐☐–☐☐☐☐ Month Day Year

____

3. Signature of Person Completing Care Planning Decision

4. ☐☐–☐☐–☐☐☐☐ Month Day Year

RESIDENT ASSESSMENT PROTOCOL TRIGGER LEGEND FOR REVISED RAPS (FOR MDS VERSION 2.0)

Key:
● = One item required to trigger
❷ = Two items required to trigger
✱ = One of these three items, plus at least one other item required to trigger
ⓐ = When both ADL triggers present, maintenance takes precedence

Proceed to RAP Review once triggered

MDS ITEM		CODE	Delirium	Cognitive Loss/Dementia	Visual Function	Communication	ADL-Rehabilitation Trigger A ⓐ	ADL-Maintenance Trigger B ⓐ	Urinary Incontinence and Indwelling Catheter	Psychosocial Well-Being	Mood State	Behavioral Symptoms	Activities Trigger A	Activities Trigger B	Falls	Nutritional Status	Feeding Tubes	Dehydration/Fluid Maintenance	Dental Care	Pressure Ulcers	Psychotropic Drug Use	Physical Restraints	
B2a	Short term memory	1		●																			B2a
B2b	Long term memory	1		●																			B2b
B4	Decision making	1,2,3		●																			B4
B4	Decision making	3						●															B4
B5a to B5f	Indicators of delirium	2	●																		●		B5a to B5f
B6	Change in cognitive status	2	●																		●		B6
C1	Hearing	1,2,3				●																	C1
C4	Understood by others	1,2,3				●																	C4
C6	Understand others	1,2,3		●		●																	C6
C7	Change in communication	2																			●		C7
D1	Vision	1,2,3			●																		D1
D2a	Side vision problem	✓			●																		D2a
E1a to E1p	Indicators of depression, anxiety, sad mood	1,2									●												E1a to E1p
E1n	Repetitive movement	1,2																			●		E1n
E1o	Withdrawal from activities	1,2								●													E1o
E2	Mood persistence	1,2									●												E2
E3	Change in Mood	2	●																		●		E3
E4aA	Wandering	1,2,3													●								E4aA
E4aA - E4eA	Behavioral symptoms	1,2,3										●											E4aA - E4eA
E5	Change in behavioral symptoms	1										●											E5
E5	Change in behavioral symptoms	2	●																		●		E5
F1d	Establishes own goals	✓								●													F1d
F2a to F2d	Unsettled relationships	✓								●													F2a to F2d
F3a	Strong id, past roles	✓								●													F3a
F3b	Lost roles	✓								●													F3b
F3c	Daily routine different	✓								●													F3c
G1aA - G1jA	ADL self-performance	1,2,3,4					●																G1aA - G1jA
G1aA	Bed mobility	2,3,4,8																		●			G1aA
G2A	Bathing	1,2,3,4					●																G2A
G3b	Balance while sitting	1,2,3																			●		G3b
G6a	Bedfast	✓																		●			G6a
G8a,b	Resident, staff believe capable	✓					●																G8a,b
H1a	Bowel incontinence	1,2,3,4																		●			H1a
H1b	Bladder incontinence	2,3,4							●														H1b
H2b	Constipation	✓																			●		H2b
H2d	Fecal impaction	✓																			●		H2d
H3c,d,e	Catheter use	✓							●														H3c,d,e
H3g	Use of pads/briefs	✓							●														H3g
I1i	Hypotension	✓																			●		I1i
I1j	Peripheral vascular disease	✓																		●			I1j
I1ee	Depression	✓																			●		I1ee
I1jj	Cataracts	✓			●																		I1jj
I1ll	Glaucoma	✓			●																		I1ll
I2j	UTI	✓																●					I2j
I3	Dehydration diagnosis	276.5																●					I3
J1a	Weight fluctuation	✓																●					J1a
J1c	Dehydrated	✓																●					J1c
J1d	Insufficient fluid	✓																●					J1d
J1f	Dizziness	✓													●						●		J1f
J1h	Fever	✓																●					J1h
J1i	Hallucinations	✓																			●		J1i
J1j	Internal bleeding	✓																●					J1j
J1k	Lung aspirations	✓																			●		J1k
J1m	Syncope	✓																			●		J1m

RESIDENT ASSESSMENT PROTOCOL TRIGGER LEGEND FOR REVISED RAPS (FOR MDS VERSION 2.0)

Key:
- ● = One item required to trigger
- ❷ = Two items required to trigger
- ✱ = One of these three items, plus at least one other item required to trigger
- ⓐ = When both ADL triggers present, maintenance takes precedence

Proceed to RAP Review once triggered

	MDS ITEM	CODE	Delirium	Cognitive Loss/Dementia	Visual Function	Communication	ADL-Rehabilitation Trigger A ⓐ	ADL-Maintenance Trigger B ⓐ	Urinary Incontinence and Indwelling Catheter	Psychosocial Well-Being	Mood State	Behavioral Symptoms	Activities Trigger A	Activities Trigger B	Falls	Nutritional Status	Feeding Tubes	Dehydration/Fluid Maintenance	Dental Care	Pressure Ulcers	Psychotropic Drug Use	Physical Restraints	
J1n	Unsteady gait	✓																			●		J1n
J4a,b	Fell	✓													●						●		J4a,b
J4c	Hip fracture	✓																			●		J4c
K1b	Swallowing problem	✓																			●		K1b
K1c	Mouth pain	✓																	●				K1c
K3a	Weight loss	1														●							K3a
K4a	Taste alteration	✓														●							K4a
K4c	Leave 25% food	✓														●							K4c
K5a	Parenteral/IV feeding	✓														●		●					K5a
K5b	Feeding tube	✓															●	●					K5b
K5c	Mechanically altered	✓														●							K5c
K5d	Syringe feeding	✓														●							K5d
K5e	Therapeutic diet	✓														●							K5e
L1a,c,d,e	Dental	✓																	●				L1a,c,d,e
L1f	Daily cleaning teeth	Not ✓																	●				L1f
M2a	Pressure ulcer	2,3,4														●							M2a
M2a	Pressure ulcer	1,2,3,4																		●			M2a
M3	Previous pressure ulcer	1																		●			M3
M4e	Impaired tactile sense	✓																		●			M4e
N1a	Awake morning	✓												❷									N1a
N2	Involved in activities	0												❷									N2
N2	Involved in activities	2,3											●										N2
N5a,b	Prefers change in daily routine	1,2											●										N5a,b
O4a	Antipsychotics	1-7																			✱		O4a
O4b	Antianxiety	1-7													●						✱		O4b
O4c	Antidepressants	1-7													●						✱		O4c
O4e	Diuretic	1-7																●					O4e
P4c	Trunk restraint	1,2													●							●	P4c
P4c	Trunk restraint	2																		●			P4c
P4d	Limb restraint	1,2																				●	P4d
P4e	Chair prevents rising	1,2																				●	P4e

RESIDENT ASSESSMENT PROTOCOL: DELIRIUM

I. PROBLEM

Delirium (acute confusional state) is a common indicator or nonspecific symptom of a variety of acute, treatable illnesses. It is a serious problem, with high rates of morbidity and mortality, unless it is recognized and treated appropriately. Delirium is never a part of normal aging. Some of the classic signs of delirium may be difficult to recognize and may be mistaken for the natural progression of dementia, particularly in the late stages of dementia when delirium has high mortality. Thus careful observation of the resident and review of potential causes is essential.

Delirium is characterized by fluctuating states of consciousness, disorientation, decreased environmental awareness, and behavioral changes. The onset of delirium may vary, depending on severity of the cause(s) and the resident's health status; however, it usually develops rapidly, over a few days or even hours. Even with successful treatment of cause(s) and associated symptoms, it may take several weeks before cognitive abilities return to pre-delirium status.

Successful management depends on accurate identification of the clinical picture, correct diagnosis of specific cause(s), and prompt nursing and medical intervention. Delirium is often caused and aggravated by multiple factors. Thus, if you identify and address one cause, but delirium continues, you should continue to review the other major causes of delirium and treat any that are found.

II. TRIGGERS

Delirium problem suggested if one or more of following present:

- Easily Distracted[a]
  [B5a = 2]
- Periods of Altered Perception or Awareness of Surroundings[a]
  [B5b = 2]
- Episodes of Disorganized Speech[a]
  [B5c = 2]
- Periods of Restlessness[a]
  [B5d = 2]
- Periods of Lethargy [a]
  [B5e = 2]
- Mental Function Varies Over the Course of the Day [a]
  [B5f = 2]
- Cognitive decline[a]
  [B6 = 2]
- Mood decline[a]
  [E3 = 2]
- Behavior decline[a]
  [E5 = 2]

---

[a] Note: All of these items also trigger on the Psychotropic Drug Use RAP (when psychotropic drug use present).

III. GUIDELINES

Detecting signs and symptoms of delirium requires careful observation. Knowledge of a person's baseline cognitive abilities facilitates evaluation.

- Staff should become familiar with resident's cognitive function by regularly observing the resident in a variety of situations so that even subtle but important changes can be recognized.

When observed in this manner, the presence of any trigger signs/symptoms may be seen as a potential marker for acute, treatable illness.

An approach to detection and treatment of the problem can be selected by reviewing the items that follow in the order presented. Also refer to the RAP KEY for guidance on the MDS items that are relevant.

DIAGNOSES AND CONDITIONS

By correctly identifying the underlying cause(s) of delirium, you may prevent a cycle of worsening symptoms (e.g., an infection-fever-dehydration-confusion syndrome) or a drug regimen for a suspected cause that worsens the condition. The most common causes of delirium are associated with circulatory, respiratory, infectious, and metabolic disorders. However, finding one cause or disorder does not rule out the possibility of additional contributing causes and/or multiple interrelated factors.

MEDICATIONS

Many medications given alone or in combination can cause delirium.

- If necessary, check doctor's order against med sheet and drug labels to avoid the common problem of medication error.
- Review the resident's drug profile with a physician.
- Review all medications (regularly prescribed, PRN, and "over-the-counter" drugs).

Number of medications. The greater the number, the greater the possibility of adverse drug reaction/toxicity.

- Review meds to determine need and benefit (ask if resident is receiving more than one class of a drug to treat a condition).
- Check to determine whether nonpharmacological interventions have been considered (e.g., a behavior management program rather than antipsychotics to address the needs of a resident who has physically or verbally abusive behavioral symptoms).

New medications.

- Review to determine whether there is a temporal relationship between onset or worsening of delirium and start of new medication.

Drugs that cause delirium.

1. PSYCHOTROPIC
   Antipsychotics
   Antianxiety/hypnotics
   Antidepressants
2. CARDIAC
   Digitalis glycosides (Digoxin),
   Antiarrhythmics, such as quinidine, procainamide (Pronestyl), disoprymide (Norpace)
   Calcium channel blockers, such as verapamil (Isoptin),
   nifedipine (Procardia), and diltiazem (Cardizem)
   Antihypertensives, such as methyldopa (Aldomet), propanolol (Inderal)
3. GASTROINTESTINAL
   H2 antagonists such as cimetidine (Tagamet) and ranitidine (Zantac)
4. ANALGESICS such as Darvon, narcotics (e.g., morphine, dilaudid)
5. ANTI-INFLAMMATORY
   Corticosteroids such as prednisone
   Nonsteroidal anti-inflammatory agents such as ibuprofin (Motrin)
6. OVER-THE-COUNTER DRUGS, especially those with anticholinergic properties
   Cold remedies (antihistamines, pseudoephedrine)
   Sedatives (antihistamines, e.g., Benadryl)
   Stay-awakes (caffeine)
   Antinauseants
   Alcohol

PSYCHOSOCIAL

After serious illness and drug toxicity are ruled out as causes of delirium, consider the possibility that the resident is experiencing psychosocial distress that may produce signs of delirium.

Isolation.

- Has the resident been away from people, objects and situations?
- Is resident confused about time, place, and meaning?
- Has the resident been in bed or in an isolated area while recuperating from an illness or receiving a treatment?

Recent loss of family/friend. Loss of someone close can precipitate a grief reaction that presents as acute confusion, especially if the person provided safety and structure for a demented resident.

- Review the MDS to determine whether the resident has experienced a recent loss of a close family member/friend.

Depression/sad or anxious mood. Mood states can lead to confusional states that resolve with appropriate treatment.

- Review the MDS to determine whether the resident exhibits any signs or symptoms of sad or anxious mood or has a diagnosis of a psychiatric illness.

Delirium RAP (3 of 5)

Restraints. Restraints often aggravate the conditions staff are trying to treat (e.g., confusion, agitation, wandering).

- Did the resident become more agitated and confused with their use?

Recent relocation.

- Has the resident recently been admitted to a new environment (new room, unit, facility)?
- Was there an orientation program that provided a calm, gentle approach with reminders and sructure to help the new resident settle into the environment?

SENSORY LOSSES

Sensory impairments often produce signs of confusion and disorientation, as well as behavior changes. This is especially true of residents with early signs of dementia. They can also aggravate a confusional state by impairing the resident's ability to accurately perceive or cope with environmental stimuli (e.g., loud noises; onset of evening). This can lead to the resident experiencing hallucinations/delusions and misinterpreting noises and images.

Hearing.

- Is hearing deficit related to easily remedied situations -- impacted ear wax or hearing aid dysfunction?
- Has sensory deprivation led to confusion?
- Has physician input been sought?

Vision.

- Has vision loss created sensory deprivation resulting in confusion?
- Have major changes occurred in visual function without the resident's being referred to a physician?

CLARIFYING INFORMATION

- Does the resident have a recent sleep disturbance?
- Does the resident have Alzheimer's or other dementia?
- Has the time of onset of the resident's cognitive and behavioral function been within the last few hours to days?

ENVIRONMENT

- Is the resident's environment conducive to reducing symptoms (e.g., quiet, well-lit, calm, familiar objects present)?
- Is the resident's daily routine broken down into smaller tasks (task segmentation) to help him/her cope?

DELIRIUM RAP KEY *(For MDS Version 2.0)*

TRIGGER — REVISION

Delirium problem suggested if one or more of following present:

- Easily Distracted[a]
  [B5a = 2]
- Periods of Altered Perception or Awareness of Surroundings[a]
  [B5b = 2]
- Episodes of Disorganized Speech[a]
  [B5c = 2]
- Periods of Restlessness[a]
  [B5d = 2]
- Periods of Lethargy [a]
  [B5e = 2]
- Mental Function Varies Over the Course of the Day [a]
  [B5f = 2]
- Deterioration in Cognitive Status[a]
  [B6 = 2]
- Deterioration in Mood[a]
  [E3 = 2]
- Deterioration in Behavioral Symptoms[a]
  [E5 = 2]

[a] Note: All of these items also trigger on the Psychotropic Drug Use RAP (when psychotropic drug use is present)

GUIDELINES

Factors that may be associated with signs and symptoms of delirium:

- **Diagnoses and Conditions.** Diabetes **[I1a]**, Hyperthyroidism **[I1b]**, Hypothyroidism **[I1c]**, Cardiac dysrhythmias **[I1e]**, CHF **[I1f]**, CVA **[I1t]**, TIA **[I1bb]**, Asthma **[I1hh]**, Emphysema/COPD **[I1ii]**, Anemia **[I1oo]**, Cancer **[I1pp]**, Dehydration **[J1c]** or Fever **[J1h]**, Myocardial infarction **[I3]**, any viral or bacterial infection **[I2]**, Surgical abdomen **[I3]**, Head trauma **[I3]**, Hypothermia **[I3]**, Hypoglycemia **[I3]**.

- **Medications**. Number of meds **[O1]**, New meds **[O2]**, Antipsychotics **[O4a]**, Antianxiety **[O4b]**, Hypnotics **[O4d]**, Analgesics (Pain meds), Cardiac meds, GI meds, Anti-inflammatory, Anticholinergics, **[from med charts]**.

- **Psychosocial**. Sad or anxious mood **[E1, E2, E3]**, Isolation **[F2e; from record]**, Recent loss **[F2f]**, Depression **[I1ee]**, Restraints **[P4c,d,e]**, Recent relocation **[AB1; A4a]**.

- **Sensory impairment**. Hearing **[C1]**, Vision **[D1]**.

Clarifying information to be considered in establishing a diagnosis: Sleep disturbance **[E1k]**. Alzheimer's **[I1q]**, Other Dementia **[I1u]**, Time of symptom onset within hours to days **[from record or observation]**;

Environment conducive to reducing symptoms: Quiet, well-lit, calm, familiar objects **[from observation]**; Task segmentation **[G7]**.

Delirium RAP Key 5 of 5

RESIDENT ASSESSMENT PROTOCOL: COGNITIVE LOSS/DEMENTIA

I. PROBLEM

Approximately 60% of residents in nursing facilities exhibit signs and symptoms of decline in intellectual functioning. Recovery will be possible for less than 10% of these residents -- those with a reversible condition such as an acute confusional state (delirium). For most residents, however, the syndrome of cognitive loss or dementia is chronic and progressive, and appropriate care focuses on enhancing quality of life, sustaining functional capacities, minimizing decline, and preserving dignity.

Confusion and/or behavioral disturbances present the primary complicating care factors. Identifying and treating acute confusion and behavior problems can facilitate assessment of how chronic cognitive deficits affect the life of the resident.

For residents with chronic cognitive deficits, a therapeutic environment is supportive rather than curative and is an environment in which licensed and nonlicensed care staff are encouraged (and trained) to comprehend a resident's experience of cognitive loss. With this insight, staff can develop care plans focused on three main goals: (1) to provide positive experiences for the resident (e.g., enjoyable activities) that do not involve overly demanding tasks and stress; (2) to define appropriate support roles for each staff member involved in a resident's care; and (3) to lay the foundation for reasonable staff and family expectations concerning a resident's capacities and needs.

II. TRIGGERS

A cognitive loss/dementia problem suggested if one or more of following are present:

- Short-term Memory Problem
  [B2a = 1]
- Long-term Memory Problem
  [B2b =1]
- Impaired Decision-making[a]
  [B4 = 1, 2, 3]
- Problem Understanding Others[(b)]
  [C6 = 1, 2, or 3]

(a) Note: These codes also trigger on the Communication RAP.
(b) Note: Code 3 also triggers on the ADL (Maintenance) RAP.

III. GUIDELINES

Review the following MDS items to investigate possible links between these factors and the resident's cognitive loss and quality of life. The four triggers identify residents with differing levels of cognitive loss. Even for those who are most highly impaired, the RAP seeks to help identify areas in which staff intervention might be useful. Refer to the RAP KEY for specific MDS and other specific issues to consider.

NEUROLOGICAL

Fluctuating Cognitive Signs and Symptoms/Neurological Status. Co-existing delirium and progressive cognitive loss can result in erroneous impressions concerning the nature of the resident's chronic limitations. Only when acute confusion and behavioral disturbances are treated, or when the treatment effort is judged to be as effective as possible, can a true measure of chronic cognitive deficits be obtained.

Recent Changes in the Signs/Symptoms of the Dementia Process. Identifying these changes can heighten staff awareness of the nature of the resident's cognitive and functional limitations. This knowledge can assist staff in developing reasonable expectations of the resident's capabilities and in designing programs to enhance the resident's quality of life. This knowledge can also challenge staff to identify potentially reversible causes for recent losses in cognitive status.

Mental Retardation, Alzheimer's Disease, and Other Adult-Onset Dementias. The most prevalent neurological diagnoses for cognitively impaired residents are Alzheimer's disease and multi-infarct dementia. But increasing numbers of mentally retarded residents are in nursing facilities, and many adults suffering from Down's syndrome appear to develop dementia as they age. The diagnostic distinctions among these groups can be useful in reminding staff of the types of long-term intellectual reserves that are available to these residents.

MOOD/BEHAVIOR

Specific treatments for behavioral distress as well as treatments for delirium, can lessen and even cure the behavioral problem. At the same time, however, some behavior problems will not be reversible, and staff should be prepared (and encouraged) to learn to live with their manifestations. In some situations where problem/distressed behavior continues, staff may feel that the behavior poses no threat to the resident's safety, health, or activity pattern and is not disruptive to other residents. For the resident with declining cognitive functions and a behavioral problem, you may wish to consider the following issues:

- Have cognitive skills declined subsequent to initiation of a behavior control program (e.g., psychotropic drugs or physical restraints)?
- Is decline due to the treatment program (e.g., drug toxicity or negative reaction to physical restraints)?
- Have cognitive skills improved subsequent to initiation of a behavior control program?
- Has staff assistance enhanced resident self-performance patterns?

CONCURRENT MEDICAL PROBLEMS

Major Concurrent Medical Problems. Identifying and treating health problems can positively affect cognitive functioning and the resident's quality of life. Effective therapy for congestive heart failure, chronic obstructive pulmonary disease, and constipation can lead, for example, to functional and cognitive improvement. Comfort (pain avoidance) is a paramount goal in controlling both acute and chronic conditions for cognitively impaired residents. Verbal reports from residents should be one (but not the only) source of information. Some residents will be unable to communicate sufficiently to pinpoint their pain.

FAILURE TO THRIVE

Cognitively impaired residents can reach the point where their accumulated health/neurological problems place them at risk of clinical complications (e.g., pressure ulcers) and death. As this level of disability approaches, staff can review the following:

- Do emotional, social, and/or environmental factors play a key role?
- If a resident is not eating, is this due to a reversible mood problem, a basic personality problem, a negative reaction to the physical and interactive environment in which eating activity occurs; or a neurological deficit such as deficiency in swallowing or loss of hand coordination?
- Could an identified problem be remedied through improved staff education -- trying an antidepressant medication, referral to OT for training or an innovative counseling program?
- If causes cannot be identified, what reversible clinical complication can be expected as death approaches (e.g., fecal impaction, UTI, diarrhea, fever, pain, pressure ulcers)?
- What interventions are or could be in place to decrease complications?

FUNCTIONAL LIMITATIONS

Extent and Rate of Change of Resident Functional Abilities. Functional changes are often the first concrete indicators of cognitive decline and suggest the need to identify reversible causes. You may find it helpful to determine the following:

- To what extent is resident dependent for locomotion, dressing and eating?
- Could the resident be more independent?
- Is resident going downhill (e.g., experiencing declines in bladder continence, locomotion, dressing, vision, time involved in activities)?

SENSORY IMPAIRMENTS

Perceptual Difficulties. Many cognitively impaired residents have difficulty identifying small objects, positioning a plate to eat, or positioning the body to sit in a chair. Such difficulties can cause a resident to become cautious and ultimately cease to carry out everyday activities. If problems are vision-based, corrective programs may be effective. Unfortunately, many residents have difficulty indicating that the source of their problem is visual. Thus, the cognitively impaired can often benefit if tested for possible visual deficits.

Ability to Communicate. Many individuals suffering from cognitive deficits seem incapable of meaningful communication. However, many of the seemingly incomprehensible behaviors (e.g., screaming, aggressive behavior) in which these individuals engage may constitute their only form of communication. By observing the behavior and the pattern of its occurrence, one can frequently come to some understanding of the needs of individuals with dementia. For example, residents who are restrained for their own safety may become noisy due to bladder or bowel urgency.

- Is resident willing/able to engage in meaningful communication?
- Does staff use non-verbal communication techniques (e.g., touch, gesture) to encourage resident to respond?

MEDICATIONS

Psychoactive and other medications can be a factor in cognitive decline. If necessary, review Psychotropic Drug Use RAP.

INVOLVEMENT FACTORS

Opportunities for Independent Activity. Staff can encourage residents to participate in the many available activities, and staff can guard against assuming an overly protective attitude toward residents. ***Decline in one functional area does not indicate the need for staff to assume full responsibility in that area nor should it be interpreted as an indication of inevitable decline in other areas.*** Review information in the MDS when considering the following issues:

- Are there factors that suggest that the resident can be more involved in his/her care (e.g., instances of greater self-performance; desire to do more independently; retained ability to learn; retained control over trunk, limbs, and/or hands)?
- Can resident participate more extensively in decisions about daily life?
- Does resident retain any cognitive ability that permits some decision making?
- Is resident passive?
- Does resident resist care?
- Are activities broken into manageable subtasks?

Extent of Involvement in Activities of Daily Life. Programs focused on physical aspects of the resident's life can lessen the disruptive symptoms of cognitive decline for some residents. Consider the following:

- Are residents with some cognitive skills and without major behavioral problems involved in the life of the facility and the world around them?
- Can modifying task demands, or the environmental circumstances under which tasks are carried out, be beneficial?
- Are small group programs encouraged?
- Are special environmental stimuli present (e.g., directional markers, special lighting)?
- Do staff regularly assist residents in ways that permit them to maintain or attain their highest predictable level of functioning (e.g., verbal reminders, physical cues and supervision regularly provided to aid in carrying out ADLs; ADL tasks presented in segments to give residents enough time to respond to cues; pleasant, supportive interaction)?
- Has the resident experienced a recent loss of someone close (e.g., death of spouse, change in key direct care staff, recent move to the nursing facility, decreased visiting by family and friends)?

COGNITIVE LOSS/DEMENTIA RAP KEY *(For MDS Version 2.0)*

TRIGGER — REVISION

A cognitive loss/dementia problem suggested if one or more of following are present:

- Short-term Memory Problem **[B2a = 1]**
- Long-term Memory Problem **[B2b =1]**
- Impaired Decision-making[(a)] **[B4 = 1, 2, 3]**
- Problem Understanding Others[(b)] **[C6 = 1, 2, or 3]**

(a) Note: Code B4=3 also triggers on the ADL (Maintenance) RAP

(b) Note: These codes also trigger on the Communication RAP.

GUIDELINES

Factors to review for relationship to cognitive loss:

- **Neurological**. MR/DD status **[AB10]**, Delirium **[B5]**, Cognitive decline **[B6]**, Alzheimer's or other dementias **[I1q,I1u]**,

Confounding Problems that may require resolution or suggest reversible causes:

- **Mood/behavior**. Depression, Anxiety, Sad mood or Mood decline **[E1, E2, E3]**, Behavioral symptoms or behavioral decline **[E4, E5]**, Anxiety disorder **[I1dd]**, Depression **[I1ee]**, Manic depressive disorder **[I1ff]**, Other psychiatric disorders **[I1gg, J1e, J1i]**.
- **Concurrent medical problems**. Constipation **[H2b]**, Diarrhea **[H2c]**, Fecal impaction **[H2d]**, Diabetes **[I1a]**, Hypothyroidism **[I1c]**, CHF **[I1f]**, Other cardiovascular disease **[I1k]**, Asthma **[I1hh]**, Emphysema/COPD **[I1ii]**, Cancer **[I1pp]**, UTI **[I2j]**, Pain **[J2]**.
- **Failure to thrive**. Terminal prognosis **[J5c]**, Low weight for height **[K2a,b]**, Weight Loss **[K3a]**, Resident status deteriorated since last assessment **[Q2]**.
- **Functional limitations**. ADL impairment **[G1]**, ADL task segmentation **[G7]**, Decline in ADL **[G9]**, Decline in continence **[H4]**.
- **Sensory impairment**. Hearing problems **[C1]**, Speech unclear **[C5]**, Rarely/never understands **[C6]**, Visual problems **[D1]**, Skin desensitized to pain/pressure **[M4e]**.
- **Medications**. Antipsychotics **[O4a]**, Antianxiety **[O4b]**, Antidepressants **[O4c]**, Diuretics **[O4e]**.
- **Involvement factors**. New admission **[AB1]**, Withdrawal from activities **[E1o]**, Participates in small group activities **[F1f, N3b, record]**, Staff/resident believe resident can do more **[G8a,b]**, Trunk, limb or chair restraint **[P4c,d,e]**.

RESIDENT ASSESSMENT PROTOCOL: VISUAL FUNCTION

I. PROBLEM

The aging process leads to a gradual decline in visual acuity: a decreased ability to focus on close objects or to see small print, a reduced capacity to adjust to changes in light and dark, and diminished ability to discriminate color. The aged eye requires about 3-4 times more light in order to see well than the young eye.

The leading causes of visual impairment in the elderly are macular degeneration, cataracts, glaucoma, and diabetic retinopathy. In addition, visual perceptual deficits (impaired perceptions of the relationship of objects in the environment) are common in the nursing home population. Such deficits are common consequence of cerebrovascular events and are often seen in the late stages of Alzheimer's disease and other dementias. The incidence of all these problems increases with age.

In 1974, 49% of all nursing home residents were described as being unable to see well enough to read a newspaper with or without glasses. In 1985, over 100,000 nursing home residents were estimated to have severe visual impairment or no vision at all. Thus vision loss is one the most prevalent losses of residents in nursing facilities. A significant number of residents in any facility may be expected to have difficulty performing tasks dependent on vision as well as problems adjusting to vision loss.

The consequences of vision loss are wide-ranging and can seriously affect physical safety, self-image, and participation in social, personal, self-care, and rehabilitation activities. This RAP is primarily concerned with identifying two types of residents: 1) Those who have treatable conditions that place them at risk of permanent blindness (e.g., Glaucoma: Diabetes, retinal hemorrhage); and 2) those who have impaired vision whose quality of life could be improved through use of appropriate visual appliances. Further, the assumption is made that residents with new acute conditions will have been referred to follow-up as the conditions were identified (e.g., sudden loss of vision; recent red eye; shingles; etc). To the extent that this did not occur, the RAP KEY follow-up questions will cause staff to ask whether such a referral should be considered.

II. TRIGGERS

An acute, reversible (R) visual function problem or the potential for visual improvement (I) suggested if one or more of following present:

- *Side Vision Problem (Reverse)*
  [D2a = checked]
- Cataracts (*Reverse*)
  [I1jj = checked]
- Glaucoma (*Reverse*)
  [I1ll = checked]
- Vision Impaired (*Improve*)
  [D1 = 1, 2, 3]

III. GUIDELINES

Visual impairment may be related to many causes, and one purpose of this section is to screen for the presence of major risk factors and to review the resident's recent treatment history. This section also includes items that ask whether the visually impaired resident desires or has a need for increased functional use of eyes.

Eye medications: Of greatest importance is the review of medications related to glaucoma (phospholine iodide, pilocarpine, propine, epinephrine, Timoptic or other Beta-Blockers, diamox, or Neptazane).

- Is the residents receiving his/her eye medication as ordered?
- Does the resident experience any side effects?

Diabetes, Cataracts, Glaucoma, or Macular Degeneration: Diabetes may affect the eye by causing blood vessels in the retina to hemorrhage (retinopathy). All these conditions are associated with decreased visual acuity and visual field deficits. If resident is able to cooperate it is very possible to test for glaucoma and retinal problems.

Exam by ophthalmologist or optometrist since problem noted:

- Has the resident been seen by a consultant?
- Have the recommendations been followed (e.g. medications, refraction [new glasses], surgery)?
- Is the recommendation compatible with the resident's wishes (e.g., medical rehab. vs. surgery)?

If neurological diagnosis or dementia exam by physician since problem noted: Check the medical record to see if a physician has examined the resident for visual/perceptual difficulties. Some residents with diseases such as myethenia gravis, stroke, and dementia will have such difficulties associated with central nervous system in the absence of diseases of the eye.

Sad or anxious mood: Some residents, especially those in a new environment, will complain of visual difficulties. Visual disorganization may improve with treatment of the sad or anxious mood.

Appropriate use of visual appliances: Residents may have more severe visual impairment when they do not use their eyeglasses. Residents who wear reading glasses when walking, for example, may misperceive their environment and bump into objects or fall.

- Are glasses labelled or color coded in a fashion that enables the resident/staff to determine when they should be used?
- Are the lenses of glasses clean and free of scratches?
- Were glasses recently lost? Were they being recently used, and now they are missing?

Functional need for eye exam/new glasses: Many residents with limited vision will be able to use the environment with little or no difficulty, and neither the resident nor staff will perceive the need for new visual appliances. In other circumstances, needs will be identified, and for residents who are capable of participating in a visual exam, new appliances, surgery to remove cataracts, etc., can be considered.

Visual Function RAP (2 of 4)

- Does resident have peripheral vision or other visual problem that impedes his/her ability to eat food, walk on the unit, or interact with others?
- Is residents's ability to recognize staff limited by a visual problem?
- If resident is having difficulty negotiating his environment or participating in self-care activities because of visual impairment has he/she been referred to low vision services?
- Does resident report difficulty seeing TV/reading material of interest?
- Does resident express interest in improved vision?
- Has resident refused to have eyes examined? How long ago did this occur? Has it occurred more than once?

Environmental modifications: Residents whose vision cannot be improved by refraction, or medical and/or surgical intervention may benefit from environmental modifications.

- Does the resident's environment enable maximum visual function (e.g., low-glare floors and table surfaces, night lights)?
- Has the environment been adapted to resident's individual needs (e.g., large print signs marking room, color coded tape on dresser drawers, large numbers on telephone, reading lamp with 300 watt bulb)? Could the resident be more independent with different visual cues (e.g., labeling items, task segmentation) or other sensory cues (e.g., cane for recognizing there are objects in path)?

Acute Problems that may have been missed: Eye pain, blurry vision, double vision, sudden loss of vision: These symptoms are usually associated with acute eye problems.

- Has resident been evaluated by a physician or ophthalmologist?

Residents with communication impairments may be very difficult to assess. Residents who are unable to understand others may have problems following the directions necessary to test visual acuity.

VISUAL FUNCTION RAP KEY *(For MDS Version 2.0)*

TRIGGER — REVISION

An acute, reversible visual function problem or the potential for visual improvement suggested if one or more of following present:

- Side Vision Problem (*Reverse*)
  [D2a = checked]
- Cataracts (*Reverse*)
  [I1jj = checked]
- Glaucoma (*Reverse*)
  [I1ll = checked]
- Vision Impaired (*Improve*)
  [D1 = 1, 2, 3]

GUIDELINES

Issues and problems to be reviewed that may suggest need for intervention:

- Eye medications **[from record]**.
- Diabetes **[I1a]**, Cataracts **[I1jj]**, Glaucoma **[I1ll]**, Macular Degeneration **[I1mm]**.
- Exam by ophthalmologist since problem noted **[from record]**.
- Neurological diagnosis or dementia **[I1q to I1cc]**.
- Indicators of Depression, Anxiety, Sad Mood **[E1]**.
- Appropriate use of visual appliances **[D3; from record, observation]**.
- Functional need for eye exam/new glasses **[from observation]**.
- Environmental modifications **[from record, observation]**.
- Other acute problems: Eye pain, blurry vision, double vision, sudden loss of vision **[from record, observation]**.

Visual Function RAP Key 4 of 4

RESIDENT ASSESSMENT PROTOCOL: COMMUNICATION

I. PROBLEM

Good communication enables residents to express emotion, listen to others, and share information. It also eases adjustment to a strange environment and lessens social isolation and depression.

EXPRESSIVE communication problems include changes/difficulties in: speech and voice production, finding appropriate words, transmitting coherent statements, describing objects and events, using nonverbal symbols (e.g., gestures), and writing. RECEPTIVE communication problems include changes/difficulties in: hearing, speech discrimination in quiet and noisy situations, vocabulary comprehension, vision, reading, and interpreting facial expressions.

When communication is limited, assessment focuses on reviewing several factors: underlying causes of the deficit, the success of attempted remedial actions, the resident's ability to compensate with nonverbal strategies (e.g., ability to visually observe nonverbal signs and signals), and the willingness and ability of staff to engage with residents to ensure effective communication. As language use recedes with dementia, both the staff and the resident must expand their nonverbal communication skills -- one of the most basic and automatic of human abilities. Touch, facial expression, eye contact, tone of voice, and posture all are powerful means of communicating with the demented resident, and recognizing and using all practical means is the key to effective communication.

II. TRIGGERS

Potential for improved communication suggested if one or more of following present:

- Hearing problem
  [C1 = 1, 2, 3]
- Problem making self understood*
  [C4 = 1, 2, 3]
- Problem understanding others
  [C6 = 1, 2, 3]

---

* Note: These codes also trigger on the Cognitive Loss/Dementia RAP.

III. GUIDELINES

The communication trigger suggests residents for whom a corrective communication treatment program may be beneficial. Specify those residents with potentially correctable problems. An effective review requires a special effort by staff to overcome any preconceived notions or fixed perceptions they may have about the resident's probable responsiveness to treatment. These perceptions may be based on the failure of prior treatment programs, as well as on assumptions that may not have been recently tested about the resident's unwillingness to begin a corrective program.

Review items listed on the RAP KEY as follows:

Confounding Problems.

As these confounding problems lessen or further decline is prevented, the resident's communication abilities should be reviewed .

Components of Communication.

Details of resident strengths and weaknesses in understanding, hearing, and expression are the direct or indirect focus of any treatment program.

Factors to be Reviewed for Possible Relationship to Communication Problems:

- For chronic conditions that are unlikely to improve, consider communication treatments or interventions that might compensate for losses (e.g., for moderately impaired residents with Alzheimer's, the use of short, direct phrases and tactile approaches to communication can be effective).
- Are there acute or transitory conditions which if successfully resolved may result in improved ability to communicate?
- Are medications in use that could cause or complicate communication deficits, where titration or substitution may result in improved ability to communicate?
- Are opportunities to communicate limited in ways that could be remedied -- e.g., availability of partners?

Clarifying Issues:
Treatment/Evaluation History.

- Has resident received an evaluation by an audiologist or speech-language pathologist? How recently?
- Has the resident's condition deteriorated since the most recent evaluation?
- If such an evaluation resulted in a plan of care, has it been followed as specified?

COMMUNICATION RAP KEY *(For MDS Version 2.0)*

TRIGGER — REVISION

Potential for improved communication suggested if one or more of following present:

- Hearing problem
  [C1 = 1, 2, 3]
- Problem making self understood
  [C4 = 1, 2, 3]
- Problem understanding others*
  [C6 = 1, 2, 3]

* Note: These codes also trigger on the Cognitive Loss/Dementia RAP.

GUIDELINES

Confounding problems that may require resolution:

- Decline in cognitive status **[B6]**
- Increased mood problems **[E3]**
- Decline in ADL status **[G9]**

Components of communication to be considered:

- Hearing **[C1]**
- Communication devices/Modes of expression **[C2, C3]**
- Decline in communication/hearing **[C7]**
- Medical status of ear — discharges, cerumen accumulation, hearing changes **[from record or exam]**
- Vision **[D1]**

Factors to be reviewed for possible relationship to communication problems:

- **Chronic Conditions.** Alzheimer's or Other dementia **[I1q, I1u]**, Aphasia **[I1r]**, CVA **[I1t]**, Parkinson's **[I1y]**, Psychiatric disorders **[I1dd to I1gg]**, Asthma **[I1hh]**, Emphysema/COPD **[I1ii]**, Cancer **[I1pp]**,
- **Transitory Conditions**. Delirium **[B5]**, Infections **[I2]**, Acute episode **[J5b]**
- **Medications**. Psychotropic **[04a-d]**, Narcotics, Parkinson's meds, Gentamycin, Tobramycin, Aspirin toxicity **[from record]**
- **Opportunities to Communicate.** Quality/quantity of communication is (or is not) commensurate with apparent ability to communicate **[staff judgement]**

Clarifying issues to be considered:

- Memory **[B2, B3]**
- Recent audiology/language pathology evaluation **[P1ba; from record]**
- Resident's condition deteriorated since last assessment **[Q2]**

Communication RAP Key 3 of 3

RESIDENT ASSESSMENT PROTOCOL: ACTIVITIES OF DAILY LIVING — FUNCTIONAL REHABILITATION POTENTIAL

I. PROBLEM

Personal mastery of ADL and mobility are as crucial to human existence in the nursing home as they are in the community. The nursing home is unique only in that most residents require help with self-care functions. ADL dependence can lead to intense personal distress -- invalidism, isolation, diminished self-worth, and a loss of control over one's destiny. As inactivity increases, complications such as pressure ulcers, falls, contractures, and muscle-wasting can be expected.

The ADL RAP assists staff in setting positive and realistic goals, weighing the advantages of independence against risks to safety and self-identity. In promoting independence staff must be willing to accept a reasonable degree of risk and active resident participation in setting treatment objectives.

Rehabilitative goals of several types can be considered:

- To restore function to maximum self-sufficiency in the area indicated;
- To replace hands-on assistance with a program of task segmentation and verbal cueing;
- To restore abilities to a level that allows the resident to function with fewer supports;
- To shorten the time required for providing assistance;
- To expand the amount of space in which self-sufficiency can be practiced;
- To avoid or delay additional loss of independence; and
- To support the resident who is certain to decline in order to lessen the likelihood of complications (e.g., pressure ulcers and contractures).

II. TRIGGERS

The two MDS trigger categories (A and B) suggest the types of residents for whom special care interventions may be most important. Such residents may have either the need and potential to improve (Rehabilitation) or the need for services to prevent decline (Maintenance).

ADL TRIGGER A (Rehabilitation)

Rehabilitation/restorative plans suggested if one or more of following present:

- Bed Mobility — not independent
  [G1aA = 1-4][(a)]
- Transfer — not independent
  [G1bA = 1-4]
- Walk in room -- not independent
  [G1cA = 1-4]
- Walk in corridor -- not independent
  [G1dA = 1-4]
- Locomotion on unit — not independent
  [G1eA = 1-4]
- Locomotion off unit — not independent
  [G1fA = 1-4]

- Dressing — not independent
  [G1gA = 1-4]
- Eating - not independent
  [G1hA = 1-4]
- Toilet Use — not independent
  [G1iA = 1-4]
- Personal Hygiene — not independent
  [G1jA = 1-4]
- Bathing — not independent
  [G2aA = 1-4]
- Resident believes he/she capable of increased independence in at least some ADLs
  [G8a = checked]
- Staff believe resident capable of increased independence in at least some ADLs
  [G8b = checked]

ADL TRIGGER B (Maintenance)

Maintenance/complication avoidance plan suggested if: [Note – when both triggers present (A & B), B takes precedence in the RAP Review]

- No ability to make decisions
  [B4 = 3][(b)]

(a) Note: Codes 2,3, and 4 also trigger on the Pressure Ulcer RAP
(b) Note: This code also triggers on the Cognitive Loss/Dementia RAP

III. GUIDELINES

Base an approach to a resident's ADL difficulty on clinical knowledge of:

- The causes of dependence;
- The expected course of the problem(s); and
- Which services work or do not work.

The MDS goal is to assist the clinician in identifying residents for whom rehabilitative/restorative goals can be reasonably established. Many ADL-restricted residents can regain partial ability for self-care. Certain types of disease-generated losses will respond to therapy. In addition, the removal of inappropriate restraints and the close monitoring of potentially toxic medications can often result in increased functioning.

Use the items in the ADL RAP KEY to consider the resident's risk of decline and chance of rehabilitation. Responses to these items permit a focused approach to specific ADL deficits (i.e., selecting and describing the specific ADL areas where decline has been observed or improvement is possible). The first thing that needs to be considered is the possible presence of ***confounding problems*** that may require resolution before rehabilitation goals can be reasonably attempted.

The second task is to clarify the resident's potential for improved functioning. The clinician might find the following sequence of questions useful in initiating an evaluation:

- Does the resident have the ability to learn? To what extent can the resident call on past memory to assist in current problem-solving situations?
- What is the resident's general functional status? How disabled is the resident, and does status vary?
- Is mobility severely impaired?
- Is trunk, leg, arm and/or hand use severely impaired?
- Are there distinct behavioral problems?

- Are there distinct mood problems?
- Is the resident motivated to work at a rehabilitative program?

Where rehabilitation goals are envisioned, use of the ***ADL Supplement*** will help care planners to focus on those areas that might be improved, allowing them to choose from among a number of basic tasks in designated areas. Part 1 of the Supplement can assist in the evaluation of all residents triggered into the RAP. Part 2 of the Supplement can be helpful for residents with rehabilitation potential (ADL Trigger A), to help plan a treatment program.

ADL Supplement (Attaining maximum possible independence).

ADL SUPPLEMENT
(Attaining maximum possible Independence)

PART 1: ADL Problem Evaluation INSTRUCTIONS: For those triggered— In areas physical help provided, indicate reason(s) for this help.	DRESSING	BATHING	TOILETING	LOCOMOTION	TRANSFER	EATING
Mental Errors: Sequencing problems, incomplete performance, anxiety limitations, etc. **Physical Limitations:** Weakness, limited range of motion, poor coordination, visual impairment, pain, etc. **Facility Conditions:** Policies, rules, physical layout, etc.						

PART 2: Possible ADL Goals If wheelchair check: ☐

INSTRUCTIONS:
For those considered for rehabilitation or decline prevention treatment—

Indicate specific type of ADL activity that might require:

1. Maintenance to prevent decline.
2. Treatment to achieve highest practical self sufficiency (selecting ADL abilities that are just above those the resident can now perform or participate in).

Dressing	Bathing	Toileting	Locomotion	Transfer	Eating
Locates/ selects/ obtains clothes	Goes to tub/ shower	Goes to toilet (include commode/ urinal at night)	Walks in room/ nearby ☐	Positions self in preparation	Opens/ pours/ unwraps/ cuts etc.
Grasps/puts on upper/ lower body	Turns on water/ adjusts temperature	Removes/ opens clothes in preparation	Walks on unit ☐	Approaches chair/bed	Grasps utensils and cups
Manages snaps, zippers, etc.	Lathers body (except back)	Transfers/ positions self	Walks throughout building (uses elevator) ☐	Prepares chair/bed (locks pad, moves covers)	Scoops/ spears food (uses fingers when necessary)
Puts on in correct order	Rinses body	Eliminates into toilet	Walks outdoors ☐	Transfers (stands/sits/ lifts/turns)	Chews, drinks, swallows
Grasps, removes each item	Dries with towel	Tears/uses paper to clean self	Walks on uneven surfaces ☐	Repositions/ arranges self	Repeats until food consumed
Replaces clothes properly	Other	Flushes	Other ☐	Other	Uses napkins, cleans self
Other		Adjusts clothes, washes hands			Other

ADL FUNCTIONAL/REHABILITATION POTENTIAL RAP KEY

(For MDS Version 2.0)

TRIGGER — REVISION

ADL TRIGGER A (Rehabilitation)

Rehabilitation/restorative plans suggested if one or more of following present:

- Bed Mobility — not independent **[G1aA = 1-4]**[a]
- Transfer — not independent **[G1bA = 1-4]**
- Walk in room -- not independent **[G1cA = 1-4]**
- Walk in corridor -- not independent **[G1dA = 1-4]**
- Locomotion on unit — not independent **[G1eA = 1-4]**
- Locomotion off unit — not independent **[G1fA = 1-4]**
- Dressing — not independent **[G1gA = 1-4]**
- Eating - not independent **[G1hA = 1-4]**
- Toilet Use — not independent **[G1iA = 1-4]**
- Personal Hygiene — not independent **[G1jA = 1-4]**
- Bathing — not independent **[G2A = 1-4]**
- Resident believes he/she capable of increased independence in at least some ADLs **[G8a = checked]**
- Staff believe resident capable of increased independence in at least some ADLs **[G8b = checked]**

ADL TRIGGER B (Maintenance)

Maintenance/complication avoidance plan suggested if: [Note -- when both triggers present (A & B), B takes precedence in the RAP Review]

- Severely impaired decision making **[B4 = 3]**[b]

(a) Note: Codes 2,3, and 4 also trigger on the Pressure Ulcer RAP

(b) Note: This code also triggers on the Cognitive Loss/Dementia RAP

GUIDELINES

Confounding problems that may require resolution:

- Delirium **[B5]**
- Persistent mood problem **[E2]**
- Decline in mood **[E3]**
- Daily behavioral symptoms **[E4]**
- Decline in behavior **[E5]**
- Unstable/acute health problem **[J5a,b]**
- Use of Psychoactive medications **[O4a,b,c,d]**
- Resident status deteriorated since last assessment **[Q2]**

Clarifying issues to be considered:

- Ability to make decisions **[B4]**
- Prior improvement in cognition, mood, behavior, or ADLs **[B6; E3, E5; G9]**
- Communication **[C]**
- Vision **[D]**
- Test for balance, functional limitation in range of motion **[G3, G4]**.

Complete ADL Supplement Part 1 for all triggered residents (see RAI Training Manual).

For a resident with rehabilitation potential, complete ADL Supplement Part 2 (see RAI Training Manual).

- Staff/resident believe resident could be more independent **[G8a,b]**

ADL/Rehabilitation Potential RAP Key 5 of 5

RESIDENT ASSESSMENT PROTOCOL: URINARY INCONTINENCE AND INDWELLING CATHETER

I. PROBLEM

Urinary incontinence is the inability to control urination in a socially appropriate manner. Nationally, 50% of nursing home residents are incontinent. Incontinence causes many problems, including skin rashes, falls, isolation, and pressure ulcers, and the potentially troubling use of indwelling catheters. In addition, continence is often an important goal to many residents, and incontinence may affect residents' psychological well-being and social interactions. Urinary incontinence is curable in many elderly residents but realistically not all will benefit from an evaluation. Catheter use increases the risk of life-threatening infections, bladder stones and cancer. Use of catheters also contributes to patient discomfort and the needless use of toxic medications often required to treat the associated bladder spasms. For many (but not all) residents, urinary incontinence is curable, and safer and more comfortable approaches are often practical for residents with indwelling catheters.

This RAP, the purpose of which is to improve incontinence, goes far beyond bladder training. Even if a patient is not believed to be a candidate for bladder training, the assessment should still be done since many other treatable conditions may be found, the treatment of which will not only improve incontinence, but the overall quality of life for the patient.

The goal of this assessment is to detect reversible causes of incontinence, such as infections and medications, and situationally induced incontinence; to identify individuals whose incontinence is caused by harmful conditions such as bladder tumors or spinal cord diseases; and to consider the appropriateness of catheter use. Staff judgment is clearly required to realize these aims. Detailed instructions are provided to facilitate this clinical process.

Continence depends on many factors. Urinary tract factors include a bladder that can store and expel urine and a urethra that can close and open appropriately. Other factors include the resident's ability (with or without staff assistance) to reach the toilet on time (locomotion), his/her ability to adjust clothing so as to toilet (dexterity), cognitive function and social awareness (e.g., recognizing the need to void in time and in an appropriate place), and the resident's motivation. Fluid balance and the integrity of the spinal cord and peripheral nerves will also have an effect on continence. Change in any one of these factors can result in incontinence, although alterations in several factors are common before incontinence develops.

II. TRIGGERS

Incontinence care plan suggested if one or more of following present:

- Incontinent 2+ times a week
  [H1b = 2, 3 or 4]
- Use of external (condom) catheter
  [H3c = checked]
- Use of indwelling catheter
  [H3d = checked]
- Use of intermittent catheter
  [H3e = checked]
- Use of pads/briefs
  [H3g = checked]

III. GUIDELINES

For residents with incontinence (including those with condom catheters), all MDS items described in Section A should be addressed, unless exclusionary criteria have been met. If incontinence persists, complete Section B and, if necessary, Section C. For residents with indwelling catheters, first complete Sections A and B and then complete Section D.

A. ITEMS NECESSARY TO EVALUATE INCONTINENCE OR NEED FOR CATHETER

Review the reversible problems listed on the RAP KEY. Virtually all are easily diagnosed, and their treatment will improve not only incontinence but functional status as well. Also, most of these factors can be identified by a nurse, but some will take a physician's order to carry out.

UTI.

Urinary tract infections are common causes of incontinence, especially new incontinence. Therefore, they should be looked for in all residents. If a clean catch urine is not feasible and the resident both has no memory recall and requires at least extensive assistance in self-transfer you may choose to forego catherization to obtain a specimen, since identification and treatment of UTIs in this population has not been shown to make a difference.

- Send a clean catch or sterile urine specimen for microscopic analysis. If >5 WBC are found, send a fresh and sterilely obtained specimen for urine culture. If UTI is found, consider treatment.
- For residents with an indwelling catheter, a new catheter should be sterilely inserted to obtain the specimen.

Fecal Impaction.

Impaction is very common and can cause incontinence by preventing the bladder from emptying well. Thus, check for impaction in all residents who are incontinent.

- To find bowel impaction, insert a gloved finger into resident's rectum.
- The finding of no stool or small amount of soft stool indicates that impaction is unlikely to be the cause of incontinence. A record demonstrating that the resident has recently passed stool is not sufficient to rule out bowel impaction.

Delirium.

If present, this is the most important problem. Often when delirium is treated, incontinence will resolve. In the meantime, regular toileting will help.

Lack of toilet access.

Daily use of restraints can result in a resident's inability to get to the toilet; quick staff response is necessary. The toilet may also be too far away for a resident who does not get adequate warning (e.g., there may not be a toilet room near the activities room). Environmental modifications such as a bedside commode, urinal, or a room closer to the toilet can be useful. To remain continent, residents may also require more staff support, such as more timely responses to requests for assistance.

Immobility.

Immobility correlates highly with incontinence in many nursing home residents. Improving the resident's ability in transferring, locomotion and toileting will often reduce incontinence, as will providing timely staff assistance when needed.

Depression.

Severe depression can result in loss of the motivation to stay dry. Prompted toileting is often helpful as a means of positive reinforcement.

Congestive Heart Failure (CHF) or Pedal Edema.

CHF and pedal edema are especially troublesome when the resident is lying down: diuresis overwhelms the bladder. Treatment of these conditions is not difficult and will improve both incontinence and functional status.

Recent Stroke.

Once the resident is stable, delirium has cleared, and locomotion has improved, continue workup if incontinence persists. Most stroke patients are continent at this point.

Diabetes Mellitus.

Diabetes with persistently high blood sugar causes fluid loss that can cause or worsen incontinence. Treatment will improve incontinence and functional status.

Medications.

Many medications can affect the bladder or urethra and result in incontinence. Physicians would usually discontinue suspect medication if possible, weighing the risks and benefits of doing so. For instance, where a calcium channel blocker is used for mild hypertension, another medication might be easily substituted; a medication for arrhythmia, however, might not have an appropriate substitute.

- Review all medications - regularly prescribed, occasional or "PRN", and any nonprescribed ("over-the-counter") medications.

Medications that can affect continence include the following classes and types of drugs:

1. Diuretics, especially those that act quickly, such as furosemide (Lasix), bumetanide (Bumex), and metolozone (Zaroxylyn), and, less frequently, thiazide agents such as hydrochlorothiazide.

2. Sedative hypnotics, i.e., sleeping pills and antianxiety drugs such as diazepam (Valium), lorazepam, Xanax, Halcion, and Dalmane.

3. Any drug with anticholinergic properties:
   - Antipsychotics (e.g., Haldol, Mellaril)
   - Antidepressants (e.g., Elavil, Triavil)
   - Narcotics (e.g., Morphine, Dilaudid, Darvon)
   - Medication for Parkinson's disease (except Sinemet and Deprenyl)
   - Disopyramide
   - Antispasmodics (e.g., Donnatal, Bentyl)
   - Antihistamines (e.g., medications for colds)

4. Calcium channel blockers (e.g., verapamil, nimodipine, nicardipine, nifedipine, and diltiazem).

5. Drugs that affect the sympathetic nervous system:
   - Alpha blockers (e.g., prazosin and phenoxybenzamine)
   - Alpha stimulants (e.g., ephedrine, pseudoephedrine, phenylpropanolamine, and nosedrops)

B. OTHER POTENTIAL CAUSES OR FACTORS CONTRIBUTING TO INCONTINENCE OR USE OF CATHETERS

Much of the information asked for above will appear in a completed MDS. However, other items of information should be obtained and reviewed if incontinence persists. Identification and treatment of these factors will frequently not only improve incontinence, but may prevent further deterioration such as paralysis. However, in the resident who both has no memory recall, requires at least extensive assistance in self-transfer, and is free of related pain, there is, as of yet, no evidence that identification and treatment of such factors would benefit the resident .

Pain

Pain in the bladder, related to urination, is a distinctly rare and abnormal symptom in the incontinent patient, and often indicates another pathological process, which may be treatable. Physician evaluation is recommended.

Excessive or Inadequate Urine Output.

If daily urine output is less than 1 liter, incontinence may worsen because of very strong, concentrated urine. A daily output over 1.5 liters can overwhelm the bladder. If present, the identification of the underlying cause of the high urine output (e.g., diabetes, high calcium, or excessive fluid intake) is required before restricting fluids.

- The amount of fluid excreted daily should be measured for 1 to 2 days. This can be done using a voiding record or, if patient is severely incontinent, by inserting a *temporary* catheter.

Atrophic Vaginitis.

Caused by reduced amount of the female hormone estrogen, this condition causes or contributes to incontinence in many women.

- Examine vagina for evidence of estrogen deficiency.

Optimally, a pelvic exam checks for signs of atrophic vaginitis.

If a resident is impaired, or appropriate equipment is not readily available, an exam may be done in the resident's bed by spreading the labia and looking inside for redness, dryness, pinpoint hemorrhages, or easy bleeding.

- Pain or irritation during the insertion of a catheter is another useful sign of the condition (catheterization normally may be uncomfortable, but should not be painful).

- Atrophic vaginitis can be treated with a low dose of oral conjugated estrogens. Contraindications to estrogen therapy include a history of breast or endometrial cancer.

Abnormal Lab Values.

Several conditions detectable only by laboratory tests can cause incontinence. These include high blood calcium or glucose and Vitamin B12 deficiency. It is also important to check the blood urea nitrogen (BUN) or creatinine because some causes of incontinence also can damage the kidneys. All of these tests should have been done within the last 60 days, except the B12, which should have been checked within the past 3 years.

Serious Conditions That Cause or Accompany Incontinence (To Be Considered By Primary Doctor).

A doctor or a nurse practitioner can identify potentially life-threatening conditions that cause or accompany urinary incontinence. These include bladder cancer or bladder stones, prostate cancer, spinal cord or brain lesions (such as slipped discs and metastatic tumors), poor bladder compliance, and tabes dorsalis.

- Bladder cancer or stones are suggested by the presence of any amount of blood in the urine (even in microscopic amounts) without evidence of UTI. To investigate for bladder cancer, the first morning urine is sent for 2 or 3 days for cytology examinations. Residents more likely to have bladder cancer are men, smokers, and those with suprapubic pain or discomfort, a history of work exposure to certain dyes, or recent onset of urge incontinence. The physician will decide who is worked up or referred to a urologist.
- Suspected prostate cancer can be detected by a rectal exam.
- Spinal cord diseases are detected by a neurological exam.
- Decreased bladder compliance can result in damage to the kidneys and should be suspected in residents with a history of conditions that result in decreased bladder compliance (pelvic radiation therapy, abdominal/pelvic resection, radical hysterectomy or prostatectomy, or spinal cord disease).
- Another cause of incontinence is tabes dorsalis (an advanced stage of syphilis), which is treatable with antibiotics.

C. FINAL EVALUATION IF INCONTINENCE PERSISTS

After the above causes of easily treatable incontinence have been eliminated and most serious underlying conditions have been investigated, conclude the evaluation with an assessment of the four causes of incontinence that are due to abnormalities within the bladder itself. The following section first describe these abnormalities and then describes the tests to detect their presence. A variety of treatment options is available for each type of incontinence, including treatment and care plans appropriate for every resident. In each case, the care plan can be tailored to the needs and characteristics of the resident with dementia, immobility, etc. Notably, bladder training and medications have been shown to significantly improve incontinence in even severely demented residents. The options are discussed in full detail in the educational material.

Exclusions: Although demented residents have been shown to benefit from targeted therapy, certain patients have a low probability of responding. Therefore, if a resident has no memory recall, is extensively dependent in self-transfer, and the facility's ability to toilet the resident on a regular schedule is imited, then the patient may not benefit from this part of the evaluation, and should be managed with pads, frequent turning and changing, or external catheters. Indications for an indwelling catheter are: the resident is in a coma or has terminal illness, a stage 3 or 4 pressure ulcer in an area affected by the incontinence, untreatable urethral blockage, the need for exact measurement of urine output, a history of being unable to void after having a catheter removed in the past, or a resident with quad/paraplegia who failed a past attempt to remove a catheter.

The bladder abnormalities can be simply understood: either (1) the bladder contracts when it should not ("uninhibited bladder"), abruptly soaking the patient ("urge incontinence"); or (2) the bladder fails to contract when it should ("atonic" or underactive bladder), so that urine builds up and spills over as "overflow incontinence." Alternatively the urethra, through which the bladder empties, is either (3) blocked by an obstruction (e.g., a large prostate) or (4) unable to close tightly enough ("stress incontinence").

By doing a "stress test" and measuring the amount of urine that remains in the bladder after voiding (Post Void Residual -- PVR) these conditions can be separated: the uninhibited bladder generally has little residual urine (<100 ml) and a negative stress test, while the atonic bladder has a much larger residual (e.g., >400 ml). Women with stress incontinence (it is rare in men) have <100 ml residual urine and a positive stress test. Men with a blocked urethra (rare in women) have >100 ml residual urine and a negative stress test.

Post-Void Residual (PVR).

The PVR (post-void residual) is the amount of urine left in the bladder after a void. Research has shown that many elderly people have large amounts left in the bladder after a void, even though they demonstrate no signs of this. That is, they do not feel full or uncomfortable, they have good urine output, and do not seem to have a large bladder by palpation or percussion. Also, in men, a high PVR can signal a variety of problems, and in both men and women, knowledge of the PVR can help guide the selection of medication. Therefore, a PVR should be determined in all patients who reach this point of the evaluation. In some cases, a physician's order may be necessary to perform a PVR. If the physician chooses not to allow this, it should be documented in the chart.

- When the resident feels relatively full, he/she should void as normally as possible into a commode, bedpan, urinal, or a toilet equipped with a collection device (hat). Measure volume voided. Within 15 minutes of voiding, under sterile conditions, insert a nonpermanent catheter to measure the residual volume (PVR). Adding the volume voided to PVR gives the Total Bladder Volume (TBV).

Attention to several points will ensure that the test is done correctly. First, if the resident cannot void intentionally, do the test after an episode of incontinence. Second, after allowing the urine to drain, apply gentle pressure with your hand to the abdomen to increase the drainage. When the urine has stopped draining, withdraw the catheter slowly, continuing to press on the lower abdomen. If possible, have the resident sit up during the catheter withdrawal. Under sterile conditions, the risk of causing an infection is under 3%. Residents with known valvular heart disease (who receive antibiotic prophylaxis for dental work) probably should receive a dose of antibiotics before the PVR is checked.

Kidney Ultrasound Test for Men With a PVR Greater Than 100 ml.

- Ultrasound of the kidneys is indicated in male residents with a PVR greater than 100 ml to rule out hydronephrosis (inability of the kidneys to drain properly), which could be due to bladder obstruction and result in preventable kidney damage.

This test has no risks (compared to the risk of the dye injection in an IVP). Evidence of urine backing into the kidneys strongly suggests the need for urologic referral; if this is not done, the resident needs chronic indwelling catheterization.

Bladder Stress Test for Female Patients.

- ***Bladder Stress Test.*** When the resident has a relatively full bladder, ***but not a strong urge to void***, have her stand or assume as upright a position as possible, relax, and cough vigorously or strain. The test is positive if there is immediate leakage similar in volume and circumstance to usual incontinence. The stress test is negative if there is a delay of more than 5 seconds, no leakage, or leakage of only a few drops, or if it is dissimilar to the usual volume and circumstance of leakage.
- Measure void plus PVR as described above (i.e., calculate Total Bladder Volume).
- ***Repeat Stress Test.*** If the bladder stress test is negative AND the Total Bladder Volume is less than 200 ml, another test is needed for verification. Insert a sterile catheter into the bladder (preferably do this while the catheter for PVR measurement is still in the bladder) and fill it with at least 200 ml of sterile water, if possible. Remove the catheter, have the patient stand up (if possible), and repeat the stress test as above.

D. FINAL EVALUATION FOR RESIDENTS WITH INDWELLING CATHETERS

After the resident with an indwelling catheter has been treated for infection and all the other treatable conditions listed above, a voiding trial can be attempted -- unless the resident has terminal illness, stage 3 or 4 pressure ulcers, or untreatable urethral blockage. This trial may reveal that the catheter is not necessary after all.

Exclusions: The resident is in a coma or has terminal illness, a stage 3 or 4 pressure ulcer in an area affected by the incontinence, untreatable blockage, the need for exact measurement of urine output, a history of being unable to void after having a catheter removed in the past, or a resident with quad/paraplegia who failed a past attempt to remove a catheter.

- If appropriate, institute a voiding trial.

(1) Before removing the catheter, record urine output every 6 hours for one or two days. Use this record to plan when to remove the catheter so that the expected urine will not be over 800 mls during the time of the voiding trial.

(2) Remove catheter and observe. For example, if the resident usually puts out 500 ml on the day shift, remove the catheter at the beginning of that shift and observe; if resident has not voided by the end of the shift, wait until the volume gets higher, but do not exceed a volume of 800 ml.

(3) If resident is able to void, check the PVR, as detailed in **Section C**.

- If volume is greater than 400 ml, reinsert indwelling catheter permanently or until resident can be referred to a urologist.
- If PVR is between 100 and 400 ml, observe resident carefully as urinary retention may redevelop over a few days to a few weeks. If not, check for presence of incontinence: if present, complete **Section C** (above).
- If PVR is less than 100 ml, check for presence of incontinence; if present, complete **Section C** (above).

(4) If resident has not voided by the time the expected volume is 800 ml, and there is no sensation of fullness, no urge to void, and no void, reinsert an indwelling catheter and record the volume. Residents who fail the voiding trial need either urologic referral, if appropriate, or permanent catheterization.

(5) If the resident has no memory recall, is unable to transfer independently, and has incontinence that is resistant to all therapy for more than 2 weeks after removing the catheter, a catheter may be reinserted if deemed appropriate by the staff.

URINARY INCONTINENCE AND INDWELLING CATHETER RAP KEY

(For MDS Version 2.0)

TRIGGER — REVISION

Incontinence care plan suggested if one or more of following present:

- Incontinent 2+ times a week
  [H1b = 2, 3 or 4]
- Use of external (condom) catheter
  [H3c = checked]
- Use of indwelling catheter
  [H3d = checked]
- Use of intermittent catheter
  [H3e = checked]
- Use of pads/briefs
  [H3g = checked]

GUIDELINES

Possible reversible problems to be reviewed in evaluating incontinence or need for catheter:

- **Conditions**: Delirium **[B5]**, Fecal Impactions **[H2d]**, Depression **[I1ee]**, UTI **[I2j]**, Edema **[J1g]**
- **Environment:** Locomotion **[G1c,d,e,f]**, Lack of access to toilet, Barriers **[observation]**, Restraints **[P4]**
- **Diagnoses**: Diabetes **[I1a]**, CHF **[I1f]**, CVA **[I1t]**, Parkinson's **[I1y]**,
- **Medications:** Diuretics **[O4e]**, Parkinson's meds, Disopyramide, Antispasmodics, Antihistamines, Drugs that stimulate or block sympathetic nervous system, Calcium channel blockers (verapamil, nifedipine, diltiazem), Narcotics **[from record]**
- **Psychoactive Medications:** Antipsychotics, Antianxiety, Antidepressants, Hypnotics,**[O4a,b,c,d]**

Other potential factors contributing to incontinence or use of catheter:

- **Conditions:** Pain **[J2]**; Excessive or inadequate urine output, Atrophic vaginitis, Cancer of bladder, prostate, brain, or spine, tabes dorsalis **[from record or exam]**
- **Abnormal Lab Values:** High blood calcium, High blood glucose, Low B_{12}, High BUN or Creatinine **[P9; from record]**

Final evaluation if incontinence persists:

- **Specific Tests:** Post Void Residual, bladder stress test for females, reflux test (kidney ultrasound for males with PVR> 100 ml.) [Note -- Tests not indicated when Comatose **[B1]** or when No memory recall **[B3e]** AND Dependent in Transfer, Locomotion **[G1b,c,d,e,f]** are both present]

Final evaluation for residents with indwelling catheter:
If indwelling catheter **[H3d]**, do Voiding Trial unless Untreatable urethral blockage **[I3]**, terminal illness **[J5c]**, or stage 3/4 pressure ulcer **[M2a]** present

Urinary Incontinence RAP Key 9 of 9

RESIDENT ASSESSMENT PROTOCOL: PSYCHOSOCIAL WELL-BEING

I. PROBLEM

Well-being refers to feelings about self and social relationships. Positive attributes include initiative and involvement in life; negative attributes include distressing relationships and concern about loss of status. On average, 30% of residents in a typical nursing facility will experience problems in this area, two-thirds of whom will also have serious behavior and/or mood problems. When such problems coexist, initial treatment is often focused on mood and behavior manifestations. In such situations, treatment for psychosocial distress is dependent on how the resident responds to the primary mood/behavior treatment regimen.

II. TRIGGERS

Well-being problem (P) or need to maintain psychosocial strengths (S) suggested if one or more of following present:

- Withdrawal from care/activities (*Problem*)*
  [E1o = 1,2]
- Conflict with staff (*Problem*)
  [F2a = checked]
- Unhappy with roommate (*Problem*)
  [F2b = checked]
- Unhappy with other resident (*Problem*)
  [F2c = checked]
- Conflict with family/friends (*Problem*)
  [F2d = checked]
- Grief Over Lost Status/Roles (*Problem*)
  [F3b = checked]
- Daily routine is very different from prior pattern in the community *(Problem)*
  [F3c = checked]

- Establishes own goals (*Strength*)
  [F1d = checked]
- Strong identification with past (*Strength*)
  [F3a = checked]

---

* Note: This item also triggers on the Mood State RAP.

III. GUIDELINES

Sequentially review the items found on the RAP KEY.

Confounding Problems.

Treatment for mood/behavior problems are often immediately beneficial to well-being.

- Does the resident have an increasing or persistently sad mood?
- Does the resident have increasing frequency or daily disturbing behavior?
- Did the mood/behavior problems appear before the reduced sense of well-being?
- Has the resident's condition deteriorated since last assessment?
- Have ongoing treatment programs been effective?

Situational Factors That May Impede Ability to Interact With Others.

Environmental and situational problems are often amenable to staff intervention without the burden of staff having to "change the resident."

- Have key social relationships been altered/terminated (e.g., loss of family member, friend or staff)?
- Have changes in the resident's environment altered access to others or to routine activities -- for example, room assignment, use of physical restraints, assignment to new dining area?

Resident Characteristics That May Impede Ability to Interact With Others.

These items focus on areas where the resident may lack the ability to enter freely into satisfying social relationships. They represent substantial impediments to easy interaction with others and highlight areas where staff intervention may be crucial.

- Do cognitive/communication deficits or a lack of interest in activities impede interactions with others?
- Does resident indicate unease in social relationships?

Lifestyle Issues.

Residents can withdraw or become distressed because they feel life lacks meaning.

- Was life more satisfactory prior to entering the nursing facility?
- Is resident preoccupied with the past, unwilling to respond to the needs of the present?
- Has the facility focused on a daily schedule that resembles the resident's prior lifestyle?

Additional Information to Clarify the Nature of the Problem.

Supplemental assessment items can be used to specify the nature of the well-being problem for residents for whom a well-being care plan is anticipated. These items represent topics around which to phrase questions and to establish a trusting exchange with the resident. Each item includes the positive and negative end of a continuum, representing the possible range that staff can use in thinking about these issues. Staff can use or not use the items in this list. For those items selected, the following issues should be considered:

- How do staff/resident perceive the ***severity*** of the problem?
- Has the resident ever demonstrated (while in the facility) ***strengths*** in the area under review?
- Are corrective strategies now being used? Have they been used in the past? To what effect?
- Is this an area that might be improved?

PSYCHOSOCIAL WELL-BEING RAP KEY *(For MDS Version 2.0)*

TRIGGER — REVISION

Well-being problem or need to maintain psychosocial strengths suggested if one or more of following present:

- Withdrawal from activities of interest (*Problem*)*
  [E1o = 1, 2]
- Conflict with staff (*Problem*)
  [F2a = checked]
- Unhappy with roommate (*Problem*)
  [F2b = checked]
- Unhappy with other resident (*Problem*)
  [F2c = checked]
- Conflict with family/friends (*Problem*)
  [F2d = checked]
- Grief Over Lost Status/Roles (*Problem*)
  [F3b = checked]
- Daily routine is very different from prior pattern in the community *(Problem)*
  [F3c = checked]

- Establishes own goals (*Strength*)
  [F1d = checked]
- Strong identification with past (*Strength*)
  [F3a = checked]

* Note: This item also triggers on the Mood State RAP.

GUIDELINES

Confounding problems:

- Increasing/persistent sad mood **[E2, E3]**
- Increasing/daily disturbing behavior **[E4, E5]**
- Resident's condition deteriorated since last assessment **[Q2]**

Situational factors that may impede ability to interact with others:

- Loss of family member, friend, or staff close to resident **[F2f, from record]**
- Initial use of physical restraints **[P4]**
- New admission **[AB1, A4a]**, Change in room assignment **[A2]**, or Change in dining location or table mates **[from record]**

Resident characteristics that may impede ability to interact with others:

- Delirium/cognitive decline **[B5, B6]**
- Communication deficit/decline **[C4, C5, C6, C7]**
- Not at ease interacting with others **[F1a]**
- Locomotion deficit/use of wheelchair **[G1c-f, G5b,c,d]**
- Diseases that impede communication — Mental retardation **[AB10]**, Alzheimer's **[I1q]**, Aphasia **[I1r]**, Other dementia **[I1u]**, Depression **[I1ee]**
- Uninvolved in activities **[N2, N4]**

Lifestyle issues:

- Incongruence of current and prior style of life **[AC, F3c]**
- Strong identification with past roles/status **[F3a]**
- Length of time problem existed **[from record]**

Supplemental problem clarification issues [from resident/family if necessary]:

- Ability to relate to others
  ___ Skill/unease in dealing with others
  ___ Reaches out/distances self
  ___ Friendly/unapproachable
  ___ Flexible/ridiculed by others
- Relationships resident could draw on
  ___ Supported/isolated
  ___ Many friends/friendless
- Dealing with grief
  ___ Moving through grief/bitter and inconsolable
  ___ Religious faith/feels punished

Psychosocial Well-Being RAP Key 3 of 3

RESIDENT ASSESSMENT PROTOCOL: MOOD STATE

I. PROBLEM

About 15% of nursing home residents will have a major depression; about 30% will exhibit noticeable symptomatic signs of a mood state problem. Such signs are often expressed as sad mood, feelings of emptiness, anxiety, or unease. They are also manifested in a wide range of bodily complaints and dysfunctions, such as loss of weight, tearfulness, agitation, aches and pains.

II. TRIGGERS

A mood problem suggested if one or more of following present:

- Resident made negative statements
  [E1a = 1,2]
- Repetitive questions
  [E1b = 1,2]
- Repetitive verbalizations
  [E1c = 1,2]
- Persistent anger with self or others
  [E1d = 1,2]
- Self deprecation
  [E1e = 1,2]
- Expressions of what appear to be unrealistic fears
  [E1f = 1,2]
- Recurrent statements that something terrible is about to happen
  [E1g = 1,2]
- Repetitive health complaints
  [E1h = 1,2]
- Repetitive anxious complaints/concerns
  [E1i = 1,2]
- Unpleasant mood in morning
  [E1j = 1,2]
- Insomnia/change in usual sleep pattern
  [E1k = 1,2]
- Sad, pained, worried facial expressions
  [E1l = 1,2]
- Crying, tearfulness
  [E1m = 1,2]
- Repetitive physical movements[(a)]
  [E1n = 1,2]
- Withdrawal from activities of interest[(b)]
  [E1o = 1,2]

- Reduced social interaction
  [E1p = 1,2]
- Mood Persistence
  [E2 = 1, 2]

(a) Note: This item also triggers on the Psychotropic Drug Use RAPs when psychotropic drug use present
(b) Note: This item also triggers on the Psychosocial Well-Being RAP.

III. GUIDELINES

Specific conditions stated below suggest the need for an altered/new care strategy. They are not exhaustive; other situations may arise in which staff decide that an altered care plan is necessary. The most obvious are instances of drug-induced side effects (addressed in Psychotropics Drug Use RAP). Residents whose mood problems do not call for care plan alterations are those with stable behavior and no unusual confounding problems.

Many of the questions and issues that follow relate to the MDS items listed on the Mood State RAP KEY. An altered care strategy is suggested when specified conditions are met.

Indicators of the need to consider a new/altered care strategy:

Has Mood Recently Declined or Problems Intensified?

- Were mood problems present 6 months ago?
- Does resident have a cyclic history of decline and improvement in mood state?
- Has loss of appetite with accompanying weight loss occurred?
- Has interest in activities declined, even though resident remains physically capable?

Mood Unimproved and Potentially Reversible Causes Present.

Resolution of delirium (fluctuating consciousness) behavioral, relationship and/or communication problems often affect a resident's mood state. Only when these conditions have been addressed can the nature of a mood problem be fully understood.

Also, consider the possible presence of other complicating factors, such as:

- Delirium
- Review recent changes in the life of the resident (e.g., death of a child, transfer to new environment, separation from loved ones, loss of functional abilities or change in body image, loss of autonomy)
- Review nature and intensity of relationship and/or behavior problems

ADL decline can be both a cause <u>and</u> a consequence of distressed mood. Reviewing the sequence of ADL and mood decline may be informative. In any case, where mood seems to impair ADL functioning, useful strategies include modifying the physical environment, separating the resident's performance of ADL activities into a series of subtasks, and using verbal reminders and cues.

- Review record to determine whether there has been a sudden onset or worsening of cognitive symptoms or communication skills following initiation of treatment (e.g., medications)
- Review to determine whether the resident is using any medications known to cause mood shifts, such as psychotropics; antihypertensives, such as clonidine (Catapres), quanethedine (Ismelin), methlydopa (Aldomet), propeneral (Inderal), reserpine; cimetidine (Tagamet); cytoxic agents; digitalis; immunosuppressives; sedatives; steroids; stimulants.

Mood Unimproved and Other Conditions to Consider

The passive resident with distressed mood may be overlooked. Such a resident may be erroneously assumed to have no mood state problem.

- Does the resident show little/no initiative?
- Does he/she remain uninvolved in activities (alone or with others)?
- Is the sad mood persistent?

Does Sad Mood Appear to Respond to Treatment (e.g., Drug Regimen)?

- Has the mood problem remained relatively unchanged for the last 90 days, or has it improved with the current treatment program?
- Have there been cycles of decline and improvement?
- Is resident receiving medications and/or psychosocial therapy?

Confounding Issues:

Are There Indications of New or Intensified Problems With Conditions That May Affect Mood Problems?

These conditions include: Alzheimer's Disease, cancer, cardiac disease, metabolic and endocrine disorders (e.g., hypercalcemia, Cushing's disease, Addison's disease, hypoglycemia, hypokalemia, porphyria). Parkinson's disease, stroke, or other neurological disease, and thyroid disease.

MOOD STATE RAP KEY *(For MDS Version 2.0)*

TRIGGER — REVISION

A mood problem suggested if one or more of following present:

- Resident made negative statements
  [E1a = 1,2]
- Repetitive questions
  [E1b = 1,2]
- Repetitive verbalizations
  [E1c = 1,2]
- Persistent anger with self or others
  [E1d = 1,2]
- Self deprecation
  [E1e = 1,2]
- Expressions of what appear to be unrealistic fears
  [E1f = 1,2]
- Recurrent statements that something terrible is about to happen
  [E1g = 1,2]
- Repetitive health complaints
  [E1h = 1,2]
- Repetitive anxious complaints/concerns
  [E1i = 1,2]
- Unpleasant mood in morning
  [E1j = 1,2]
- Insomnia/change in usual sleep pattern
  [E1k = 1,2]
- Sad, pained, worried facial expressions
  [E1l = 1,2]
- Crying, tearfulness
  [E1m = 1,2]
- Repetitive physical movements[a]
  [E1n = 1,2]
- Withdrawal from activities of interest[b]
  [E1o = 1,2]
- Reduced social interaction
  [E1p = 1,2]
- Mood Persistence
  [E2 = 1, 2]

(a) Note: This item also triggers on the Psychotropic Drug Use RAPs when psychotropic drug use present

(b) Note: This item also triggers on the Psychosocial Well-Being RAP.

GUIDELINES

Indicators of the need to consider a new/altered care strategy:

- Mood decline **[E3]**
- Mood unimproved **[E3]** AND reversible conditions present
  - — Recent move into/within facility **[AB1, Record]**
  - — Delirium **[B5]** Cognitive decline **[B6]**; Delusions **[J1e]**, Hallucinations **[J1i]**,
  - — Communication decline **[C7]**
  - — Grief due to loss **[F2f]**
  - — ADL decline **[G9]**
  - — Use of meds known to cause mood shifts (e.g., antihypertensives, cimetidine, clonidine, cytoxic agents, digitalis, guanethidine, immunosuppressive, methyldopa, nitrates, propranolol, reserpine, steroids, stimulants) **[from record]**

- Mood unimproved **[E3]** AND indication of problem with cognitive ability/memory, decision-making ability, and ability to understand **[B2, B4; C6]** AND ANY of following:
  - — Little or no initiative shown **[F1]**
  - — Little or no involvement in activities **[N2]**
  - — No psychotropic medications **[O4a,b,c]**
  - — No psychological therapy **[P1be]**

- Behavioral or Relationship problems present **[E4; F2]**

Confounding issues to be considered:

- Communication skills **[C4, C5, C6]**
- **Diseases:** Thyroid disease **[I1b,c]**, Cardiac Disease **[I1d - I1k]**, Neurological disease **[I1q to cc]**, Anxiety **[I1dd]**, Depression **[I1ee]**, Manic depression **[I1ff]**, Schizophrenia **[I1gg]**, Cancer **[I1pp]**, Other Psychosis **[I3]**, Hypercalcemia, Cushing's, Addison's, Hypoglycemia, Hypokalemia, Porphyria **[I3]**

Mood State RAP Key 4 of 4

RESIDENT ASSESSMENT PROTOCOL: BEHAVIORAL SYMPTOMS

I. PROBLEM

Between 60% and 70% of residents in a typical nursing facility exhibit emotional, social, and/or behavior disorders; about 40% have purely behavioral symptoms (i.e., wandering, verbal abuse, physically aggressive and/or socially inappropriate behaviors). Residents with behavioral symptoms also frequently have other related problems. Over 80% of those who have behavioral symptoms will have some type of cognitive deficit; about 75% will have mood and/or relationship problems.

Behavioral symptoms are often seen as a source of danger and distress to the residents themselves and sometimes to other residents and staff. Nursing facilities often find such residents difficult to cope with, and physicians often seem unaware of the wide range of available treatment and management options. As a result, overuse of physical restraints or psychotropic drugs is not uncommon. About one-half of residents who exhibit "problem" behaviors will be physically restrained, and about one-half will receive psychoactive medications - antipsychotics (neuroleptics), antianxiety agents, and, to a lesser extent, antidepressants. These interventions, however, have potentially serious negative side-effects, and many nurses in nursing facilities report being uncomfortable using only physical restraints and/or psychotropics to manage residents with behavioral symptoms. As a result, there is an increasing trend toward using other interventions and treatments in addressing behavioral symptoms.

II. TRIGGERS

The MDS trigger items identify two types of residents for whom further review is suggested: residents who exhibit the behavioral symptoms of wandering, being verbally abusive, being physically aggressive and/or exhibiting socially inappropriate behavioral symptoms AND residents who have improved behavioral symptoms but who are receiving treatment or intervention that might mask manifestations of the behavior (e.g., decreased wandering because resident restrained).

Review of behavior status suggested if one or more of following present:

- Wandering*
  [E4aA = 1,2,3]
- Verbally abusive
  [E4bA = 1,2,3]
- Physically abusive
  [E4cA = 1,2,3]
- Socially inappropriate
  [E4dA = 1,2,3]
- Resists Care
  [E4eA = 1,2,3]
- Behavior improved
  [E5 = 1]

---

* Note — This Item also triggers on the Fall RAP

Behavioral Symptoms RAP (1 of 6)

III. GUIDELINES

The items in this RAP (and in the RAP KEY) begin with those items that help to draw the distinction between serious behavioral symptoms and others that can be more easily accommodated. This is followed by a section on potential causes or factors involved in the manifestation of problem behaviors the resolution of which might reduce or eliminate the behavior(s).

EVALUATING THE SERIOUSNESS OF BEHAVIORAL SYMPTOMS

The first trigger identifies residents who currently exhibit some type of behavioral symptoms for which additional or new treatment programs may be considered. Not all behaviors need an extensive intervention. Some behaviors neither endanger nor distress the resident or others. For example, many hallucinations and delusions (when <u>not</u> a sign of psychosis or an acute condition such as delirium) are benign. Residents with such behavioral manifestations may be accommodated (e.g., tolerated, behavior rechanneled or redirected) within the environment of the nursing facility. Thus, determining whether a particular behavioral manifestation <u>is</u> a problem is an important step and involves determining the nature and severity of the behavior(s) in question and the effects of the behavior(s).

Observing Specific Behavioral Manifestations in the Most Recent 7-Day Period.

- Review to determine the intensity, duration, and frequency of behavior problems over the last 7-day and 14-day periods. Did these changes vary over time?
- Is there a pattern to the behavior manifestations based on observations over a 7-14 day time period? (Consider such factors as time of day, nature of the environment, what the resident and others were doing at the time the problem behavior was manifested.)

Identifying Stability/Change in the Nature of Behavioral Problems.

Identifying patterns of behaviors over time may help clarify the underlying causes of problem behaviors. For example, such a review may reveal a pattern in which a resident's catastrophic reactions typically occur only in the presence of a particular combination of stressors (e.g., a person who can tolerate large groups for singing but not for meals). Similarly, observing a resident over time may reveal that a resident's seemingly random behaviors are associated with particular events (e.g., yelling/screaming associated with objecting to someone changing the channel during a favored television program; wandering associated with the need to toilet). Addressing the causes of such patterns may reduce or eliminate the behavior.

- How did behavior develop over time? Were problem signs evident earlier in the resident's stay or even earlier in the resident's life?
- Has resident experienced recent changes (e.g., movement to a new unit, assignment of new nonlicensed direct care staff to the unit, change in medication, withdrawal from a treatment program, decline in cognitive status)?

Determine the Ways in Which Behavior Problems Impinges on Other Functioning.

Understanding that a behavior can - but does not always - interfere with a resident's self-performance and treatment regimens is useful in considering the need for interventions. This view can also help to ensure that aggressive treatments or interventions (e.g., physical restraints or antipsychotics) are not introduced simply to keep the resident "looking normal."

- Does the behavior endangered the resident? Others? If so, in what ways does it endanger the resident or others?
- Are behavior problems related to daily variations in functional performance? If so, how?
- Does behavior problem lead to resistance to care?
- Does it lead to difficulties dealing with people and coping in the facility?

REVIEW OF POTENTIAL CAUSES OF BEHAVIORAL SYMPTOMS

Many behaviors, however, are problematic for the resident or others. Many are directly associated with acute health conditions, neurological diseases, or psychiatric conditions. Still others originate in the resident's reaction to external factors, such as psychotropic medications, the use of physical restraints, and stressors in the environment (e.g., loud noises, changes in familiar routines). Identifying the various factors involved in the manifestation of behavioral symptoms is critical. Such a process may reveal conditions that can be resolved, thus eliminating or reducing the behavioral symptoms. Further, distinguishing among potential causes or interrelationships is essential to developing an appropriate care plan (e.g., distinguishing between behaviors originating with a neurological condition as contrasted to a psychotic syndrome). Consideration of the items in the Behavioral Symptoms RAP KEY (as well as in related RAPs as indicated) should facilitate this process.

Cognitive Status Problem Interactions.

Decision-making ability is a key indicator of effective cognitive skills. Resolving acute confusional state or delirium, a potentially reversible problem, can be critical to behavior management. (See Delirium RAP if a diagnosis or signs and symptoms of delirium are present.)

For many residents with chronic progressive dementia, certain behaviors may continue in spite of remedial treatments or interventions. In some instances, the behaviors will be distressing; however, in many instances behaviors can be accommodated. For example, many residents who wander can be accommodated without restraints in a hazard-free environment. Similarly, the needs and patterns of demanding residents or those with catastrophic reactions can often be anticipated or the most disrupting reactions to the distress alleviated. The Cognitive Loss/Dementia RAP refers to several issues that can be considered for such residents. Thus, that RAP should be completed prior to this RAP on Behaviors for residents who have cognitive problems.

Presence of Mood and/or Relationship Problem Interactions.

Mood and relationship problems often produce disturbed behavioral symptoms. If the underlying problems are resolved, the behavior may lessen or stop.

- Does the resident have an unresolved mood state or relationship problem that may lead to behavioral symptoms (e.g., anxiety disorder and agitation; depression or isolation and verbally abusive behavior)? Refer to the Psychosocial Well-Being RAP and to the Mood State RAP.

- Is there an association among mood state, relationship, and behavioral symptoms?
- Can a cause and effect relationship be determined?
- Does the resident experience a sense of frustration because of rejection by family? If so, does this frustration result in the resident verbally abusing staff or other residents?

Relationship Difficulties That May Affect Behavior.

- Does the presence or absence of other persons precipitate an event?
- Was a combative act prompted by paranoid delusions about another's motives or actions?
- Did recent loss of loved one, change in staff, an intrafacility move, or placement with a roommate with whom the resident cannot communicate lead to disruptive behavioral symptoms?

Environmental Conditions.

A review of the resident's behaviors over time may, as noted earlier, reveal a pattern of behaviors that helps identify the causes of the behaviors. Because environmental conditions often have a profound effect on residents' behaviors, these factors should be given special consideration.

- Are staff sufficiently responsive? Do they recognize stressors for the resident and early warning signs of problem behavior?
- Do staff follow the resident's familiar routines?
- Do noise, crowding or dimly lit areas affect resident's behavior?
- Are other residents physically aggressive?

Illness/Conditions.

Sometimes, the onset of acute illnesses and/or the worsening of a chronic illness produces disturbed behaviors. Often identification and treatment of the illness will resolve the problem behavior. In addition, a resident with certain chronic conditions, particularly difficulties in making his/her needs understood or in understanding others may also exhibit problem behaviors that can be eliminated or reduced if more effective methods of communication are adopted by staff and families. Sensory impairments (vision,hearing) may also produce disruptive behaviors that would lessen or disappear if the underlying condition were addressed.

- Can physical health factors close in time to the disturbed behavior be identified (e.g., pain or discomfort from physical conditions such as arthritis, constipation, or headache)?
- Can the observed behavior be associated with an acute illness(e.g., urinary tract infection, other infections, fever, hallucinations/delusions, sleep deprivation, fall with physical trauma, nutritional deficiencies, weight loss, dehydration/insufficient fluids, electrolyte disorder, or acute hypotension)?
- Can the observed behavior be associated with the worsening of a chronic illness (e.g., congestive heart failure, diabetes, psychoses, Alzheimer's disease or other dementia, CVA, or hypoglycemia for a diabetic)?
- What was the role of impaired hearing, vision, or ability to communicate or understand others?

Current Treatment/Management Procedures: Positive and Negative Consequences.

A number of treatment or management interventions may affect a resident's behavior. Some may have had a positive effect, while others may exacerbate existing behavioral symptoms - or produce new problems. Both are important to consider in reaching a decision about whether to proceed with a care plan intervention. For example, review the resident's interest in, use of, or participation in psychological treatment program(s). This review will be especially important for residents who have recently experienced improved behavioral status. For some residents and some management programs, continuation of treatments may be central to maintaining their new-found control. In other cases, either the interventions can be reduced (at least on a trial basis), or the side effects of the intervention may be so severe that alterations in the treatment regimen should be considered. For example, a drug or restraint program may result in increased confusion and agitation, reduced ADL self-performance, a decline in mood, or a general decrease in the quality of life for the resident. On the other hand, breaking tasks of daily life down into smaller steps that the resident can comprehend and perform may reduce stress and prevent problem behavior.

- Has the resident been evaluated by a psychiatrist, etc.? When?
- Are there indicators that treatments have helped resident gain increased control over life? What were they?
- Can improvement be attributed to an identifiable treatment?
- If behavioral symptoms have decreased, can medication or behavior management programs be withdrawn?
- Is the onset or change of behaviors associated with the start of (or change in prescription of) a medication(s)?
- Is the behavior associated with the use of a physical restraint (e.g., increased agitation and anger)?
- Has the resident received care in a specially designed therapeutic unit?
- Are there special staff training/support programs that focus on managing behavioral symptoms?
- What disciplines are involved? How frequent/consistent is the training?
- Has task segmentation been used to maximize resident involvement?

BEHAVIORAL SYMPTOMS RAP KEY *(For MDS Version 2.0)*

TRIGGER — REVISION

Review of behavior status suggested if one or more of following present:

- Wandering*
  [E4aA = 1,2,3]
- Verbally abusive
  [E4bA = 1,2,3]
- Physically abusive
  [E4cA = 1,2,3]
- Socially inappropriate
  [E4dA = 1,2,3]
- Resists Care
  [E4eA = 1,2,3]
- Behavior improved
  [E5 = 1]

* Note — This Item also triggers on the Fall RAP

GUIDELINES

Review and describe behavioral symptom:

- **Evaluating the seriousness and stability/change of behavioral symptoms.** Review of intensity, duration, frequency and, if any, pattern of behaviors, their development over time, and their effect on the resident and others **[E4aB, E4bB, E4cB, E4dB, E4eB, from record]**.

Review potential causes that could be addressed or resolved:

- **Cognitive status problems.** Delirium **[B5]**, Alzheimer's Disease **[I1q]** or other dementia **[I1u]**, Effects of stroke **[C4, C5, C6; G5, G6; I1r, I1t]**.

- **Mood or relationship problems.** Sad or anxious mood **[E1]**, Unsettled relationships **[F2]**, Psychiatric diagnosis **[I1dd, I1ee, I1ff, I1gg]**

- **Environmental conditions.** Departure from resident's normal routines prior to entering facility **[F3c]**, Staff responses, presence of stressful conditions of physically aggressive resident **[from record, interviews with staff, resident]**

- **Illness/conditions.** Onset of acute illness, worsening of chronic illness **[J5a,b]**, and other related problems, such as Constipation **[H2b]**, Diabetes **[I1a]**, CHF **[I1f]**, Pneumonia **[I2e]**, Septicemia **[I2g]**, UTI **[I2j]** or other infection **[I2, I3]**, Fever **[J1h]**, Delusions **[J1e]**, Hallucinations **[J1i]**, Pain **[J2]**, Fall with physical trauma to head **[J4a,b; I1cc]**

- **Communication deficits.** Difficulty making self understood **[C4]** or Understanding others **[C6]**

- **Sensory impairments.** Hearing problem **[C1]**, Visual problem **[D1]**, Visual Limitations **[D2]**

- **Treatment/management procedures.** Antipsychotics, antianxiety, antidepressants, hypnotics **[O4a,b,c,d]**, Behavior management program **[P2]**, Trunk, limb or chair restraints **[P4c,d,e]**

Behavioral Symptoms RAP Key 6 of 6

RESIDENT ASSESSMENT PROTOCOL: ACTIVITIES

I. PROBLEM

The Activities RAP targets residents for whom a revised activity care plan may be required to identify those residents whose inactivity may be a major complication in their lives. Resident capabilities may not be fully recognized: the resident may have recently moved into the facility or staff may have focused too heavily on the instrumental needs of the resident and may have lost sight of complications in the institutional environment.

Resident involvement in passive as well as active activities can be as important in the nursing home as it was in the community. The capabilities of the average resident have obviously been altered as abilities and expectations change, disease intervenes, situational opportunities become less frequent, and extended social relationships less common. But something that should never be overlooked is the great variability within the resident population: many will have ADL deficits, but few will be totally dependent; impaired cognition will be widespread, but so will the ability to apply old skills and learn new ones; and sense may be impaired, but some type of two-way communication is almost always possible.

For the nursing home, activity planning is a universal need. For this RAP, the focus is on cases where the system may have failed the resident, or where the resident has distressing conditions that warrant review of the activity care plan. The types of cases that will be triggered are: (1) residents who have indicated a desire for additional activity choices; (2) cognitively intact, distressed residents who may benefit from an enriched activity program; (3) cognitively deficient, distressed residents whose activity levels should be evaluated; and (4) highly involved residents whose health may be in jeopardy because of their failure to "slow down."

In evaluating triggered cases, the following general questions may be helpful:

- Is inactivity disproportionate to the resident's physical/cognitive abilities or limitations?
- Have decreased demands of nursing home life removed the need to make decisions, to set schedules, to meet challenges? Have these changes contributed to resident apathy?
- What is the nature of the naturally occurring physical and mental challenges the resident experiences in everyday life?
- In what activities is the resident involved? Is he/she normally an active participant in the life of the unit? Is the resident reserved, but actively aware of what is going on around him/her? Or is he/she unaware of surroundings and activities that take place?
- Are there proven ways to extend the resident's inquisitive/active engagement in activities?
- Might simple staff actions expedite resident involvement in activities? For example: Can equipment be modified to permit greater resident access of the unit? Can the resident's location or position be changed to permit greater access to people, views, or programs? Can time and/or distance limitations for activities be made less demanding without destroying the challenge? Can staff modes of interacting with the resident be more accommodating, possibly less threatening, to resident deficits?

II. TRIGGERS

ACTIVITIES TRIGGER A (Revise)

Consider revising activity plan if one or more of following present:

- Involved in activities little or none of time
  [N2 = 2, 3]
- Prefers change in daily routine
  [N5a = 1,2]
  [N5b = 1,2]

ACTIVITIES TRIGGERS B (Review)

Review of activity plan suggested if both of following present:

- Awake all or most of time in morning
  [N1a = checked]
- Involved in activities most of time
  [N2 = 0]

III. GUIDELINES

The followup review looks for factors that may impede resident involvement in activities. Although many factors can play a role, age as a valid impediment to participation can normally be ruled out. If age continues to be linked as a major cause of lack of participation, a staff education program may prove effective in remedying what may be overprotective staff behavior.

Issues to be Considered as Activity Plan is Developed.

Is Resident Suitably Challenged, Overstimulated? To some extent, competence depends on environmental demands. When the challenge is not sufficiently demanding, a resident can become bored, perhaps withdrawn, may resort to fault-finding and perhaps even behave mischievously to relieve the boredom. Eventually, such a resident may become less competent because of the lack of challenge. In contrast, when the resident lacks the competence to meet challenges presented by the surroundings, he or she may react with anger and aggressiveness.

- Do available activities correspond to resident lifetime values, attitudes, and expectations?
- Does resident consider "leisure activities" a waste of time - he/she never really learned to play, or to do things just for enjoyment?
- Have the resident's wishes and prior activity patterns been considered by activity and nursing professionals?
- Have staff considered how activities requiring lower energy levels may be of interest to the resident - e.g., reading a book, talking with family and friends, watching the world go by, knitting?
- Does the resident have cognitive/functional deficits that either reduce options or preclude involvement in all/most activities that would otherwise have been of interest to him/her?

Confounding Problems to be Considered.

Health-related factors that may affect participation in activities. Diminished cardiac output, an acute illness, reduced energy reserves, and impaired respiratory function are some of the many reasons that activity level may decline. Most of these conditions need not necessarily incapacitate the resident. All too often, disease-induced reduction of activity may lead to progressive decline through disuse, and further decrease in activity levels. However, this pattern can be broken: many activities can be continued if they are adapted to require less exertion or if the resident is helped in adapting to a lost limb, decreased communication skills,new appliances, and so forth.

- Is resident suffering from an acute health problem?
- Is resident hindered because of embarrassment/unease due to presence of health-related equipment (tubes, oxygen tank, colostomy bag, wheelchair)?
- Has the resident recovered from an illness? Is the capacity for participation in activities greater?
- Has an illness left the resident with some disability (e.g., slurred speech, necessity for use of cane/walker/wheelchair, limited use of hands)?
- Does resident's treatment regimen allow little time or energy for participation in preferred activities?

Other Issues to be Considered.

Recent decline, in resident status — cognition, communication, function, mood, or behavior. When pathologic changes occur in any aspect of the resident's competence, the pleasurable challenge of activities may narrow. Of special interest are problematic changes that may be related to the use of psychoactive medications. When residents or staff overreact to such losses, compensatory strategies may be helpful - e.g., impaired residents may benefit from periods of both activity and rest; task segmentation can be considered; or available resident energies can be reserved for pleasurable activities (e.g., using usual stamina reserves to walk to the card room, rather than to the bathroom) or activities that have individual significance (e..g, sitting unattended at a daily prayer service rather than at group activity program).

- Has staff or the resident been overprotective? Or have they misread the seriousness of resident cognitive/functional decline? In what ways?
- Has the resident retained skills, or the capacity to learn new skills, sufficient to permit greater activity involvement?
- Does staff know what the resident was like prior to the most recent decline? Has the physical/other staff offered a prognosis for the resident's future recovery, or change of continued decline?
- Is there any substantial reason to believe that the resident cannot tolerate or would be harmed by increased activity levels? What reasons support a counter opinion?
- Does resident retain any desire to learn or master a specific new activity? Is this realistic?
- Has there been a lack of participation in the majority of activities which he/she stated as preference are as even though these types of activities are provided?

Environmental factors. Environmental factors include recent changes in resident location, facility rules, season of the year, and physical space limitations that hinder effective resident involvement.

- Does the interplay of personal, social, and physical aspects of the facility's environment hamper involvement in activities? How might this be addressed?
- Are current activity levels affected by the season of the year or the nature of the weather during the MDS assessment period?
- Can the resident choose to participate in or to create an activity? How is this influenced by facility rules?
- Does resident prefer to be with others, but the physical layout of the unit gets in the way? Do other features in the physical plant frustrate the resident's desire to be involved in the life of the facility? What corrective actions are possible? Have any been taken?

Changes in availability of family/friends/staff support. Many residents will experience not only a change in residence but also a loss of relationships. When this occurs, staff may wish to consider ways for resident to develop a supportive relationship with another resident, staff member or volunteer that may increase the desire to socialize with others and/or to participate in activities with this new friend.

- Has a staff person who has been instrumental in involving a resident in activities left the facility/been reassigned?
- Is a new member in a group activity viewed by a resident as taking over?
- Has another resident who was a leader on the unit died or left the unit?
- Is resident shy, unable to make new friends?
- Does resident's expression of dissatisfaction with fellow residents indicate he/she does not want to be a part of an activities group?

Possible Confounding Problems to be Considered for Those Now Actively Involved in Activities. Of special interest are cardiac and other diseases that might suggest a need to slow down.

ACTIVITIES RAP KEY *(For MDS Version 2.0)*

TRIGGER — REVISION

ACTIVITIES TRIGGER A (Revise)

Consider revising activity plan if one or more of following present:

- Involved in activities little or none of time **[N2 = 2, 3]**
- Prefers change in daily routine **[N5a = 1,2]** **[N5b = 1,2]**

ACTIVITIES TRIGGERS B (Review)

Review of activity plan suggested if both of following present:

- Awake all or most of time in morning **[N1a = checked]**
- Involved in activities most of time **[N2 = 0]**

GUIDELINES

Issues to be considered as activity plan is developed:

- Time in facility **[AB1]**
- Cognitive status **[B2, B4]**
- Walking/locomotion pattern **[G1c,d,e,f]**
- Unstable acute/chronic health conditions **[J5a,b]**
- Number of treatments received **[P1]**
- Use of Psychoactive medications **[O4a,b,c,d]**

Confounding problems to be considered:

- Performs tasks slowly and at different levels (reduced energy reserves) **[G8c,d]**
- Cardiac dysrhythmias **[I1e]**
- Hypertension **[I1h]**
- CVA **[I1t]**
- Respiratory diseases **[I1hh,I1ii]**
- Pain **[J2]**

Other issues to be considered:

- Customary routines **[AC]**
- Mood **[E1, E2]** and Behavioral Symptoms **[E4]**
- Recent loss of close family member/friend or staff **[F2f; from record]**
- Whether daily routine is very different from prior pattern in the community **[F3c]**

Activities RAP Key 5 of 5

RESIDENT ASSESSMENT PROTOCOL: FALLS

I. PROBLEM

Falls are a common source of serious injury and death among the elderly. Each year, 40% of nursing home residents fall. Up to 5% of falls result in fractures; an additional 15% result in soft tissue injuries. Moreover, most elders are afraid of falling, and this fear can limit their activities.

In about one-third of falls, a single potential cause can be identified; in two-thirds, more than one risk factor will be involved. Risk factors that are internal to the resident include the resident's physical health and functional status. External risk factors include medication side effects, the use of appliances and restraints, and environmental conditions. Identification and assessment of those who have fallen and those who are at high risk of falling are the goals of this RAP.

II. TRIGGERS

Potential for Additional Falls [A] or Risk of Initial Fall [R] suggested if one or more of following present:

- *Fell in past 30 days (Additional)* [c]
  [J4a = checked]
- Fell in past 31-180 days (*Additional*) [c]
  [J4b = checked]

- Wandering [a] *(Risk)*
  [E4aA = 1,2,3]
- Dizziness (*Risk*) [c]
  [J1f = checked]
- Use of trunk restraint (*Risk*) [b]
  [P4c = 1,2]
- Use of Antianxiety drugs (*Risk*)[d]
  [O4b = 1-7]
- Use of Antidepressant drugs (*Risk*)[d]
  [O4c = 1-7]

(a) Note: This item also triggers on the Behavior Symptom RAP.
(b) Note: Code 2 also triggers on the Pressure Ulcer RAP. Both codes trigger on the Physical Restraint RAP.
(c) Note: This item also triggers on the Psychotropic Drug Use RAP (when psychotropic drugs present).
(d) When present with specific condition, this item is part of trigger on Psychotropic Drug Use RAP.

III. GUIDELINES

To reach a decision on a care plan, begin by reviewing whether one or more of the major risk factors listed on the RAP KEY are present. Clarifying information on the nature of the risk or type of issue to be considered for the RAP KEY items follows.

Multiple Falls: Is There a Previous History of Falls, or was the Fall an isolated Event?

Refer to the MDS, reports of the family, and incident reports.

Internal Risk Factors.

Review to determine whether the items listed on the RAP KEY under the following headings are present. Each of these represents an underlying health problem or condition that can cause falls and may be addressed so as to prevent future falls.

- *Cardiovascular*
- *Neuromuscular/functional*
- *Orthopedic*
- *Perceptual*
- *Psychiatric or cognitive*

External Risk Factors.

These risk factors can often be modified to reduce the resident's risk of falls.

Medications. Certain drugs can produce falls by causing related problems (hypotension, muscle rigidity, impaired balance, other extrapyramidal side effects [e.g., tremors], and decreased alertness). These drugs include: antipsychotics, antianxiety/hypnotics, antidepressants, cardiovascular medications, and diuretics.

- Were these medications administered prior to or after the fall?
- If prior to the fall, how close to it were they first administered?

Appliances and Devices.

- If the resident who falls (or is at risk of falling) uses an appliance observe his/her use of the appliance for possible problems.
- Review the MDS and the resident's record to determine whether restraints were used prior to the fall and might have contributed to the fall, (e.g., causing a decline function or an increase in agitation).

Environmental/Situational Hazards. *Many easily modifiable hazards (e.g., poor lighting, patterned* carpeting, poorly arranged furniture) in the environment may cause falls both in relatively healthy and in frail elderly residents.

For Those Who Have Fallen Previously, Review the Circumstances Under Which the Fall Occurred.

Attempt to gather information on most recent fall. Needed information includes:

- Time of day, time since last meal.
- Was resident doing usual or unusual activity?
- Was he/she standing still or walking? Reaching up or down? Not reaching?
- Was resident in a crowd of people? Responding to bladder/bowel urgency?
- Was there glare or liquid on floors? Foreign objects in walkway? New furniture placement or other changes in environment?
- Is there a pattern of falls in any of the above circumstances?
- If you know what the resident was doing during the fall, have her/him perform that activity and observe (protect resident to ensure that a fall does not occur during this test).

Take necessary vital signs:

- At time of fall, obtain supine and upright blood pressure and heart rate, IF the resident does not have a serious injury such as a fracture of the hip or lower extremity.
- When reproducing circumstances of a fall (e.g., if the resident fell 10 minutes after eating a large meal, take vital signs 10 minutes after the residents eats).
- Measure blood pressure and heart rate when the resident is supine AND 1 and 3 minutes after standing; note temperature and respiratory rate.

For Residents At Risk of Future Falls, Review Environmental/Situational Factors to Determine Whether Modifications Are Needed

- Observe resident's usual pattern of interaction with his/her environment – the way he/she gets out of bed, walks, turns, gets in and out of chairs, uses the bathroom. Observations may reveal environmental solutions to prevent falls.
- Observe him/her get out of bed, walking 20 feet, turn in a 360° circle, standing up from a chair without pushing off with his/her arms (fold arms in front), and using the bathroom.

FALLS RAP KEY *(For MDS Version 2.0)*

TRIGGER — REVISION

Potential for Additional Falls or Risk of Initial Fall suggested if one or more of following present:

- Fell in past 30 days (*Additional*) [c]
  [J4a = checked]
- Fell in past 31-180 days (*Additional*) [c]
  [J4b = checked]

- Wandering [a] *(Risk)*
  [E4aA = 1,2,3]
- Dizziness (*Risk*) [c]
  [J1f = checked]
- Use of trunk restraint (*Risk*) [b]
  [P4c = 1,2]
- Use of Antianxiety drugs (*Risk*)[d]
  [O4b = 1-7]
- Use of Antidepressant drugs (*Risk*)[d]
  [O4c = 1-7]

(a) Note: This item also triggers on the Behavior Symptom RAP.

(b) Note: Code 2 also triggers on the Pressure Ulcer RAP. Both codes trigger on the Physical Restraint RAP.

(c) Note: This item also triggers on the Psychotropic Drug Use RAP (when psychotropic drugs present).

(d) When present with specific condition, this item is part of trigger on Psychotropic Drug Use RAP

GUIDELINES

Review risk factors for falls to identify problems that may be addressed/resolved:

- **Multiple Falls. [J4a, J4b]**

- **Internal Risk Factors.**
  - -- *Cardiovascular:* Cardiac dysrhythmia **[I1e]**
  - -- *Neuromuscular/functional:* Loss of arm or leg movement **[G4b,d]**, Decline in functional status **[G9]**, Incontinence **[H1]**, Hypotension **[I1i]**, CVA **[I1t]**, Hemiplegia/Hemiparesis **[I1v]**, Parkinson's **[I1y]**, Seizure disorder **[I1aa]**, Syncope **[J1m]**, Chronic/acute condition makes unstable **[J5a, J5b]**, Unsteady gait **[J1n]**,
  - -- *Orthopedic:* Joint pain **[J3g]**, Arthritis **[I1l]**, Fracture of the hip **[I1m, J4c]**, Missing limb (e.g., amputation) **[I1n]**, Osteoporosis **[I1o]**
  - -- *Perceptual:* Impaired hearing **[C1]**, Impaired vision **[D1, D2]**, Dizziness/vertigo **[J1f]**
  - -- *Psychiatric or cognitive*: Delirium **[B5]**, Decline in cognitive skills **[B6]**, Manic depression **[I1ff]**, Alzheimer's **[I1q]**, Other Dementia **[I1u]**

- **External Factors**
  - -- *Medications*: Psychotropic meds **[O4a,b,c,d]** Cardiovascular meds **[from record]** and Diuretics **[O4e]**
  - -- *Appliances/devices* (time started): Pacemaker **[from record]**; Cane/walker/crutch **[G5a]**; Devices and restraints **[P4a,b,c,d,e]**
  - -- ***Environmental/situational hazards and, if relevant, circumstances of recent fall(s):*** **[Review of situation and environment]** glare; poor illumination; slippery floors; uneven surfaces; patterned carpets; foreign objects in walkway; new arrangement of objects; recent move into/within facility; proximity to aggressive resident; time of day; time since meal; type of activity; standing still/walking in a crowded area/ reaching/not reaching; responding to bladder/bowel urgency.

FALLS RAP Key 4 of 4

RESIDENT ASSESSMENT PROTOCOL: NUTRITIONAL STATUS

I. PROBLEM

Malnutrition is not a response to normal aging; it can arise from many causes. Its presence may signal the worsening of a life-threatening illness, and it should always be seen as a dramatic indicator of the resident's risk of sudden decline. Severe malnutrition is, however, relatively rare, and this RAP focuses on signs and symptoms that suggest that the resident may be at risk of becoming malnourished. For many who are triggered, there will be no obvious, outward signs of malnutrition. Prevention is the goal, and early detection is the key.

Early problem recognition can help to ensure appropriate and timely nutritional intervention. For many residents, simple adjustments in feeding patterns may be sufficient. For others, compensation or correction for food intake problems may be required.

Within a nutrition program, food intake is best accomplished via oral feedings. Tube (enteral) feeding is normally limited to residents who have a demonstrated inability to orally consume sufficient food to prevent major malnutrition or weight loss. Parenteral feeding is normally limited to life-saving situations where both oral and enteral feeding is contraindicated or inadequate to meet nutrient needs. Oral feeding is clearly preferred. Depending on the nature of the problem, residents can be encourage to use finger foods; to take small bites; to use the tongue to move food in the mouth from side to side; to chew and swallow each bite; to avoid food that causes mouth pain, etc. Therapeutic programs can also be designed to review for the need for adaptive utensils to compensate for problems in sucking, closing lips, or grasping utensils; to help the confused resident maintain a fixed feeding routine, etc.

II. TRIGGERS

Malnutrition problem suggested if one or more of following observed

- Weight loss
  [K3a = 1]
- Taste alterations
  [K4a = checked]
- Leaves 25% or more food uneaten at most meals
  [K4c = checked]
- Parenteral/IV feeding[(a)]
  [K5a = checked]
- Mechanically altered diet
  [K5c = checked]
- Syringe (oral feeding)
  [K5d = checked]
- Therapeutic diet
  [K5e = checked]
- Pressure ulcer[(b)]
  [M2a = 2, 3, or 4]

[(a)] Note: These items also trigger on the Dehydration/Fluid Maintenance RAP.
[(b)] Note: These items also trigger on the Pressure Ulcer RAP

Nutritional Status RAP (1 of 4)

III. GUIDELINES

RESIDENT FACTORS THAT MAY IMPEDE ABILITY TO CONSUME FOOD

Reduced ability to feed self

Reduced ability to feed self can be due to arthritis, contractures, partial or total loss of voluntary arm movement, hemiplegia or quadriplegia, vision problems, inability to perform activities of daily living without significant assistance, and coma.

Chewing problems

Residents with oral abscesses, ill-fitting dentures, teeth that are broken, loose, carious or missing, or those on mechanically altered diets frequently cannot eat enough food to meet their calorie and other nutrient needs. Significant weight loss can, in turn, result in poorly fitting dentures and infections that can lead to more weight loss.

Losses from diarrhea or an ostomy

Swallowing problems

Swallowing problems arise in several contexts: the long-term result of chemotherapy, radiation therapy, or surgery for malignancy (including head and neck cancer); fear of swallowing because of COPD/emphysema/asthma; stroke; hemiplegia or quadriplegia; Alzheimer's disease or other dementia; and ALS.

Possible Medical Causes

Numerous conditions and diseases can result in increased nutrient requirements (calories, protein, vitamins, minerals, water, and fiber) for residents. Among these are cancer and cancer therapies, Parkinson's disease with tremors, septicemia, pneumonia, gastrointestinal influenza, fever, vomiting, diarrhea and other forms of malabsorption including excessive nutrient loss from ostomy, burns, pressure ulcers, COPD/emphysema/asthma, Alzheimer's disease with concomitant pacing or wandering, and hyperthyroidism.

Malignancy and nutritional consequences of chemotherapy, radiation therapy/surgery. For the resident undergoing therapy aimed at remission or cure, aggressive nutritional support is necessary to achieve the goal; for the resident with incurable malignancy who is undergoing palliative therapy or is not responding to curative therapy, aggressive nutritional support is often medically inappropriate.

- Have the wishes of the resident and family concerning aggressive nutritional support been ascertained?

Anemia (nutritional deficiency, not malnutrition). A hematocrit of less than 41% is predictive of increased morbidity and mortality for residents.

- Are shortness of breath, weakness, paleness of mucous membranes and nailbeds, and/or clubbing of nails present?

Chronic COPD increases calorie needs and can be complicated by an elevated fear of choking when eating or drinking.

Shortness of breath (frequently seen with congestive heart failure, hypertension, edema, and COPD/emphysema/asthma). This is another condition that can cause a fear of eating and drinking, with a consequent reduction in food intake.

Constipation/intestinal obstruction/pain can inhibit appetite

Drug-induced anorexia often causes decreased or altered ability to taste and smell foods.

Delirium

PROBLEMS TO BE REVIEWED FOR POSSIBLE RELATIONSHIP TO NUTRITIONAL STATUS PROBLEM (Causal link)

Mental problems.

Mental retardation, Alzheimer's or other dementia, depression, paranoid fears that food is poisoned, and mental retardation can all lead to anorexia, resulting in significant amounts of uneaten food and subsequent weight loss.

Behavior patterns and problems.

Residents who are fearful, who pace or wander, withdraw from activities, cannot communicate, or refuse to communicate, often refuse to eat or will eat only a limited variety and amount of foods. Left untreated, behavior problems that result in refusal to eat can cause significant weight loss and subsequent malnutrition.

- Does resident use food to gain staff attention?
- Is resident unable to undertand the importance of eating?

Inability to Communicate.

For most residents, enjoying food and mealtimes crucially affects quality of life. Inability to make food and mealtime preferences known can result in a resident eating poorly, losing weight, and being unhappy. Malnutrition due to poor communication usually indicates substandard care. Early correction of communication problems, where possible, can prevent malnutrition.

- Does the area in which meals are served lend itself to socialization among residents? Is it a place where social communication can easily take place?
- Has there been a failure to provide adequate staff and/or adequate time in feeding or assisting residents to eat?
- Has there been a failure to recognize the need and supply adaptive feeding equipment for residents who can be helped to self-feed with such assistance?
- Is the resident capable of telling staff that he/she has a problem with the food being served- e.g., finds it to be unappetizing or unattractively presented?

Amputation

Weight loss may be due to an amputation.

NUTRITIONAL STATUS RAP KEY *(For MDS Version 2.0)*

TRIGGER — REVISION

Malnutrition problem suggested if one or more of following observed

- Weight loss
  [K3a = 1]
- Complains about taste of many foods
  [K4a = checked]
- Leaves 25% or more food uneaten at most meals
  [K4c = checked]
- Parenteral/IV feeding[(a)]
  [K5a = checked]
- Mechanically altered diet
  [K5c = checked]
- Syringe (oral feeding)
  [K5d = checked]
- Therapeutic diet
  [K5e = checked]
- Pressure ulcer[(b)]
  [M2a = 2, 3, or 4]

GUIDELINES

Factors that impede ability to consume foods:

- Reduced ability to feed self **[G1h]**
- Ostomy losses **[H3i]**,
- Chewing problems **[K1a]**
- Swallowing problems **[K1b]**
- **Possible medical causes:** Diarrhea **[H2c]**, Anemia **[I1oo]**, Cancer **[I1pp]**, Pneumonia **[I2e]**, Fever **[J1h]**, Shortness of breath **[J1l]**, Chemotherapy **[P1a]**, and nutrient/medication interactions (e.g., antipsychotics **[O4a]**, cardiac drugs, diuretics **[O4e]**, laxatives, antacids) **[from record]**

Problems to be reviewed for possible relationship to nutritional status problem:

- **Mental problems**: Mental retardation **[AB10]**, Fear that food is poisoned **[from record; E1]**; Alzheimer's Disease **[I1q]**, Other dementia **[I1u]**; Anxiety disorders **[I1dd]**; Depression **[I1ee]**;
- **Behavior problems:** Pacing **[E1n]**, Withdrawal from activities of interest **[E1o]**, Wandering **[E4a]**, Throwing food **[E4d]**, Slowness in self feeding **[G8c]**, Leaves 25% or more food uneaten **[K4c]**
- **Inability to communicate**: Comatose **[B1]**, Unable to make food and mealtime preferences known **[C3g]**, and Difficulty making self understood **[C4]**, Difficulty understanding others **[C6]**, Aphasia **[I1r]**
- **Functional problems:** Loss of upper extremity use **[G4a,b,c]**, Amputation **[I1n]**

(a) Note: These items also trigger on the Dehydration/Fluid Maintenance RAP

(b) Note: These items also trigger on the Pressure Ulcer RAP

RAP Key 4 of 4

RESIDENT ASSESSMENT PROTOCOL: FEEDING TUBES

I. PROBLEM

The efficacy of tube feedings is difficult to assess. When the complications and problems are known to be high and the benefits difficult to determine, the efficacy of tube feedings as a long-term treatment for individuals requires careful evaluation.

Where residents have difficulty eating and staff have limited time to assist them, insertion of feeding tubes for the convenience of nursing staff is an unacceptable rationale for use. The only rationale for such feedings is demonstrated medical need to prevent malnutrition or dehydration. Even here, all possible alternatives should be explored prior to using such an approach for long-term feeding, and restoration to normal feeding should remain the goal throughout the treatment program.

Use of nasogastric and nasointestinal tubes can result in many complications including, but not limited to: agitation, self-extubation (removal of the tube by the patient), infections, aspiration, unintended misplacement of the tube in the trachea or lungs, inadvertent dislodgment, and pain.

This RAP focuses on reviewing the status of the resident using tubes. The Nutritional Status and Dehydration/Fluid Maintenenace RAPs focus on resident needs that may warrant the use of tubes. To help clarify the latter issue, the following guidelines indicate the type of review process required to ensure that tubes are used in only the exceptional and acceptable situation. As a general rule, residents unable to swallow or eat food and unlikely to eat within a few days due to physical problems in chewing or swallowing (e.g., stroke or Parkinson's disease) or mental problems (e.g., Alzheimer's depression) should be assessed regarding the need for a nasogastric or nasointestinal tube or an alternative feeding method. In addition, if normal caloric intake is substantially impaired with endotracheal tubes or a tracheostomy, a nasogastric or nasointestinal tube may be necessary. Finally, tubes may be used to prevent meal-induced hypoxemia (insufficient oxygen to blood), which occurs with patients with COPD or other pulmonary problems that interfere with eating (e.g., use of oxygen, broncholdilators, tracheostomy, endotracheal tube with ventilator support).

1. Assess causes of poor nutritional status that may be identified and corrected as a first step in determining whether a nasogastric tube is necessary (see Nutritional Status RAP).

   (a) Eating, swallowing and chewing disorders can negatively affect nutritional status (low weight in relation to height, weight loss, serum albumin level, and dietary problems) and the initial task is to determine the potential causes and period of time such problems are expected to persist. Recent lab work should also be reviewed to determine if there are electrolyte imbalances, fluid volume imbalances, BUN, creatinine, low serum albumin, and low serum protein levels before treatment decisions are made. Laboratory measurement of sodium and potassium tell whether or not an electrolyte imbalance exists. Residents taking diuretics may have potassium losses requiring potassium supplements. If these types of imbalances cannot be corrected with oral nutrition and fluids or intravenous feedings, then a nasogastric or nasointestinal tube may be considered.

   (b) Determine whether fluid intake and hydration problems are short-term or long-term.

   (c) Review for gastrointestinal distention, gastrointestinal hemorrhage, increased gastric acidity, potential for stress ulcers, and abdominal pain.

(d) Identify pulmonary problems (e.g., COPD and use of endotracheal tubes, tracheostomy, and other devices) that interfere with eating or dehydration.

(e) Review for mental status problems that interfere with eating such as depression, agitation, delirium, dementia, and mood disorders.

(f) Review for other problems such as cardiovascular disease or stroke.

2. Determine the need for such a tube. Examine alternatives.

Alternatives to nasogastric and nasointestinal tubes should always be considered. Intravenous feedings should be used for short-term therapy as a treatment of choice or at least a first option. Jejunostomy may have some advantages for long-term therapy, although may increase the risk for infection. A gastrostomy is better tolerated by agitated patients and those requiring prolonged therapy (more than 2 weeks). Gastrostomy with bolus feedings is preferable to nasogastric or nasointestinal tubes for long-term therapy for comfort reasons and to prevent the dislodgement and complications associated with nasal tubes. It is also less disfiguring as it can be completely hidden under clothing when not in use.

3. Assure informed consent and right to refuse treatment. Informed consent is essential before inserting a nasogastric or nasointestinal tube. Potential advantages, disadvantages, and potential complications need to be discussed. Resident preference are normally given the greatest weight in decisions regarding tube feeding. State laws and judicial decisions must also be taken into account. If the resident is not competent to make the decision, a durable power of attorney or living will may determine who has the legal power to act on the resident's behalf. Where the resident is not competent or no power of attorney is in effect, the physician may have the responsibility for making a decision regarding the use of tube feeding. In any case, when illness is terminal and/or irreversible, technical means of providing fluids and nutrition can represent extraordinary rather than ordinary means of prolonging life.

4. Monitor for complications and correct/change procedures and feedings when necessary. Periodic changing of the nasogastric and intestinal tubes is necessary, although the appropriate interval for changing tubes is not clear. Assessment and determination of continued need should be completed before the tube is reinserted. Specific written orders by the physician are required.

Individuals at risk of pulmonary aspiration (such as those with altered pharyngeal reflexes or unconsciousness) should be given a nasointestinal tube rather than a nasogastric tube, or other medical alternative. Those at risk for displacement of a nasogastric tube, such as those with coughing, vomiting, or endotracheally intubated, should also be given a nasointestinal tube rather than a nasogastric tube or other medical alternative.

II. TRIGGER

Consider efficacy and need for feeding tubes if:

- Feeding Tube present *
  [K5b = checked]

---

* Note: This item also triggers on the Dehydration RAP

Feeding Tubes RAP (2 of 5)

III. GUIDELINES

COMPLICATIONS OF TUBE FEEDING

To reiterate, serious potential negative consequences include agitation, depression, mood disorders, self-extubation (removal of the tube by the patient), infections, aspirations, misplacement of tube in trachea or lungs, pain, and tube dysfunction. Abnormal lab values can be expected and should be reviewed.

Infection in the trachea or lungs. Gastric organisms grow as a result of alkalizing (raising) the gastric pH. Gastric colonization results in transmission of gastric organisms to the trachea and the development of nosocomial pneumonia. In one study, colonization in 89% of patients within 4 days in ventilated patients with enteral nutrition was found with nosocomial respiratory infection in 62% of the patients studied. Symptoms of respiratory infections to be monitored include coughing, shortness of breath, fever, chest pain, respiratory arrest, delirium, confusion, and seizures.

Aspiration of gastric organisms into the trachea and the lungs. The incidence is difficult to determine, but most studies suggest it is relatively high.

Inadvertent respiratory placement of the tube is the most common side effect of tube placement. In one study, 15% of small-bore nasogastric tubes and 27-50% of nasointestinal tubes were found to be out of their intended position upon radiographic examination without any other evidence of displacement. Respiratory placement can occur in any patient, but is most likely in those who are neurologically depressed, heavily sedated, unable to gag, or endotracheally intubated. Detecting such placement is difficult; the following comments address this issue:

- Radiologic detection is the most definitive means to detect tube displacement. Under this procedure, pneumothorax and inadvertent placement in the respiratory tract can be avoided by first placing the feeding tube in the esophagus with the tip above the xiphoid process and then securing the tube and confirming placement with a chest x-ray. Then the tube may be advanced into the stomach and another x-ray taken to confirm the position. The stylet can then be removed and tube feeding begun. Unfortunately, nursing homes are highly unlikely to have appropriate radiological technology and it is normally unreasonable to expect them to make arrangements to have patients transported to available radiology.

- pH testing of gastric aspirates to determine whether a tube is in the gastric, intestine, or the respiratory area is a promising method for testing feeding tube placement. However, parameters for various secretions from the three areas have not yet been clinically defined.

- Aspiration of visually recognizable gastrointestinal secretions, although a frequently used method of determining placement of tubes, is of questionable value as the visual characteristics of secretions can be similar to those from the respiratory tract.

- Ausculatory method: although "shooshing" or gurgling sounds can indicate placement in the stomach, the same sounds can occur when feeding tubes are inadvertently placed in the pharynx, esophagus and respiratory tract. Although small-bore tubes make the ausculatory method more difficult to use, large-bore nasogastric tubes may also be placed inadvertently in the respiratory tract producing false gurgling.

Inadvertent dislodgement of the tubes. Nonweighted tubes appear to be more likely to be displaced than weighted tubes (with an attached bolus of mercury or tungsten at the tip).

Other complications include: pain, epistaxis, pneumothorax, hydrothorax, nasal alar necrosis, nasopharyngitis, esophagitis, eustachitis, esophageal strictures, airway obstruction, pharyngeal and esophageal perforations. Symptoms of respiratory infections are to be reviewed.

Complications of gastric tract infections and gastric problems. Symptoms include abdominal pain, abdominal distention, stress ulcers, and gastric hemorrhage. There is also a need to monitor for complications including diarrhea, nausea, abdominal distention, and asphyxia. Such complications signal the need for a change in the type of formula or diagnostic work for other pathology.

Complications for the cardiovascular systems. Symptoms of cardiac distress or arrest to be monitored include chest pain, loss of heart beat, loss of consciousness, and loss of breathing.

Periodic tests to assure positive nitrogen balance during enteral feeding. Where positive balance is not achieved, a formula with high nitrogen density is needed. The absorptive capacity is impaired in many elderly patients so that serum fat and protein should be monitored. Effective nutrients should result in positive nitrogen balance, maintenance or increases in body weight, triceps skinfold and midarm muscle circumference maintenance, total iron binding capacity maintenance, and serum urea nitrogen level maintenance. Caloric intake and resident weight should be monitored on a regular basis.

FEEDING TUBES STATUS RAP KEY *(For MDS Version 2.0)*

TRIGGER

Consider efficacy and need for feeding tubes if:

- Feeding Tube present *
  [K5b = checked]

GUIDELINES

Factors that may impede removal of tube:

- Comatose **[B1]**
- Failure to eat **[K4c]** **AND** Resists assistance in eating **[E4e]**
- **Diagnoses:** CVA **[I1t]**, Gastric ulcers **[I3]**,
- Gastric bleeding **[from record]**
- Chewing problem **[K1a]**
- Swallowing problem **[K1b]**
- Mouth pain **[K1c]**
- Length of time feeding tube has been in use **[from record]**

Potential complications of tube feeding:

- **Diagnostic conditions:** Delirium **[B5]**, Repetitive physical movements **[E1n]**, Anxiety **[I1dd]**, Depression **[I1ee]**, Recurrent lung aspirations **[J1k]**
- Self-extubation (removal of tube by resident) **[from record]**
- Limb restraints in use to prevent self-extubation **[P4d]**
- **Infections in lung/trachea:** Pneumonia **[I2e]**, Fever **[J1h]**, Shortness of breath **[J1l]**, Placement or dislodgement of tube into lung **[from exam, record]**
- **Side-effects of enteral feeding solutions:** Constipation **[H2b]**, Diarrhea **[H2c]**, Fecal impaction **[H2d]**, Abdominal distention or pain **[exam]**, Dehydrated **[J1c]**
- **Respiratory problems:** Pneumothorax, hydrothorax, airway obstruction, acute respiratory distress, respiratory distress **[I3; from observation, record]**
- **Cardiac distress/arrest:** Chest pain **[J3c]**, loss of heart beat, loss of consciousness, loss of breathing **[from observation, record]**
- Abnormal lab values **[P9]**

* Note: This item also triggers on the Dehydration RAP

Feeding Tube Status RAP Key 5 of 5

RESIDENT ASSESSMENT PROTOCOL: DEHYDRATION/FLUID MAINTENANCE

I. PROBLEM

On average, one can live only four days without water. Water is necessary for the distribution of nutrients to cells, elimination of wastes, regulation of body temperature, and countless other complex processes.

Dehydration is a condition in which water or fluid loss (output) far exceeds fluid intake. The body becomes less able to maintain adequate blood pressure, deliver sufficient oxygen and nutrients to the cells, and rid itself of wastes. Many distressing symptoms can originate from these conditions, including:

- **Dizziness on sitting/standing** (blood pressure insufficient to supply oxygen and glucose to brain);
- **Confusion or change in mental status** (decreased oxygen and glucose to brain);
- **Decreased urine output** (kidneys conserve water);
- **Decreased skin turgor**, dry mucous membranes (symptoms of dryness);
- **Constipation** (water insufficient to rid body of wastes); and
- **Fever** (water insufficient to maintain normal temperature).

Other possible consequences of dehydration include: decreased functional ability, predisposition to falls (because of orthostatic hypotension), fecal impaction, predisposition to infection, fluid and electrolyte disturbances, and ultimately death.

Nursing home residents are particularly vulnerable to dehydration. It is often difficult or impossible to access fluids independently; the perception of thirst can be muted; the aged kidney can have a decreased ability to concentrate urine; and acute and chronic illness can alter fluid and electrolyte balance.

Unfortunately, many symptoms of this condition do not appear until significant fluid has been lost. Early signs and symptoms tend to be unreliable and nonspecific; staff will often disagree about the clinical indicators of dehydration for specific cases; and the identification of the most crucial symptoms of the condition are most difficult to identify among the aged. Early identification of dehydration is thus problematic, and the goal of this RAP is to identify any and all possible high risk cases, permitting the introduction of programs to prevent the condition from occurring.

When dehydration is in fact observed, treatment objectives focus on restoring normal fluid volume, preferably orally. If the resident cannot drink between 2500-3000 cc's every 24 hours, water and electrolyte deficits can be made up via other routes. Fluids can be administered intravenously, subcutaneously, or by tube until resident is adequately hydrated and can take and retain sufficient fluids orally.

II. TRIGGERS

Dehydration suggested if one or more of following present:

- Dehydration
  [J1c = checked]
- Insufficient fluid/did not consume all liquids provided
  [J1d = checked]

- UTI
  [I2j = checked]
- Dehydration diagnosis
  [I3 = 276.5]
- Weight fluctuation of 3+ pounds
  [J1a = checked]
- Fever
  [J1h = checked]
- Internal bleeding
  [J1j = checked]
- Parenteral/IV [(a)]
  [K5a = checked]
- Feeding tube [(b)]
  [K5b = checked]
- Taking diuretic
  [O4e = 1-7]

(a) Note: This item also triggers on the Nutritional Status RAP
(b) Note: This item also triggers on the Feeding Tube RAP

III. GUIDELINES

RESIDENTS FACTORS THAT MAY IMPEDE ABILITY TO MAINTAIN FLUID BALANCE

Moderate/severely impaired decision-making ability.

- Has there been a recent unexplainable change in mental status?
- Does resident seem unusually agitated or disoriented?
- Is resident delirious?
- Is resident comatose?
- Does dementia, aphasia or other condition seriously limit resident's understanding of others, or how well others can understand the resident?

Comprehension/Communication problems.

Body control problems.

- Does resident require extensive assistance to transfer?
- Does resident freely move on the unit?
- Has there been recent ADL decline?

Hand dexterity problem.
- Can resident grasp cup?

Bowel problems.
- Does the resident have constipation or a fecal impaction that may be interfering with fluid intake?

Swallowing problems.

- Does resident have mouth sore(s)/ulcer(s)?
- Does resident refuse food, meals, meds?
- Can resident drink from a cup or suck through a straw?

Use of Parenteral/IV.

Are feeding tubes in use?

RESIDENT DEHYDRATION RISK FACTORS

Dehydration risk factors can be categorized in terms of whether they decrease **fluid intake** or **increase fluid loss**. The higher the number of factors, the greater the risk of dehydration. Ongoing fluid loss through the lungs and skin occurs at a normal rate of approximately 500 cc/day and increases with rapid respiratory rate and sweating. Therefore, **decreased fluid intake** for any reason can lead to dehydration.

Purposeful Restriction of Fluid Intake.

- Has there been a decrease in thirst perception?
- Is resident unaware of the need to intake sufficient fluids?
- Has resident or staff restricted intake to avoid urinary incontinence?
- Are fluids restricted because of diagnostic procedure or other health reason?
- Does sad mood, grief, or depression cause resident to refuse foods/liquids?

Presence of infection, fever, vomiting/diarrhea/nausea, excessive sweating (e.g., a heat wave).

Frequent use of laxatives, enemas, diuretics.

Excessive urine output (polyuria).

Excessive urine output (polyuria) may be due to:

- Drugs (e.g., lithium, phenytoin), alcohol abuse
- Disease (e.g., diabetes mellitus, diabetes insipidus)
- Other conditions (e.g., hypoaldosteronism, hyperparathyroidism)

Other test results.

Relevant test result to be considered:

- Does systolic/diastolic blood pressure drop 20 points on sitting/standing?
- On inspection, do oral mucous membranes appear dry?
- Does urine appear more concentrated and/or decreased in volume?

DEHYDRATION/FLUID MAINTENANCE STATUS RAP KEY *(For MDS Version 2.0)*

TRIGGER — REVISION

Dehydration suggested if one or more of following present:

- Dehydrated
  [J1c = checked]
- Insufficient fluid/did not consume all liquids provided
  [J1d = checked]
- UTI
  [I2j = checked]
- Dehydration diagnosis
  [I3 = 276.5]
- Weight fluctuation of 3+ pounds
  [J1a = checked]
- Fever
  [J1h = checked]
- Internal bleeding
  [J1j = checked]
- Parenteral/IV [a]
  [K5a = checked]
- Feeding tube [b]
  [K5b = checked]
- Taking diuretic
  [O4e = 1-7]

[a] Note: This item also triggers on the Nutritional Status RAP

[b] Note: This item also triggers on the Feeding Tube RAP

GUIDELINES

Resident Factors that May Impede Ability to Maintain Fluid Balance:

- Indicators of Delirium **[B5]**
- Moderate/severely impaired decision-making ability **[B4]**
- Comprehension/communication problem **[C4, C6]**
- Body control problems **[G3, G4]**
- Hand dexterity problem **[G4c]**
- Constipation **[H2b]**
- Fecal impaction **[H2d]**
- Swallowing problem **[K1b]**
- Recent (within 7 days) deterioration in ADLs **[observe, ask Direct Care Staff]**

Resident Dehydration Risk Factors:

- Purposeful restriction of fluids **[J1d; from record]**
- Diarrhea **[H2c]**, Presence of infection **[I2]**, Fever **[J1h]**, Vomiting **[J1o]**, Nausea **[from record]**, Excessive sweating **[from record, exam]**
- Frequent laxative/enema/diuretic use **[from record; H3h, O4e]**
- Excessive urine output **[from record, exam]**
- Other tests: Standing/sitting blood pressure, Status of oral mucous membranes, Urine output volume **[from record]**

RAP Key 4 of 4

RESIDENT ASSESSMENT PROTOCOL: DENTAL CARE

I. PROBLEM

Having teeth/dentures that function properly is an important requisite for nutritional adequacy. Having teeth/dentures that are clean and attractive can promote a resident's positive self-image as well as personal appearance thereby enhancing social interactions among residents, residents and staff, and residents and visitors. Good oral health can decrease a resident's risk of oral discomfort and in some instances, systemic illness from oral infections/cancer. Residents at greatest risk due to impaired abilities are primarily those with multiple medical conditions and medications, functional limitations in self-care, and communication deficits. Also at risk are more self-sufficient residents who lack motivation or have no consistent history of performing oral health functions. Residents with a history of alcohol and/or tobacco use have a greater risk of developing chronic oral lesions.

II. TRIGGERS

Dental Care or Oral Health problem suggested if:

- Mouth Debris *(Dental Care)*
  [L1a = checked]
- Less Than Daily Cleaning of Teeth/Dentures *(Dental Care)*
  [L1f = not checked]

- Mouth Pain *(Oral Health)*
  [K1c = checked]
- Some/All natural teeth lost and does not have or does not use dentures *(Oral Health)*
  [L1c = checked]
- Broken, Loose or Carious Teeth *(Oral Health)*
  [L1d = checked]
- Inflamed Gums, Oral Abscesses, Swollen/Bleeding Gums, Ulcers, Rashes *(Oral Health)*
  [L1e = checked]

III. GUIDELINES

CONFOUNDING PROBLEMS

Debris on teeth, gums, and oral tissues may consist of food and bacteria-laden plaque that can begin to decay teeth or cause foul denture odors if not removed at least once daily. The purpose of this section is to examine confounding problems (from the MDS) which may be prohibiting a resident from adequately removing oral debris.

Impaired cognitive skills.

- Does the resident need reminders to clean his/her teeth/dentures?
- Does he remember the steps necessary to complete oral hygiene?
- Would he benefit from task segmentation or supervision?

Impaired ability to understand:

- Can the resident follow verbal directions or demonstrations for mouth care?
- If the resident has language difficulties, does he/she know what to do when handed a toothbrush/toothpaste and placed at the bathroom sink?

Impaired vision.

- Is resident's vision adequate for performing mouth care or checking its adequacy?

Impaired personal hygiene.

- Did the resident receive supervision or assistance with oral/dental care during the last 7 days?
- Has he/she been assessed to see if he/she could do it independently?
- Does the resident have partial/total loss of voluntary arm movement or impaired hand dexterity that inteferes with self-care?
- What would the resident need to be more independent?

Resists ADL assistance:

- Does the resident resist mouth care? If so, why (e.g., would rather do own care, painful mouth, apathy related to depression, not motivated - never cared for teeth/mouth, approach of staff, fear)?

Motivation/Knowledge of resident who is independent in oral/dental care but still has debris or performs care less than daily.

- Is he/she brushing adequately?
- Does he/she know that it is most important to brush near the gumline?
- Does he/she need to be shown how or be given reinforcement for maintaining good hygiene?

Adaptive equipment for oral hygiene.

- Has the resident tried or would he/she benefit from using a built-up, long-handled, or electric toothbrush, or suction brush for cleaning teeth?
- If resident has dentures, does he/she have denture cleaning devices (e.g., denture brush, soaking bath)?

Dental Care RAP (2 of 5)

Dry mouth from dehydration or medications.

- Dry mouth can contribute to the formation of debris. Is the resident's lips, tongue, or mouth dry, sticky, or coated with film?
- Is the resident taking enough fluids? Is lip balm being applied to resident who has painful, cracking or bleeding lips?
- Is he/she taking any medications that can cause dry mouth (e.g., decongestants, antihistamines, diuretics, antihypertensives, antidepressants, antipsychotic, antineoplastics)?
- If these medications are necessary, has the resident tried saliva substitutes to stimulate moisture?

TREATMENT HISTORY AND OTHER RELEVANT FACTORS

Mouth pain or sensitivity can be related to either minor and easily treatable (e.g., gum irritation from ill-fitting dentures, localized periodontal problem) or more serious problems (e.g., oral abscess, cancer, advanced tooth decay or periodontal disease). The presence of pain may prevent the resident from eating adequately.

Residents with cognitive impairment and/or those who have difficulty making their needs known are difficult to assess. They may not complain specifically of mouth pain but may instead have decreased food intake or changes in behavior.

The presence of lesions, ulcers, inflammation, bleeding, swelling, or rashes may be representative of a minor probelm (e.g., irritation from wearing dentures for 24 hours/day), which resolves when the cause is alleviated (e.g., combination of mouth care and leaving dentures out.) However, these signs may also indicate more serious problems, even dental emergencies (e.g., infection). If the problem does not resolve with specific local treatment after a couple of days OR if these signs are accompanied by pain, fever, lymphadenopathy (swollen glands) and/or signs of local infection (e.g., redness), chewing or swallowing problems, or changes in mental status or behavior, a dental consult should be considered.

Review mouth for Candidiasis (white areas that appear to be removable anywhere in mouth, (mostly on tongue) for lethargic residents who have one or more of following diagnoses: stroke, Alzheimer's, Parkinson's, anxiety disorder, depression, diabetes, osteoporosis, or septicemia.

Broken, loose, or carious teeth may progress to more severe problems (e.g., dislodging a decayed tooth and swallowing or aspirating it). Although, not emergencies, a dental consult should be considered.

If a resident has lost some or all of his/her natural teeth and does not have dentures (or partial plates) staff should consider if the resident has the cognitive ability and motivation to wear dentures.

- Has a dentist evaluated resident for dentures?
- Why doesn't resident use his/her dentures (or partial plates)?
- Are teeth in good repair?
- Do they fit well?
- Are they comfortable to wear when eating or talking?
- Does the resident like the way he/she looks when wearing them?
- Has a dentist evaluated resident for dentures?
- Has a dental hygienist interviewed and made recommendations regarding oral hygiene care?

Exam by dentist since problem noted. When evaluating a resident with mouth pain or the presence of any of the other trigger signs, check the record to see if a dentist has examined the resident since the problem was first noted.

- Was the current problem addressed?
- What were the recommendations?

Use of anticoagulants.

- Is the resident on coumadin or heparin that would put him/her at risk for bleeding if dental work is necessary?
- Is it noted on the medical record?

Valvular heart disease or prosthesis (e.g., heart valve, false hip, etc.).

- Are either of these conditions present?
- If so are they clearly noted in the medical record so that necessary precautious be taken prior to dental work?

DENTAL CARE RAP KEY *(For MDS Version 2.0)*

TRIGGER — REVISION

Dental Care or Oral Health problem suggested if one or more of the following present:

- Mouth Debris (*Dental Care*)
  [L1a = checked]
- Less Than Daily Cleaning of Teeth/Dentures (*Dental Care*)
  [L1f = not checked]
- Mouth Pain (*Oral Health*)
  [K1c = checked]
- Some/All natural teeth lost and does not have or does not use dentures *(Oral Health)*
  [L1c = checked]
- Broken, Loose or Carious Teeth (*Oral Health)*
  [L1d = checked]
- Inflamed Gums, Oral Abscesses, Swollen/Bleeding Gums, Ulcers, Rashes (*Oral Health)*
  [L1e = checked]

GUIDELINES

Confounding problems to be considered:

- Impaired cognitive skills **[B1, B4]**
- Impaired ability to understand **[C1, C6]**
- Impaired vision **[D1]**
- Resists ADL assistance **[E4e]**
- Impaired personal hygiene **[G1j]**
- Motivation/knowledge **[from observation]**
- Adaptive equipment for oral hygiene **[from record]**
- Dry mouth from dehydration **[J1c,d]** or from medications **[from medication sheet]**

Treatment history/relevant factors:

- Mouth pain or sensitivity **[K1c]**
- Presence of lesions, ulcers, inflammation, bleeding, swelling or rashes **[L1e]**
- Broken, loose or carious teeth **[L1d]**
- Natural teeth lost/ no dentures **[L1c]**
- Exam by dentist/dental hygienist since problem noted **[from record]**
- Use of anticoagulants **[from record]**
- Valvular heart disease or valvular appliance **[I3]**

DENTAL RAP Key 5 of 5

RESIDENT ASSESSMENT PROTOCOL: PRESSURE ULCERS

I. PROBLEM

Between 3% and 5% (or more) of residents in nursing facilities have pressure ulcers (pressure sores, decubitus ulcers, bedsores). Sixty percent or more of residents will typically be at risk of pressure ulcer development. Pressure ulcers can have serious consequences for the elderly and are costly and time consuming to treat. However, they are one of the most common, preventable and treatable conditions among the elderly who have restricted mobility. Successful outcomes can be expected with preventive and treatment programs.

Assessment goals are: (1) to ensure that a treatment plan is in place for residents with pressure ulcers; and (2) to identify residents at risk for developing a pressure ulcer who are not currently receiving some type of preventive care program.

II. TRIGGERS

Pressure ulcer present or there is a risk for occurrence if one or more of following present (risk):

- Pressure Ulcer(s) Present *(Present)* [a]
  [M2a = 1,2,3,4]
- Bed mobility problem *(Risk)*
  [G1aA = 2,3,4,8] [b]
- Bedfast *(Risk)*
  [G6a = checked]
- Bowel Incontinence *(Risk)*
  [H1a = 1,2,3,4]
- Peripheral Vascular Disease *(Risk)*
  [I1j = checked]
- Previous Pressure Ulcer *(Risk)*
  [M3 = 1]
- Skin desensitized to pain or pressure *(Risk)*
  [M4e = checked]
- Daily Trunk Restraint *(Risk)* [c]
  [P4c = 2]

(a) Note: Codes 2, 3, and 4 also trigger on the Nutritional Status RAP
(b) Note: Codes 2, 3, and 4 also trigger on the ADL RAP
(c) Note: This code also triggers on the Falls RAP and Physical Restraints RAP

III. GUIDELINES

Review the MDS items listed on the RAP KEY for relevance in understanding the type of care that may be required.

Diagnoses, Conditions and Treatments that Present Complications.

Consider carefully whether the resident exhibits conditions or is receiving treatments that may either place the resident at higher risk of developing pressure ulcers or complicate their treatment. Such conditions include:

Diabetes, Alzheimer's Disease and other dementias. An impairment in cognitive ability, particularly in severe end-stage dementia, can lead to immobility.

Edema. The presence of extravascular fluid can impair blood flow. If prolonged or excess pressure is applied to an area with edema, skin breakdown can occur.

Antidepressants and antianxiety/hypnotics. These medications can produce or contribute to lessened mobility, worsen incontinence, and lead to or increase confusion.

Interventions/Programs to Consider if the Resident Develops a New Pressure Ulcer, or an Ulcer Being Treated is not Resolved.

A variety of factors may explain this occurrence; however, they may suggest the need to evaluate current interventions and modifications of the care plan.

- Review the resident's medical condition, medications, and other risk factors to determine whether the care plan (for prevention or cure) addresses all potential causes or complications.
- Review the care plan to determine whether it is actually being followed (e.g., is the resident being turned often enough to prevent ulcer formation).

Things to Consider If The Resident Is At Risk For Pressure Ulcers But Is Not Receiving Preventive Skin Care.

Even if pressure ulcers are not present, determine why this course of prevention is not being provided to a resident with risk factors.

- Is the resident new to the unit?
- Do few or many risk factors for the development of pressure ulcers apply to this resident?
- Are staff concentrating on other problems (e.g., resolution of behavior problems) so that the risks pressure of ulcers are masked?

PRESSURE ULCERS RAP KEY *(For MDS Version 2.0)*

TRIGGER — REVISION

Pressure ulcer present or risk for occurrence if one or more of following present:

- Pressure Ulcer(s) Present *(Present)* [a]
  [M2a = 1,2,3,4]
- Bed mobility problem *(Risk)*
  [G1aA = 2,3,4,8] [b]
- Bedfast *(Risk)*
  [G6a = checked]
- Bowel Incontinence *(Risk)*
  [H1a = 1,2,3,4]
- Peripheral Vascular Disease *(Risk)*
  [I1j = checked]
- Previous Ulcer *(Risk)*
  [M3 = 1]
- Skin desensitized to pain or pressure *(Risk)*
  [M4e = checked]
- Daily Trunk Restraint *(Risk)* [c]
  [P4c = 2]

[a] Note: Codes 2, 3, and 4 also trigger on the Nutritional Status RAP

[b] Note: Codes 2, 3, and 4 also trigger on the ADL RAP

[c] Note: This code also triggers on the Falls RAP and Physical Restraints RAP

GUIDELINES

Other factors that address or may complicate treatment of pressure ulcers or risk of ulcers:

- **Diagnoses or conditions:**

  Diabetes **[I1a]**, Alzheimer's disease **[I1q]**, Other dementia **[I1u]**, Hemiplegia/Hemiparesis **[I1v]**, Multiple Sclerosis **[I1w]**, Edema **[J1g]**

- **Interventions/Programs:**
  - — Pressure relieving chair/beds **[M5a, M5b]**
  - — Turning/repositioning **[M5c]**
  - — Nutrition or hydration program to manage skin care problems **[M5d]**
  - — Ulcer care **[M5e]**
  - — Surgical wound care/treatment **[M5f]**
  - — Application of dressings (with or without topical medications) other than to feet **[M5g]**
  - — Application of ointment/medications (other than to feet) **[M5h]**
  - — Preventative or protective skin care (other than to feet) **[M5i]**
  - — Preventive or protective foot care **[M6e]**
  - — Application of dressings to feet (with or without topical medications) **[M6f]**
  - — Use of restraints **[P4c,d,e]**

- **Medications:**

  Antipsychotics **[O4a]**
  Antianxiety **[O4b]**
  Antidepressants **[O4c]**
  Hypnotics **[O4d]**

Pressure Ulcers RAP Key 3 of 3

RESIDENT ASSESSMENT PROTOCOL: PSYCHOTROPIC DRUG USE

I. PROBLEM

Psychotropic drugs are among the most frequently prescribed agents for elderly nursing home residents. Studies in nursing facilities suggest that 35% to 65% of residents receive psychotropic medications.

When used appropriately and judiciously, these medications can enhance the quality of life of residents who need them. However, all psychotropic drugs have the potential for producing undesirable side effects or aggravating problematic signs and symptoms of existing conditions. An important example is postural hypotension, a condition associated with serious and life-threatening side effects. Severity of delirium side effects is dependent on: the class and dosage of drug, interactions with other drugs, and the age, and health status of the resident.

Maximizing the resident's functional potential and well-being while minimizing the hazards associated with drug side effects are important goals of therapy. In reviewing a psychotropic drug regimen there are several rules of thumb:

- Evaluate the need for the drug (e.g., consider amount and type of distress, response to nonpharmacologic interventions, pros and cons of drug side effects in relation to distress without the drug). Distinguish between treating specific diagnosed psychiatric disorders and treating symptoms. Specific psychiatric disorders (e.g., schizophrenia, major depression) have specific drug treatments with published guidelines for dosage and duration of treatment. However, a recorded diagnosis of a psychiatric disorder does not necessarily require drug treatment if symptoms are inactive.

- Start low, go slow. If needed, psychotropic drugs should be started at lowest dosage possible. To minimize side effects, doses should be increased slowly until either there is a therapeutic effect, side effects emerge, or the maximum recommended dose is reached.

- Each drug has its own set of actions and side effects, some more serious than others; these should be evaluated in terms of each user's medical-status profile, including interaction with other medications.

- Consider symptoms or decline in functional status as a potential side effect of medication.

II. TRIGGERS

TO BE TRIGGERED, RESIDENT MUST FIRST USE A PSYCHOTROPIC DRUG [Antipsychotic, antidepressant, or antianxiety] [O4a,b, or c = 1-7]. If used, go to RAP review if one or more of following present:

PSYCHOTROPIC TRIGGER A

Potential for Drug-Related Hypotention or gait disturbances if:

- Repetitive physical movement[a]
  [E1n = 1,2]
- Balance While Sitting
  [G3b = 1,2,3]
- Hypotension
  [I1i = checked]
- Dizziness/Vertigo[b]
  [J1f = checked]
- Syncope
  [J1m = checked]
- Unsteady Gait
  [J1n = checked]
- Fell in past 30 days[b]
  [J4a = checked]
- Fell in past 31-180 day[b]
  [J4b = checked]
- Hip fracture
  [J4c = checked]
- Swallowing problem
  [K1b = checked]

Potential for Drug-Related Cognitive/Behavioral Impairment if: [c]

- Delirium/Disordered Thinking
  - Easily distracted
    [B5a = 2]
  - Periods of altered perception or awareness of surroundings
    [B5b = 2]
  - Episodes of disorganized speech
    [B5c = 2]
  - Periods of restlessness
    [B5d = 2]
  - Periods of lethargy
    [B5e = 2]
  - Mental function varies over the course of the day
    [B5f = 2]
- Deterioration in Cognitive Status [c]
  [B6 = 2]
- Deterioration in Communication
  [C7 = 2]
- Deterioration in Mood [c]
  [E3 = 2]
- Deterioration in Behavioral Symptoms [c]
  [E5 = 2]

Psychotropic Drug Use RAP (2 of 11)

- Depression
  [I1ee = checked]
- Hallucinations
  [J1i = checked]

Potential for Drug Related Discomfort if:

- Constipation
  [H2b = checked]
- Fecal Impaction
  [H2d = checked]
- Lung Aspiration
  [J1k = checked]

(a) Note: This item also triggers on the Mood RAP
(b) Note: These items also trigger on Falls RAP
(c) Note: All of these items also trigger on the Delirium RAP

III. GUIDELINES

If any of the triggered conditions are present complete the following:

Step One.

Conduct the following reviews:

1. Drug review [from record]

- Length of time between when the drug was first taken and onset of problem
- Dose of drug and how frequently taken
- Number of classes of psychotropics taken
- Reason drug prescribed

2. Review resident's conditions that impair drug metabolism/excretion

- Impaired liver/renal function
- Acute condition(s)
- Dehydration

3. Review behavior/mood/psychiatric status

- Current problem status
- Recent changes in mood and behavior
- Behavior management program
- Psychiatric conditions

Step Two.

Compare the drugs the resident is currently taking with common side effects listed below. Refer to Tables A, B, and C for clarification.

POTENTIAL PSYCHOTROPIC DRUG-RELATED SIDE EFFECTS

Clarifying Information if Hypotension present

Postural (orthostatic) hypotension (decrease in blood pressure upon standing) is one of the major risk factors for falls related to psychotropic drugs. It is commonly seen with the low-potency antipsychotic drugs (chlorpromazine, thioridizene) and with tricyclic antidepressants. Both classes of drugs have anticholinergic properties. Within each class, drugs with the most potent anticholinergic properties also seem to produce the greatest hypotensive effects. Symptoms of dizziness/vertigo upon sitting or standing from a lying position, syncope (fainting), and falls/fractures, should be seriously considered as potential indicators of psychotropic-drug-induced hypotension. In addition, these symptoms may be due to a disturbance of heart rhythm, which could be aggravated by a tricyclic antidepressant. The occurrence of any of the aforementioned symptoms requires assessment of postural vital signs and heart rhythm.

- ***Measurement of postural vital signs.*** Measure blood pressure and pulse when the resident is lying down. Remeasure blood pressure and pulse after the resident has been on his/her feet for one to five minutes (if unable to stand, measure after the resident has been sitting). Occasionally, further drops in blood pressure occur after the person has been up for some time. While a drop of more than 20 mm Hg systolic is always abnormal, it is particularly significant if accompanied by dizziness, loss of balance, or a standing blood pressure of less than 100 mm Hg. A large drop may be clinically significant even if the lower pressure is not abnormally low, particularly in residents who have some degree of cerebrovascular disease.

Clarifying Information if Movement Disorder Present

High fever AND/OR muscular rigidity. Antipsychotic drugs can interfere with temperature regulation, which can lead to the potentially fatal problem of hyperthermia. Also, when high fever is accompanied by severe muscular rigidity, "neuroleptic malignant" syndrome must be suspected. Fever above 103 degrees in a resident on an antipsychotic drug is a medical emergency because of the disturbed temperature regulation. Even lesser degrees of fever, if accompanied by severe muscular rigidity, are medical emergencies. Temperature must therefore be monitored especially closely in residents on psychotropic drugs with anticholinergic properties. In addition, nonantipsychotic drugs with anticholinergic properties, such as antidepressants, may aggravate fever by impairing sweating.

Parkinson's disease. This condition is known to be aggravated by all antipsychotic drugs. At times, it is difficult to know whether parkinsonian symptoms (e.g., tremors, especially of hands; pill-rolling of hands; muscle rigidity of limbs, necks, trunk) are due to Parkinson's disease or to present or recent antipsychotic drug therapy. There should be a strong bias in favor of reducing or eliminating antipsychotic drugs in residents with Parkinson's disease unless there are compelling behavioral or psychotic indications. Antiparkinson drugs should be considered when antipsychotic drugs are clinically necessary in residents with Parkinson's disease.

Five movement disorders are commonly encountered in residents on antipsychotic drugs. All of these disturbances can adversely affect a resident's quality of life as well as increase his/her risk of accidents. The triggered MDS items in Group 2 are signs/symptoms of these disorders. To clarify whether the resident is suffering from one of these disorders, all residents on antipsychotic drugs should be periodically screened for the following conditions:

Parkinsonism. As with Parkinson's disease, this condition may involve ANY combination of tremors, postural unsteadiness, and rigidity of muscles in the limbs, neck, or trunk. Although the most common is a pill-rolling or alternating tremor of the hands, other kinds of tremors are occasionally seen. At times, a resident with Parkinsonism will have no tremor, only rigidity and shuffling gait. Symptoms respond to antiparkinson drugs, but not always completely. Dosage reduction or substitution of nonantipsychotic drug, when feasible, is the preferred management.

Akinesia. This condition is characterized by marked decrease in spontaneous movement, often accompanied by nonparticipation in activity and self-care. It is managed by reducing the antipsychotic drug or adding an antiparkinson drug.

Dystonia. This disorder is marked by holding of the neck or trunk in a rigid, unnatural posture. Usually the head is either hyperextended or turned to the side. The condition is uncomfortable and prompt treatment with an antiparkinson drug can be helpful.

Akathisia — the inability to sit still. The resident with this disorder is driven to constant movement, including pacing, rocking, or fidgeting, which can, at times persist for weeks, even after the antipsychotic drug is stopped. The condition responds occasionally to antiparkinson drugs, but less consistently than parkinsonism or dystonia. Sometimes benzodiazepines or beta-blockers are helpful in treating the symptom, although dosage reduction is the most desirable treatment when possible.

Tardive dyskinesia — persistent, sometimes permanent movements induced by long-term antipsychotic drug therapy. Most typical are thrusting movements of the tongue, movements of the lips, or chewing or puckering movements. These involuntary movements can clearly interfere with chewing and swallowing. When they do, the dyskinesia can be suppressed by raising the dose of the antipsychotic drug, **but this will make the problem more permanent**. When possible, it is usually preferable to reduce or eliminate the antipsychotic drug, because the symptoms of dyskinesia will often decrease over time after drug discontinuation.

Other variations of tardive dyskinesia include abnormal limb movements, such as peculiar and recurrent postures of the hands and arms, or rocking or writhing trunk movements. There is no consistently effective treatment. Withdrawal of the antipsychotic drug leads to eventual reversal of the symptoms over many months, in about 50% of cases.

Clarifying Information if Gait Disturbance Present (Other Than That Induced by Antipsychotics)

Long-acting benzodiazepine antianxiety drugs have been implicated in increasing the risk of falls and consequent injury by producing disturbances of balance, gait, and positioning ability. They also produce marked sedation, often manifested by short-term memory loss, decline in cognitive abilities, slurred speech, drowsiness in the morning/daytime sedation, and little/no activity involvement. If an antianxiety drug is needed to treat an anxiety disorder, a short-acting benzodiazepine or buspirone would be preferable to a long-acting benzodiazepine. Buspirone is nonsedating and takes several weeks to work. Dosage should be increased slowly.

Clarifying Information if Cognitive/Behavior Impairment Present

Acute confusion/delirium. The MDS items which tap the syndrome of acute confusion or delirium, can all be caused or aggravated by psychotropic drugs of any of the major classes. If the resident does not have acute confusion related to a medical illness or severe depression consider the psychotropic drug as a

cause. The most helpful information in establishing a relationship is the linkage between starting the drug and the occurrence of the change in cognitive status.

Depression. Both anti-anxiety and antipsychotic drugs may cause symptoms of depression as a side effect, or may aggravate depression in a resident with a depressive disorder who receives these drugs rather than specific antidepressive therapy.

Hallucinations/delusions. While these are often symptoms of mental illness, all of the major classes of psychotropic drugs can actually produce or aggravate hallucinations. The antidepressant drugs, the more anticholinergic antipsychotic drugs, and the shorter-acting benzodiazepines such as triazolam and lorazepam are most implicated in causing visual hallucinations. Visual hallucinations in the aged are virtually always indicative of brain related disturbance (e.g., delirium) rather than a psychiatric disorder.

Major differences in AM/PM self-performance. All classes of psychotropic drugs can have an effect on a resident's ability to perform activities of daily living. Establishing a link between the time a drug is taken and the change in self-performance is helpful in evaluating the problem.

Decline in cognition/communication. Decline in these areas signals the possibility that the decline is drug-induced and the need to review the relationship of the decline with initiation or change in drug therapy. All major classes of psychotropics can cause impairment of memory and other cognitive skills in vulnerable residents. While memory loss in nursing facility residents is caused primarily by dementing disorders and other neurologic disease, psychotropic drugs, particularly those with anticholinergic side effects, and long-acting benzodiazepines, definitely contribute to memory impairment. In contrast, treatment of depression or psychosis can actually improve usable memory, which is very much disrupted by severe psychiatric illness. If memory worsens after initiating or increasing the dose of a psychotropic drug, consider reducing or discontinuing the drug, or substituting a less anticholinergic drug. For a resident with anxiety, a short-acting benzodiazepine or buspirone is preferable to a long-acting benzodiazepine.

Decline in mood. (See reference to Depression above.)

Decline in behavior. Problem behaviors may be aggravated and worsened by psychotropic drugs as they can contribute to confusion, perceptual difficulties, and agitation.

Decline in ADL status. Drug side effects must always be considered if a resident becomes more dependent in ADLs. In addition, psychotropic drugs can precipitate or worsen bladder incontinence either through a change in cognition or through a direct action on bladder function.

Clarifying Issues if Drug-Related Discomfort Present

Dehydration; Reduced dietary bulk; Lack of exercise.

Constipation/fecal impaction. Any psychotropic drug with anticholinergic effects can cause or aggravate constipation; the effects are pronounced with tricyclic antidepressants and with low-potency antipsychotic drugs such as chlorpromazine or thioridizine. Milder cases of constipation can be treated with stool softeners, bulk-forming agents, and increased fluid; more severe constipation is best managed by substituting a less anticholinergic agent, or decreasing or discontinuing the psychotropic drug if possible. Antianxiety drugs can contribute to constipation if they sedate the resident to the point that fluid intake or exeresis is impaired. The problem can be handled by switching to a less sedating drug, decreasing dosage, or discontinuing the drug if possible.

Urinary retention. This condition may be manifested by the inability to urinate, or new onset or worsening of urinary incontinence (caused by overflow of urine from a full bladder that cannot empty properly). Any psychotropic drug with anticholinergic properties can produce or aggravate urinary retention. The problem is best managed by substituting a less anticholinergic agent, or decreasing or discontinuing the psychotropic drug if possible.

Dry mouth. This symptom is a common side effect of any psychotropic drug with anticholinergic properties. Dry mouth can aggravate chewing and swallowing problems. Substituting a less anticholinergic drug may be helpful. Other remedies include artificial saliva or sugar-free mints or candies (sugar contributes to cavity formation).

WHEN TO DISCONTINUE DRUG TREATMENT

1. Drug treatment that is ineffective after a reasonable trial should be discontinued or changed. The definition of a reasonable trial depends on the drug class and therapeutic indication.

2. When a medication is effective, but produces troublesome side effects, either the dose should be reduced or the medication should be replaced by a therapeutically equivalent agent less likely to cause the problematic side effect. If this is not feasible, or if doing it leads to a recurrence of symptoms, specific medical therapy for the troublesome side effects should be considered. For example, if the best drug for treating a resident's depression causes constipation, stool softeners, laxatives, or bulk-forming agents can be prescribed.

3. When a medication is effective and does not cause troublesome side effects, it should be continued for a defined period, and then efforts should be made to taper and eventually discontinue the drug.

4. Psychotropic medication should be prescribed on a permanent basis only if symptoms have recurred on at least two previous attempts to taper the medication after a defined period of therapy.

COMMONLY PRESCRIBED PSYCHOTROPIC DRUGS AND THEIR SIDE EFFECTS

TABLE A. ANTIPSYCHOTIC (NEUROLEPTIC) DRUGS

Generic Name	Brand Name	Incidence of Side Effects			
		Sedation	Hypotension	Anticholinergic Symptoms[1]	Extrapyramidal Symptoms[2]
Chlorpromazine	Thorazine	Marked	Marked	Marked	Mild
Thioridazine	Mellaril	Marked	Marked	Marked	Mild
Acetophenazine	Tindal	Mild	Mild	Moderate	Mild
Perphenazine	Trilafon	Mild	Mild	Moderate	Moderate
Loxapine	Loxitane	Mild	Mild	Moderate	Moderate
Molindone	Moban	Mild	Mild	Moderate	Moderate
Trifluoperazine	Stelazine	Mild	Mild	Mild	Marked
Thiothixene	Navane	Mild	Mild	Mild	Marked
Fluphenazine	Prolixin	Mild	Mild	Mild	Marked
Haloperidol	Haldol	Minimal	Minimal	Mild	Marked

TABLE B. ANTIDEPRESSANT DRUGS

Generic Name	Brand Name	Incidence of Side Effects		
		Sedation	Hypotension	Anticholinergic Symptoms[1]
Cyclic antidepressants				
Imipramine	Tofranil	Mild	Moderate	Mod-strong
Desipramine	Norpramin	Mild	Mild-mod	Mild
Doxepin	Adapin Sinequan	Mod-strong	Moderate	Strong
Amitriptyline	Elavil Triavil	Strong	Moderate	Very Strong
Nortriptyline	Aventyl Pamelor	Mild	Mild	Moderate
Maprotiline	Ludiomil	Mod-strong	Moderate	Moderate
Amoxapine*	Asendin	Mild	Moderate	Moderate
Fluoxetine	Prozac	Variable	Nil	Nil
Triazolopryridine Antidepressant				
Trazodone	Desyrel	Mod-strong	Moderate	Mild
MAO inhibitors[+]				
Phenelzine	Nardil	Mild	Moderate	Mild
Tranylcypromine	Parnate	Mild	Moderate	Mild
Other				
Bupropion	Wellbutrin	None May cause agitation High incidence of seizures	Nil	Nil

COMMONLY PRESCRIBED PSYCHOTROPIC DRUGS AND THEIR SIDE EFFECTS (cont.)

TABLE C. ANTIANXIETY AND HYPNOTIC DRUGS

Generic Name	Brand Name	Duration of Action
Benzodiazepines		
Triazolam	Halcion	Very short
Oxazepam	Serax	Short
Temazepam	Restoril	Short
Lorazepam	Ativan	Short
Alprazolam	Xanax	Medium
Chlordiazepoxide	Librium	Long
Diazepam	Valium	Long
Clorazepate	Tranxene	Long
Flurazepam	Dalmane	Very long
Barbiturates		
Antihistamines		
Diphenhydramine	Benadryl	Moderate
Hydroxyzine	Vistaril	Moderate
Chloral hydrate	Noctec	Long
Other		
Buspirone	BuSpar	Not meaningful

* Also a neuroleptic drug with all the neuroleptic side effects.

\+ Special diet required; many drug interactions.

1 Anticholinergic symptoms include: dry mouth, constipation, urinary retention, blurred vision, confusion, disorientation, short-term memory loss, hallucinations, insomnia, agitation and restlessness, picking behaviors, fever.

2 Extrapyramidal symptoms include: movement disorder, such as Parkinsonism, dyskinesias, and akathisia (described in text).
Antidepressants (except Amoxapine) and antianxiety/hypnotics do not produce extrapyramidal side effects.

PSYCHOTROPIC DRUG USE RAP KEY *(For MDS Version 2.0)*

TRIGGER — REVISION

TO BE TRIGGERED, MUST FIRST USE PSYCHOTROPIC DRUG **[Antipsychotic, antidepressant, or antianxiety] [O4a,b, or c = 1-7]. If used, go to RAP review if one or more of following present:**

Potential for Drug-Related Hypotension or gait disturbances

- Repetitive physical movements[a]
  [E1n = 1,2]
- Balance While Sitting
  [G3b = 1,2,3]
- Hypotension
  [I1i = checked]
- Dizziness/Vertigo[b]
  [J1f = checked]
- Syncope
  [J1m = checked]
- Unsteady Gait
  [J1n = checked]
- Fell in past 30 days[b]
  [J4a = checked]
- Fell in past 31-180 day[b]
  [J4b = checked]
- Hip fracture
  [J4c = checked]
- Swallowing problem
  [K1b = checked]

Potential for Drug-Related Cognitive/Behavioral Impairment if: [c]

- Delirium/Disordered Thinking
  - Easily distracted
    [B5a = 2]
  - Periods of altered perception or awareness of surroundings
    [B5b = 2]

---

[a] Note: This item also triggers on the Mood RAP

[b] Note: These items also trigger on Falls RAP

[c] Note: All of these items also trigger on the Delirium RAP

GUIDELINES

If resident is triggered, review the following:

- **Drug review [from record]**
  - Length of time between when drug first taken and onset of problem;
  - Doses of drug and how frequently taken;
  - Number of classes of psychotropics taken;
  - Reason drug prescribed

- **Review resident's condition that affect drug metabolism/excretion**

  Impaired liver/renal function **[I1qq, I3]**; Acute condition **[J5b]**; Dehydration **[J1c]**

- **Review Behavior/Mood Status:** Current problem status **[E1, E2, E4]**, Recent changes **[E3, E5]**, Behavior management program **[P1be, P2]**; Psychiatric Diagnoses **[I1dd,ee,ff,gg]**

Clarifying Information if Hypotension present:

- Postural changes in vital signs **[from exam]**
- Drugs with marked anticholinergic properties **[from record]**

Clarifying Information if Movement Disorder present:

- High Fever **[J1h]** AND/OR Muscular rigidity **[from record, observation]**
- Tremors, especially of hands; pill-rolling of hands; muscle rigidity of limbs, neck, trunk (Parkinsonism) **[I1y; from record, observation]**
- Marked decrease in spontaneous movement (Akinesia) **[from record, observation]**
- Rigid, unnatural, uncomfortable posture of neck or trunk (Dystonia) **[from record, observation]**
- Restlessness, inability to sit still (Akathisia) **[from record, observation]**
- Persistent movements of the mouth (e.g., thrusting of tongue, movements of lips, chewing/puckering) **AND/OR** peculiar and recurrent postures of limbs, trunk (Tardive Dyskinesia) **[from record, observation]**

Psychotropic Drug Use RAP Key **10 of 11**

PSYCHOTROPIC DRUG USE RAP KEY (continued)

TRIGGER — REVISION

- — Episodes of disorganized speech
  [B5c = 2]
- — Periods of restlessness
  [B5d = 2]
- — Periods of lethargy
  [B5e = 2]
- — Mental function varies over the course of the day
  [B5f = 2]

- Deterioration in Cognitive Status [(c)]
  [B6 = 2]
- Deterioration in Communication
  [C7 = 2]
- Deterioration in Mood [(c)]
  [E3 = 2]
- Deterioration in Behavioral Symptoms [(c)]
  [E5 = 2]
- Depression
  [I1ee = checked]
- Hallucinations
  [J1i = checked]

Potential for Drug Related Discomfort if:

- Constipation
  [H2b = checked]
- Fecal Impaction
  [H2d = checked]
- Lung Aspiration
  [J1k = checked]

GUIDELINES

Clarifying Information if Gait Disturbances present:

- Long-acting benzodiazepines **[from med record]**
  — Recent dosage increase **[from med record]**
- Short-term memory loss; Decline in cognition **[B6]**; Slurred speech **[C5]**
- Decreased AM wakefulness **[E1k; N1a]**; Little/no activity involvement **[N2]**

Clarifying Information if Cognitive/Behavioral Impairment present:

If neither of following are present, psychotropic drug side effects can be considered as a major cause of problem:

- Acute confusion (delirium) related to medical illness **[B5]**
- Depression **[I1ee]**

Clarifying Issues if Drug-Related Discomfort present:

- Dehydration **[J1c]**; Reduced dietary bulk; Lack of exercise **[from record]**, Constipation **[H2b]**, Fecal impaction **[H2d]**, Urinary retention **[I3; from record]**
- Other potential drug-related discomforts that may require resolution: Dry mouth, if on antipsychotic or antidepressant **[observation]**

Psychotropic Drug Use RAP Key 11 of 11

RESIDENT ASSESSMENT PROTOCOL: PHYSICAL RESTRAINTS

I. PROBLEM

Studies of nursing homes show that between 30 and 40% of residents are physically restrained. This is quite serious since negative effects of restraint use include declines in residents' physical functioning (e.g., ability to ambulate) and muscle condition, contractures, increased incidence of infections, and development of pressure sores, delirium, agitation, and incontinence. Moreover, restraints have been found in some cases to increase the incidence of falls and other accidents (e.g., strangulation). Finally, residents who are restrained face the loss of autonomy, dignity and self-respect. In effect, the use of physical restraints undercuts the major goals of long-term care — to maximize independence, functional capacity, and quality of life. Thus, the goal of minimizing or eliminating restraint use has become central to both clinical practice and federal law.

The primary reason given for applying restraints is to protect residents from falls and accidents. Facilities are also concerned about potential lawsuits and malpractice claims that might result if residents should fall. Other reasons cited for restraint use include to provide postural support or positioning for residents, to facilitate treatment (e.g., preventing residents from pulling out IV lines or NG tubes), and to manage behaviors such as wandering or physical aggressiveness.

The experience of many health care providers suggests that facility goals can often be met without the use of physical restraints and their negative side effects. In part, this involves identifying and treating health, functional, or psychosocial problems that may be causing the condition for which restraints were ordered (e.g., falls, wandering, agitation). Minimizing use of restraints also involves care management alternatives, such as: modifying the environment to make it safer; maintaining an individual's customary routine; using less intrusive methods of administering medications and nourishment; and recognizing and responding to residents' needs for psychosocial support, responsive health care, meaningful activities, and regular exercise.

II. TRIGGERS

***Definition*:** Physical restraints are any manual method or physical or mechanical device, material, or equipment attached or adjacent to the resident's body that the resident cannot easily remove and that restricts freedom of movement or normal access to his/her body.

- Use of trunk restraint [a]
  [P4c = 1,2]
- Use of limb restraint
  [P4d = 1,2]
- Use of chair that prevents rising
  [P4e = 1,2]

[a] Note: Code 2 also triggers on the Pressure Ulcer RAP. Both codes trigger on the Falls RAP

III. GUIDELINES

In evaluating and reconsidering the use of restraints for a resident, consider needs, problems, conditions, or risk factors (e.g., for falls) which, if addressed, could eliminate the need for using restraints. Refer to the RAP KEY for specific MDS items to consider as you review the following issues.

Physical Restraints RAP (1 of 5)

WHY ARE RESTRAINTS USED?

The first step in determining whether use of a restraint can be reduced or eliminated is to identify the reasons a restraint was applied.

- Review the resident's record and consult primary caregivers to determine reason for use.

Ask the following questions:

- ***Why*** is the resident restrained?
- ***What type(s)*** of restraint is used?
- ***During what time of day*** is each type(s) used?
- ***Where*** is the resident restrained (e.g., own room in bed, chair in hallway)?
- ***How long*** is the resident restrained each day?
- ***Under what circumstances*** (e.g., when left alone, after family leave, when not involved in structured activity, when eating)?
- ***Who*** suggested that the resident be restrained (e.g., staff, family, resident)?

CONDITIONS ASSOCIATED WITH RESTRAINT USE.

It may be possible to identify and resolve health/functional/psychosocial needs, risks, or problems that caused restraints to be used. By addressing the underlying condition(s) and cause(s), the facility may eliminate the apparent need for the restraint(s). In addition, a review of underlying needs, risks, or problems may help to identify other potential kinds of treatments. After determining why and how a restraint is used, review the appropriate areas described below.

Problem Behavioral Symptoms.

To determine presence of a behavioral symptom, review the MDS. If the behavioral symptom for which the resident is restrained was not exhibited in the last 7 days, was it because the restraint prohibited the behavior from occurring (e.g., resident was restrained and could not wander)? If a behavioral symptom was present during the last 7 days or the resident was restrained to prevent a behavioral symptom, consider the resident to have a behavioral symptom and review Behavioral Symptom RAP as indicated.

Risk of Falls.

Although restraints have ***<u>not</u>*** been shown to safeguard residents from injury, one of the most common reasons given by facilities for restraining residents is to prevent falls. In some instances, restraints have been reported to contribute to falls and injuries. Because of the complications associated with restraint use, many physicians and geriatric clinicians recommend exploring alternatives for preventing falls, such as treating health problems and making environmental modifications.

- Review risk factors for falls on RAP KEY. Refer to Falls RAP if these risks are present or if the restraint is being used to prevent falls.

Conditions and Treatments.

Another reason facilities give for using restraints is to prevent a resident from removing tubes.

If the resident is being restrained to manage resistance to any type of tube or mechanical device (e.g., indwelling/external catheter, feeding tube, intravenous line, oxygen mask/cannula, wound dressing), review the following to facilitate decision-making:

- Is the tube/mechanical device used to treat a life-threatening condition?
- Does the resident actually need a particular intervention that may be potentially burdensome to him/her? Are there less intrusive treatment options?
- Why is the resident reacting to the tube/mechanical device with resistance? (e.g., Does the device produce discomfort or irritation? Is the resident really resisting or is the device just something to fidget with? Is the treatment compatible with the resident's wishes? Does the resident understand the reason for the method of treatment? Has the resident/family been informed about the risks and benefits of treatment options?)

HCFA Guideline: "If there are medical symptoms which are life threatening (such as dehydration, electrolyte imbalance, urinary blockage) then a restraint may be used temporarily to provide necessary lifesaving treatment. Physical restraints may be used for brief periods to allow medical treatment to proceed, if there is documented evidence of resident or legal approval of the treatment."

- If an indwelling or external catheter is present, review the Urinary Incontinence RAP for alternatives.
- If a feeding tube is present, review the Feeding Tube RAP

ADL Self-Performance.

In rare instances, a restraint can enhance a resident's ability to be more self-sufficient, IF the restraint use is supportive and time-limited.

Review the MDS, to determine if the restraint contributes to the resident's self-performance of an activity (e.g., wheelchair belt supports trunk while resident wheels self, geri-chair used only at meals enables wandering resident to attend to feeding self).

Confounding problems to be considered:

Many problem behaviors are manifestations of unmet health, functional, and/or psychosocial needs that can often be reduced, eliminated, or managed by addressing the conditions that produced them. (See RAP on Behavioral Symptoms). Conditions associated with behavioral symptoms and restraint use include:

- Delirium (acute confusional state)
- Impaired cognition
- Impaired communication (e.g., difficulty making needs/wishes understood or understanding others)

- Unmet psychosocial needs (e.g., social isolation, disruption of familiar routines, anger with family members)
- Sad or anxious mood
- Resistance to treatment, medication, nourishment
- Psychotropic drug side effects (e.g., motor agitation, confusion, gait disturbance)
- If a behavior management program is in place, does it adequately address the causes of the resident's particular problem behaviors?

Other Factors to be Considered.

Resident's Response to Restraints

In evaluating restraint use, it is important to review the resident's reaction to restraints (e.g., positive and negative, such as passivity, anger, increased agitation, withdrawal, pleas for release, calls for help, constant attempts to untie/release self). This will help determine whether presumed benefits are outweighed by negative side effects.

Review MDS items on other potential negative effects of restraint use, such as declines in functional self-performance, body control, skin condition, mood and cognition, since restraints have been in use.

Alternatives to Restraints

Many interventions may be as effective or even more effective than restraints in managing a resident's needs, safety risks, and problems. To be effective the intervention must address the underlying problem.

- Review resident's record and confer with staff to determine whether alternatives to restraints have been tried.
- If alternatives to restraints have been tried, what were they?
- How long were the alternatives tried?
- What was the resident's response to the alternatives at the time?
- If the alternative(s) attempted were ineffective, what else was attempted?
- How recently were alternatives other than restraints attempted?

Philosophy and Attitudes

In reconsidering the use of restraints for a resident, consider the philosophy, values, attitudes, and wishes of the resident regarding restraint use, as well as those of his family/significant others, and caregivers. Consider the impact of restraints on facility environment and morale.

- Is there consensus or differences among affected parties in choosing between resident independence and freedom in favor of presumed safety?

PHYSICAL RESTRAINTS RAP KEY *(For MDS Version 2.0)*

TRIGGER — REVISION

Review for efficacy, side effects and alternatives if one or more of the following:

- Use of trunk restraint [a]
  [P4c = 1,2]
- Use of limb restraint
  [P4d = 1,2]
- Use of chair that prevents rising
  [P4e = 1,2]

(a) Note: Code 2 also triggers on the Pressure Ulcer RAP. Both codes trigger on the Falls RAP

GUIDELINES

Review factors and complications associated with restraint use:

- **Behavioral Symptoms**: Repetitive physical movements **[E1n]**, Any behavioral symptoms **[E4]**, Part of behavior management program **[P1be, P2; from record]**
- **Risk of Falls**: Dizziness **[J1f]**; Falls **[J4a, J4b]**;
  Antianxiety **[O4b]**; Antidepressant **[O4c]**
- **Conditions and Treatments:** Catheter **[H3c,d]**; Hip fracture **[J4c, I1m]**; Unstable/acute condition **[J5a,b]**; Parenteral/IV and/or feeding tube **[K5a,b]**; Wound care/treatment **[M5f,g,h,i]**; IV meds **[P1ac]**; Respirator/Oxygen **[P1ag, P1al]**
- **ADL Self performance [G1]**
- **Confounding problems to be considered:**
  — Delirium **[B5]**
  — Cognitive loss/dementia **[B2, B4]**
  — Impaired communication **[C4, C6]**
  — Sad/anxious mood **[E1, E2]**
  — Resistance to treatment/meds/ nourishment **[E4e]**
  — Unmet psychosocial needs **[F1, F2, F3]**
  — Psychotropic drug side effects **[see record, J1e,f,h,i,m,n]**
- **Other factors to be considered:** Resident's response to restraint(s); use of alternatives to restraints; resident/family/staff philosophy, values, wishes, attitudes about restraints **[record, observation, discussion]**

Physical Restraints RAP Key 5 of 5

APPENDIX D

INTERVIEWING TECHNIQUES

Performing an accurate and comprehensive assessment requires that the assessor communicate effectively with a number of individuals. The following suggestions can be used by an individual assessor to obtain information from residents, facility staff and resident families. There are other possible models for resident data collection and interviewing, especially when conducted by a team, which you may want to consider in your specific facility.

When conducting any interview to collect information in the RAI process, there are some general concepts that you should consider.

First, emphasize to all individuals that you interview (i.e., residents, families and staff) that the RAI process is a way to "get to know the resident". You should explain that the RAI assessment provides valuable information that will be used by facility staff to develop the resident's care plan. This is an opportunity to bring residents and families into the assessment and care-planning process.

Second, be flexible as to how you conduct the RAI process with each resident. It is not necessary for you to complete the assessment in the same order sequence as sections appear on the MDS form. The MDS is not a questionnaire; it is a set of common items and definitions for assessment, which provides a structure for systematically recording the information you obtain. You should let the resident's needs guide you during the assessment process.

You may wish to use the following general techniques, if appropriate, when conducting interviews:

To elicit complete and satisfactory answers, you will often need to ask neutral or nondirective questions. **Examples are:**

"What do you mean?"
"Tell me what you have in mind."
"Tell me more about that."
"Please be more specific."
"Give me an example."

Repeat a question if you think it has been misunderstood or misinterpreted.

Pause or hesitate to indicate that you are listening and need more or better information. This is a good technique to use while you are determining the individual's response pattern.

Some items will require special sensitivity during the questioning process (e.g., the MDS items in Section B dealing with memory), and you should note the instructions in Chapter 3 on how to assess each item or gather the information to respond to each item.

Some respondents may be eager to talk with you and will stray from the topic at hand. When a person strays, you should gently guide the conversation back to the topic. For example you may say:

"That's interesting." "Now I need to know..." "Let's get back to..."
"Tell me about..."

Validate your understanding of what a respondent is saying. Be careful that you do not appear to be challenging a respondent when clarifying a statement. For example you may say:

"I think I hear you saying that..."
"Let's see if I understood you correctly. You said ... Is that right?"

When respondents (resident/family/caregivers) disagree or when a resident (who you believe is capable of rational judgment) says something contrary to information contained in the record, you should clarify the information. Ultimately, use your best clinical judgment to weigh all information.

Consider developing and using a printed questionnaire to help residents and families contribute important information (e.g., Customary Routine).

Finally and most importantly, validate with the resident, through observations or interview, what you have heard from other facility staff, family members or what you have read in the record.

When collecting information from facility staff there are other important considerations which may make the process easier and more efficient.

You should respect the professional status of staff. Consider their need to perform their other duties in addition to providing necessary assessment information for you. The following suggestions may assist you when conducting facility staff interviews:

1. Post a schedule of residents who are being assessed during a given period (e.g., month) so that staff can prepare to participate in the assessment.

2. Provide prior notice to other staff members that an assessment is due, giving direct care staff an opportunity to gather their thoughts about residents. You may wish to provide a worksheet that staff (e.g., nursing assistants) could use to note particular resident information (e.g., ADLs).

3. Schedule interviews in advance, at mutually convenient times; avoid busy work load times.

4. Know what you want to cover. Leave a few minutes for staff to provide open-ended comments that may pertain to the well-being of the resident.

5. Provide other staff members with a list of areas you wish to cover to expedite the process.

6. Key your questions to the time period for which resident performance is being assessed.

You will often need to discuss a resident with more than one facility staff member. For example, an individual staff member who has been on a 3 week vacation may recall the resident's function a month ago instead of during the last 7 days. A nurse that floats from unit to unit may not know the residents well enough to respond appropriately. If a facility staff respondent struggles with answers or seems vague in referring to the time period in question, you should consider seeking another respondent.

Reinforce to all staff at the onset of the interview that you are gathering information to learn as much about the resident as possible to best plan for the resident's care. Reassure any staff that your purpose is the RAI process and not an evaluation of their job performance.

APPENDIX E

Commonly Prescribed Medications by Category by Brand (generic)

Antipsychotics
Clozaril (Clozapine)
Compazine (Prochlorperazine)
Haldol (Haloperidol)
Inapsine (Droperidol)
Loxitane (Loxapine)
Mellaril (Thioridazine)
Moban (Molindone)
Navane (Thiothixene)
Orap (Pimozide)
Prolixin (Fluphenazine)
Serentil (Mesoridazine)
Sparine (Promazine)
Stelazine (Trifluoperazine)
Taractan (Chlorprothixene)
Thorazine (Chlorpromazine)
Tindal (Acetophenazine)
Trilafon (Perphenazine)
Vesprin (Triflupromazine)

Antidepressants
Adapin (Doxepin)
Asendin (Amoxapine)
Aventyl, Pamelor (Nortriptyline)
Desyrel (Trazodone)
Elavil (Amitriptyline)
Lithonate, Lithane (Lithium)
Ludiomil (Maprotiline)
Marplan (Isocarboxazid)
Nardil (Phenelzine)
Norpramin (Desipramine)
Pamelor (Nortriptyline)
Parnate (Tranylcypromine)
Prozac (Fluoxetine)
Sinequan (Doxepin)
Surmontil (Trimipramine)
Tofranil (Imipramine)
Vivactil (Protriptyline)
Wellbutrin (Bupropion)
Zoloft (Sertraline)

Antianxiety
(Phenobarbital)
Anytal (Amobarbital)
Atarax (Hydroxyzine)
Ativan (Lorazepam)
Buspar (Buspirone)
Centrax (Prazepam)
Doriden (Glutethimide)
Equanil, Miltown (Meprobamate)
Librium (Chlordiazepoxide)
Noctec (Chloral Hydrate)
Noludar (Methyprylon)
Paxipam (Halazepam)
Serax (Oxazepam)Tranxene (Clorazepate)
Tranxene (Clorazepate)
Valium (Diazepam)
Vistaril (Hydroxyzine)
Xanax (Alprazolam)

Hypnotics
Alurate (Aprobarbital)
Dalmane (Flurazepam)
Doral (Quazepam)
Halcion (Triazolam)
Nembutal (Pentobarbital)
Placidyl (Ethchlorvynol)
ProSom (Estazolam)
Restoril (Temazepam)
Seconal (Secobarbital)

Diuretics

This list inlcudes examples of diuretics (brand name and generic equivalents) likely to be seen in a nursing home population. This list is not inclusive; consult your pharmacist, the resident's physician, or a drug reference manual, as necessary.

Brand (generic)

Aldactazide (spironolactone/hydrochlorothiazide
Aldactone (Spironolactone)
Aqua-Ban
Aquatensen (Methyclothiazide)
Bumex (Bumetanide)
Diamox (Acetazolamide)
Diuril (Chlorothiazide)
Dyazide (Triamterene/hydrochlorothiazide)
Dyrenium (Triamterene)
Edecrin (Ethacrynic Acid)
Enduron (Methyclothiazide)
Esidrix (Hydrochlorothiazide)
Hydrodiuril (Hydrochlorothiazide)
Hydromox (Quinethazone)
Hygroton (Chlorthalidone)
Lasix (Furosemide)
Lozol (Indepamide)
Mannitol (Mannitol)
Maxzide (Triameterene/hydrochlorothiazide)
Midamor (Amiloride)
Moduretic (Amiloride HC1/hydrochlorothiazide)
Neptazane (Methazolamide)
Oretic (Hydrochlorothiazide)
Zaroxolyn (Metolazone)

APPENDIX F

CPS SCORING RULES
Impairment Count
(Number of the following):
- Decision Making: Not Independent=1-2
- Understood: Not Independent=1-3
- Short-Term Memory: Not OK=1
Severe Impairment Count
(Number of the following):
- Decision Making: Mod. Impaired=2
- Understood: Sometimes/Never=2-3
All Residents
Coma?
No (0)
Yes (1)
Decision-Making
Severely Impaired (3)
Not Severely Impaired (0-2)
Impairment Count?
0
2 or 3
1
Total Dependent Eating?
No (0-3)
Yes (4)
Severe Impairment Count
0
1
2
(0) Intact
(1) Boarderline Intact
(2) Mild Impairment
(3) Moderate Impairment
(4) Mod. Severe Impairment
(5) Severe Impairment
(6) Very Severe Impairment
Average mini mental score in field trial where 30 is best and 0 is worst
24.9
21.9
19.2
15.4
6.9
5.1
0.4
Reference: Morris, JN, Fries, BF, et al MDS Performance Scale. J. Gerontology 1994; 49, m174-m182

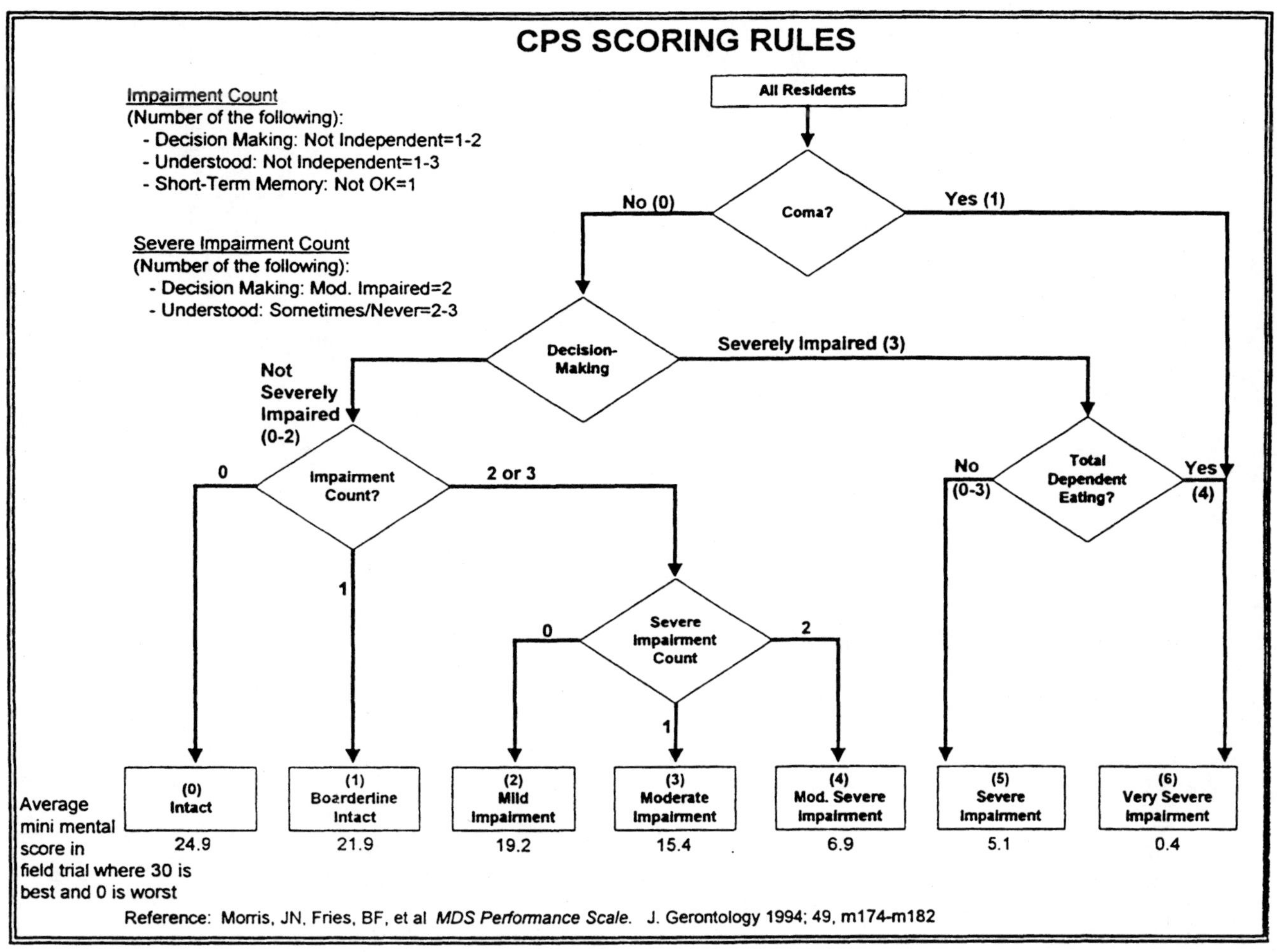

APPENDIX G

STATUTORY AND REGULATORY REQUIREMENTS FOR LONG TERM CARE FACILITIES - RESIDENT ASSESSMENT AND CARE PLANNING

The following table displays the statutory requirements and the Federal regulations related to the Resident Assessment Instrument (RAI), the Minimum Data Set (MDS) and care planning for Medicare or Medicaid certified long term care facilities.

Section 1819 of the Social Security Act is the Federal law regarding the requirements for skilled nursing facilities (SNFs) participating in the Medicare program. Section 1919 of the Social Security Act is the Federal law regarding the requirements for nursing facilities (NFs) participating in the Medical Assistance program.

Part 483 of Title 42 of the code of Federal Regulations (CFR) are the requirements for Long Term Care Facilities (SNFs and NFs). "F" tags are Health Care Financing Administration (HCFA) data tags assigned to each of the requirements in 42 CFR 483.

REQUIREMENT AREA	STATUTORY REQUIREMENT (MEDICARE)	STATUTORY REQUIREMENT (MEDICAID)	FEDERAL REGULATION/ HCFA "F" TAG
Specification of MDS Core Elements	1819 (f)(6)(A)	1919 (f)(6)(A)	
Designation of RAI Instruments	1819 (f)(6)(B)	1919 (f)(6)(B)	
Services to be Provided in Accordance with Plan of Care	1819 (b)(2)	1919 (b)(2)	42 CFR 483.20 (d)(1-3) F 279, F 280, F 281
Requirement for Resident Assessments	1819 (b)(3)(A)	1919 (b)(3)(A)	42 CFR 483.20 (a-b) F 271, F 272

Certification of Resident Assessment i. Completion and Signature(s) ii. Penalty for Falsification iii. Use of Independent Assessors	1819 (b)(3)(B)	1919 (b)(3)(B)	42 CFR 483.20 (c)(1-2) F 278 42 CFR 483.20 (c)(3) F 278 42 CFR 483.20 (c)(4) F 278
Frequency of Assessments	1819 (b)(3)(C)	1919 (b)(3)(C)	42 CFR 483.20 (b)(4-5) F 273, F 274, F 275, F 276
Use of Assessments	1819 (b)(3)(D)	1919 (b)(3)(D)	42 CFR 483.20 (c)(6) (Refer to F 279)
Coordination with State-Required Preadmission Screening Program	1819 (b)(3)(E)	1919 (b)(3)(E)	42 CFR 483.20 (c)(7) F 277
State Specification of Resident Assessment Instrument	1819 (e)(5)	1919 (e)(5)	
Clinical Record Requirements for Resident Assessment and Plan of Care	1819 (b)(6)(C)	1919 (b)(6)(C)	42 CFR 483.75 (n)(6) F 516

Table of Contents

Note: In some instances, questions seemed suited to more than one section of this document. Where this overlap existed, the question was placed under the Section heading to which it was best suited.

Questions on the Basic Assessment Tracking Form and Face Sheet

1: Are facilities required to complete the Basic Assessment Tracking Form (Section AA) at the current time or only after HCFA's MDS automation requirements are effective?

A: A paper or hard copy of the Basic Assessment Form must accompany each Full, Quarterly, or State required assessment, effective as of the date of MDS 2.0 implementation. The User's Manual reference for this question is on page 3-1. The reference on page 2-13 of the User's Manual is incorrect.

2: In Section AA #7, is the Medicaid Number intended to capture the <u>case number</u> or the <u>recipient number</u>?

A: The number in Section AA #7 is the Medicaid Recipient Number. This is a 14 digit code that tracks the person across all provider types. The Recipient Number is a unique identifier number assigned by the State Medicaid office. Questions regarding the Medicaid number can be referred to the State Medicaid office or the State RAI Coordinator.

3: Is a reentry form required when a resident returns from a hospital if they were not discharged from the nursing facility?

A: Yes, a Discharge Tracking form should have been completed when the resident was transferred to the hospital. Upon return, complete the Reentry form. See the User's Manual reference on page 3-12.

4: When must the Face Sheet be submitted? Does the Face Sheet need to be updated to Version 2.0 or will the old one suffice?

A: When HCFA's MDS automation requirements are effective, Face Sheet information on Version 2.0 must be submitted with the first assessment record that is submitted. For residents admitted prior to implementation of Version 2.0 of the MDS, use information on the original Face Sheet to complete the Version 2.0 Face Sheet (i.e., crosswalk data from original Face Sheet items measuring the same thing on Version 2.0). Three new items appear on the Version 2.0 Face Sheet (i.e., AB4-Zip Code; AB7-Education, and AB11-Date Background Information completed). These should be completed prior to submission. For residents admitted after implementation of Version 2.0, the Face Sheet information should be submitted with the first assessment record that is required after HCFA's MDS automation requirements are effective.

5: The Briggs forms have a Face Sheet attached to every MDS. Is a Face Sheet required on every MDS?

A: No. The Face Sheet is completed once, when the resident first enters the facility. The Face Sheet is also required if the person re-enters the facility after a discharge where return had not been previously expected. If MDS forms are purchased in a "set", discard the Face Sheet page or draw a line through it when it does not apply to the current assessment.

6: What are the time frames for completion of the Basic Assessment Tracking form?

A: It must be completed within the same time frame as the required assessment (e.g., within 14 days after admission).

7: How long is the Face Sheet (Section AB, AC, and AD) to be kept in the active record?

A: The Face Sheet is completed once and is to remain a permanent part of the resident's record. While part of HCFA's original RAI Training Manual, this statement was inadvertently omitted in the User's Manual for Version 2.0. If the resident is permanently discharged, (without expectation of return), and then comes back to the facility, a new Face Sheet must be completed. The User's Manual reference for this question is on page 3-14.

8: What is the reason for requiring a signature at Section AD?

A: The signature at AD covers Sections AB and AC, which is maintained in the active record throughout the resident's stay. The signature at R2 applies to information entered in Sections A through R. Sections A through R can be thinned after 15 months, thereby separating the R2 signature from Sections AB and AC. Sections AB and AC remain in the chart.

9: Regarding MDS item AB2, "Admitted From (at Entry)", which code is most appropriately used for a licensed residential facility?

A: Use code 3, "Board and care/assisted living/group home".

10: Regarding item AB8a, "Primary Language", if a resident spoke English as a second language, but reverted to the original language due to their present condition (cognitive deficit, CVA, etc...), do you code the language the resident is currently speaking, or the language they used to speak, prior to the onset of their current condition?

A: Code as primary the language the resident currently speaks or understands.

11: On page 3-21 of the User's Manual which refers to item AB9, what is meant by "major life activities"?

A: The language used is adapted from PASARR. Refer to 42 CFR Subpart C 483.102 b (ii), for a definition of "level of impairment", which discusses functional limitations in "major life activities" according to (A) Interpersonal function, (B) Concentration, persistence and pace and (C) Adaptation to change.

12: What is the purpose of the Basic Assessment Tracking forms?

A: The Basic Assessment Tracking form identifies the resident in a computerized environment. The Discharge and Reentry Tracking forms provide key information to identify and track the movement of residents in and out of the facility.

13: Is the Reentry Tracking Form kept with the MDS or computer information only?

A: Keep the Discharge and Reentry Tracking forms along with all RAI information (MDS, Quarterly reviews, RAP Summary forms) for a 15-month period. It is not necessary to maintain a hard copy in facilities where the **entire** clinical record is stored electronically, (see manual, page 2-19 for related criteria). The User's Manual reference for this response is on page 2-18.

14: How soon must the Discharge Tracking form be completed, and where is it kept?

A: The User's Manual reference for this response is on page 3-2. The Discharge Tracking form is completed when the resident is discharged from the facility (i.e., stays overnight or is admitted to another health care facility). It is not completed for therapeutic or social leave. The Discharge Tracking form must always be completed at the time of any discharge from the nursing home and must be maintained in the active clinical record along with the required 15 months of RAI information. Once HCFA's MDS automation requirements are effective, it is anticipated the facilities will have to encode this information within 7 days after the resident's discharge from the facility. The 7-day time frame will also apply to encoding of the Reentry Tracking information for residents who return to the facility.

15: Does the Discharge Tracking form apply to outpatient or 23 hour observation stays when the resident is not actually discharged from the facility?

A: No. The Discharge Tracking form is completed only when the resident is out of the facility for an overnight stay, except for a temporary visit home. This applies regardless of the facility's policy and procedure for discharge or opening and closing records.

16: In reference to #8 on the MDS, Reason for Assessment, please explain "discharged--return not anticipated."

A: The User's Manual reference for this response is on page 3-11, #6 (see form on page B-16, Section AA., #8, a6). This code is used on the **Discharge Tracking Form only** and applies when a resident is permanently discharged from a nursing home (as opposed to situations in which the record is closed, temporarily discharging the resident from the facility, during a brief absence such as a hospitalization). This provides a means of "closing" the record of any resident at the point of discharge from the facility (when return is not anticipated).

17: What is the intent of the statement "skip if not discharged" on the Discharge Tracking form, Section R?

A: Please disregard this statement, which was inadvertently left on the final version of the form. This line may be deleted by forms manufacturers and software vendors.

18: Is it necessary to keep blank Discharge and Reentry forms in the resident's clinical record until they are needed?

A: No. Include in the active record once completed.

19: If Reentry forms are not required until HCFA's computerization requirements are effective, what forms are required to indicate return to the facility after a hospital stay?

A: The MDS Version 2.0 Discharge and Reentry Tracking forms are only required in States that require submission of MDS data. Otherwise, facilities are not required to complete any Assessment form when a resident returns from a hospital stay, unless the resident has experienced a significant change in status. Upon return, the resident's status should be evaluated for possible Significant Change.

20: How soon after discharge or reentry must the Discharge or Reentry Form be completed?

A: Complete these forms no later than 7 days after the event.

21: How is Section AB dated when additional information in AB and AC is received late?

A: As the "Background Information" items are not repeated in subsequent assessments, this is the only place where additional information can be added or changed after the original assessment completion date.

In a paper system, fill out a new form with the new information and date of the assessment in AB11. Facilities may also fill in the missing information on the previously completed form, with the entries identified with the new date and signature of the assessor. In a computer system, the new information should be entered and a new print-out generated. Item AB11 is used to indicate when this information is entered. The User's Manual reference for this question is on page 3-22 and 3-23.

Questions on Items in MDS Sections A Through G

22: On the Quarterly and Annual Assessments, what is the information on Item A3a used for?

A: Item A3a is a critical concept. All Assessments must have an Assessment Reference Date that indicates the period of common observation for all assessment items. This Assessment Reference Date is the designated endpoint of the observation period for that particular Quarterly or Full assessment. All MDS items are coded by observing the resident's status or performance back in time from this point. For example, if the Assessment Reference Date for an Annual assessment is May 27, the period of common observation for 7-day items is May 21-27. For 14-day items, the common observation period is May 14-27, and so on. The User's Manual reference for this question is on page 3-30.

23: The top of each page of the MDS form contains the wording "Numeric Identifier", followed by a blank line. What is this used for?

A: This is an optional item that the facility may use to identify a resident as they gather information on the MDS. In a paper environment where pages may be separated, this item could aid the facility in gathering the form together. See the example shown on pages 4-24 through 4-30 in the User's Manual. This is not a HCFA requirement.

24: Should documents supporting advance directives be maintained in the resident's active clinical record for surveyor review?

A: 42 CFR 483.10 requires facilities to protect and promote the rights of each resident, including the right to "formulate an advanced directive". There is no regulatory text specifying a location for advanced directive information. Unless there are State codes or regulations regarding this matter, the method of communicating the information is up to the facility. If documentation is not available in the resident's clinical record, facility staff should be the source of this information, and surveyors will assess whether the staff knowledge and actions are in agreement with resident/family wishes. Some facilities elect to maintain the information in the resident's clinical record. For advanced directives to be included in item A10, the User's Manual (page 3-39) indicates that documentation must be available in the record.

25: Where would evidence of task segmentation, (item G7) be found? If scored "yes", is further evaluation required?

A: This information may be documented anywhere in the clinical record (e.g., nurse's notes or therapy notes), or it may not be documented at all, as the MDS is considered a primary source document. Since item G7 is not part of the RAP trigger, assessment is not necessarily required. It makes sense however, that staff should be knowledgeable about how to break down task(s) for individual residents (i.e., based upon that individual's needs) so that they may integrate task segmentation into the resident's care.

26: I have advised facilities that the reliability of entering the data in the ADL section is considerably improved by completing the Self Performance column first for all items and then returning to the top and completing the Support column because of the differences in the scales to score these two columns. Facility staff say that computer programs will not let them complete the form in the manner I've suggested. Is that a problem?

A: Your suggestion may be of value to staff who are new to the process and who are completing a paper form of the MDS 2.0. Studies have shown that reliability is indeed improved by using this method. However, HCFA cannot direct software vendors to make this change. If desired, facilities should contact their software support representative who may alter your system to meet the facility's needs.

27: If a resident demonstrates a behavior after the assessment observation period is ended, we document this in the clinical record and address the behavior on the care plan. How is this behavior reflected in the RAI assessment?

A: The facility maintains a responsibility to address issues and behaviors relevant to a resident whether or not they occur during the MDS observation period. Such information should be documented in the clinical record and referenced as necessary to support decisions of whether and how to care plan. Although an event may not occur during the MDS observation period (and therefore will not be coded on the MDS), the assessor has the professional responsibility to make a decision regarding the review of RAPs that did not trigger. Ongoing assessment, planning and evaluation are basic components of clinical practice. Refer to the problem identification model addressed in chapter 1 of the RAI User's Manual.

28: During the MDS assessment observation period, a resident is assessed as needing medical evaluation and treatment for depression, and the facility alerts the physician about this need. The evaluation is completed and treatment is begun after the MDS observation period is over. How is this reflected in our assessment and care planning?

A: The assessment process in ongoing. Changes in the resident's status and plan of care (i.e. physician's orders, delivery of care and services, the resident's response to care and treatment provided, etc.) should be documented clearly in the clinical record after the RAI is completed. Revisions should be made to the care plan as a result of an ongoing assessment and evaluation process and as appropriate for the individual situation, whenever changes occur.

29: In the example on page 4-26 in the User's Manual, is the date at MDS item A3a correct?

A: No. A3a in this example should be dated 09-01-1995. This was previously acknowledged by HCFA and sent out as a correction.

30: What is the significance of item A3b?

A: This item was originally designed to allow for correction in a computer environment. However, HCFA's current correction policy (refer to the RAI User's Manual, page 2-25), does not allow the item to be used. Additional changes may be forthcoming when HCFA's ADP requirements are published.

31: For item A4a on the Quarterly and the Annual Assessment, if a resident has not been hospitalized do we leave the item blank?

A: For both the Full and Quarterly Assessments, if the resident has not been hospitalized in the past 90 days, leave this item blank. The Users Manual reference for this question is on page 3-31.

32: Please define item A7h, "Medicaid resident liability or Medicare co-payment".

A: This is the beneficiary's liability for PART A coinsurance.

33: Regarding the intent of Item C6 - Ability to Understand Others: Is writing an acceptable substitute for verbal communication?

A: Yes. According to the intent as described on page 3-53 of the RAI Version 2.0 User's Manual, information may be communicated to the resident orally, in writing, or in sign language or braille. When coding the item, be sure to follow the processes described on page 3-53. The resident may definitely be able to understand others when the information is presented to the resident in a way that he or she is most able to receive it. However, not all persons who interact with the resident will share information in the same way. If the resident needs to receive information in writing because he is highly hearing impaired but others (e.g., a roommate, visitors, other residents, etc.) do not present the information in writing, you must take this into consideration in coding the response that best reflects the resident's objective ability to understand information as it is presented to him.

34: Under Section E1, if "verbal expression" occurs five times during 30 days, but not daily, how is it coded?

A: The answer to this question is "1". By definition, code "2" applies to daily, or almost daily behavior. The User's Manual reference for coding this question is on page 3-60.

35: If a resident was showing signs of depression for six days in one week (but less than six days for each of the other weeks during the 30-day period), how would I code Section E1?

A: The behavior in this example would be coded as "1". For more coding information, refer to the response to the previous question.

36: Should the response to MDS item E4e, "Resists Care" include instances where the resident exercised his/her right to refuse treatment?

A: No. The item includes resistance to taking medications/injections, ADL assistance or help with eating. This category does not include instances where the resident has made an informed choice not to follow a course of care (e.g., resident has exercised his or her right to refuse treatment, and reacts negatively as staff try to re-institute treatment). Refer to the User's Manual, page 3-63.

37: "Change in Behavioral Symptoms", MDS item E5, asks for a comparison to behavioral status 90 days ago. Does this comparison include the entire 90 day period, or a snapshot of today versus a one-day snapshot of 90 days ago?

A: Item E5 asks for a snapshot of "today" as compared to 90 days ago (i.e., a comparison of two points in time). The intent of the item is to document whether the behavioral symptoms or resistance to care exhibited by the resident remained stable, increased or decreased in frequency of occurrence or alterability as compared to the resident's status of 90 days ago. By definition, this refers to the status (new onset, improvement, worsening) of any of the symptoms described in item E4. If the resident is a new admission to the facility, review changes during the period prior to admission and score the resident at the time of the observation period, as compared to the resident's status 90 days ago. Refer to the User's Manual, pages 3-66 through 3-68. Behavioral symptoms for the entire 90 day period should be reviewed however, for care planning purposes.

38: Why do F1b, "Establishes own goals" and F3a, "Strong identification with past roles and life status" trigger the Psychosocial RAP?

A: Both are new as trigger elements and were added in response to providers and consumer advocacy groups' desires to use the triggers to help staff focus on areas of resident strengths. This helps in staffs' efforts to assist the resident reach his or her highest practicable level of well-being. Data indicated that triggers needed to be more inclusive for this RAP.

39: Regarding MDS items F2 and F3, the guidelines in the User's Manual on page 3-70 (process paragraph) state to observe "over the past seven days". This was not stated for MDS item F1. The observation periods for F1, 2 and 3 are not noted on the MDS. Please clarify the expected observation period for F1.

A: Items for which observation periods are not specifically listed on the MDS are always 7 days. Use "over the past seven days" as the observation period for F1. This is stated in the "process" paragraph on page 3-69 in the manual.

40: Regarding the concept of weight bearing support in Item G1A (ADL Self-Performance), Code "3", Extensive Assistance: Does weight bearing support refer to staff "taking some of the resident's weight?"

A: Yes.

41: How should items G1c and d, (pertaining to locomotion on and off unit), be coded for a resident who propels his wheelchair, but does not make it to a destination without assistance?

A: Code the items according to the amount and frequency of assistance received, using the ADL Self-Performance and Support code instructions provided in the User's Manual, Section G.

42: If a resident is bed bound and does not walk, do you code them as an "8"?

A: Assuming this question is in reference to Section G, items 1e and 1f (locomotion on and off the unit), the User's Manual reference for this response begins on page 3-73. If the resident is bed bound and does not walk and there was no locomotion via bed, wheelchair or other means, then you would code as "8". However, if the bed is moved in order to provide locomotion on or off the unit, then you would code according to the definitions provided in Section G., 1A & B. If this question refers to G1c and 1d (walk in room/corridor), code as an 8.

43: Is standing balance (MDS item G3b) coded for standing only? How is the item coded for residents who can stand, but who cannot get to a standing position without physical assistance?

A: Refer to the User's Manual, page 3-91. "DO NOT attempt to test residents who cannot stand by themselves". Code these residents as "3", "Not able to attempt test without physical help".

44: Can a Restorative Aide do the testing necessary to code items G4 (A) and (B)?

A: No. A therapist or nurse should conduct the evaluation.

45: Regarding G4 (A), "Limitation in Range of Motion", in the example in the User's Manual on page 3-98, the resident has a bilateral limitation in neck range of motion, yet the item is coded "1", which is defined as a limitation on one side of the body. Is this correct?

A: This example contains a coding error. The item should be coded "2", limitation on both sides of the body.

46: The coding instructions for G4 (B), "Loss of Voluntary Movement", on page 3-98 of the User's Manual do not include a coding option for a resident who has full loss on one side of the body, and full range on the other. How would this be coded? Also, how should we code for partial loss on one side and full loss on the other?

A: Code both situations "1" for Partial Loss of Voluntary Movement.

47: Regarding Section G, item 4cB, how do you code a resident who has arthritis in both hands, but is able to dress self?

A: There is not enough information provided to code the question. A diagnosis of arthritis does not necessarily impact function. To determine the code, you must consider two parameters: completion of the task (i.e., not interfering with daily functions) and coordination of movements. You have already determined that the resident is functionally able to complete the task of self-dressing, which would rule out code 2. If the resident has full ROM in both hands, use code 0. Next determine coordination of movements: select code 0 if the resident's movements were smooth and coordinated; code 1 if the resident's movements were slow and uncoordinated. Refer to the coding instructions in the User's Manual on page 3-98.

48: Regarding Section G, explain the intent of code 8, particularly regarding walking and eating.

A: Code 8 is reserved for use when an ADL did not occur in the 7 day observation period. For example, use code 8 when the resident did not walk in the past 7 days, (in room/in corridor), for both the self performance and the support columns. Refer to the guidelines, definitions and examples in the User's Manual, beginning on page 3-73.

The eating item for G1h, is a little more complex. If in the past 7 days the resident truly did not receive any nourishment, the item would be coded 8. It should go without saying that this is a serious issue. Be careful not to confuse total dependence with eating (code 4) with the activity itself (in this case, receiving nourishment and fluids). Keep in mind that a resident who is fed via tube, and manages the tube feeding independently is coded as independent (code 0). G1h includes receiving IV fluids. For a resident who is receiving fluids for hydration, and is totally dependent, this is coded as 4, rather than 8.

49: When is code 8 appropriate for ADL items?

A: Code 8 means the activity did not occur in the past 7 days. A resident who has not been out of bed in the past 7 days could be coded 8 for (A) & (B) in MDS Sections G1b-f, unless the bed was moved (locomotion on/off unit). Other ADL's are considered individually. Refer to the ADL coding guidelines in the User's Manual on pages 3-77 through 3-82. Also refer to the bottom of page 2-24.

50: If a resident lacks all ability to perform ROM (range of motion) exercises on request due to impaired cognition, and has no limitations in ROM, how should G4a & b be coded? A Physical therapist told me that active assistive ROM cannot be done with mentally impaired residents because they cannot follow the instructions the User's Manual suggests.

A: This is a good question because many residents in nursing facilities are cognitively impaired. These items are coded based on the resident's ability to perform range of motion and voluntary movement. For G4a, a resident who is unable to follow your verbal instructions or a demonstration of movements can be actively assisted in range of motion exercises to assess for limitations. Move the resident's joints through slow, active assisted ROM by providing support and direction with each activity. In this section, you can also use observations, by the staff, of what the resident can do. Refer to the User's Manual, page 3-96.

51: How would item G4, column B be coded for the example in the User's Manual on page 3-97?

A: There is not enough information to score G4 in this example. The assessor would have to utilize available information pertaining to the individual resident in order to score this item.

52: When a resident cannot/does not have voluntary ROM due to impaired cognition, yet at other times, strikes out or makes movements considered ROM, how is this coded?

A: You can use staff observations of the ROM activity to determine whether a resident can actually perform the activity, regardless of whether the movement was "on command", provided the movement fits the criteria on page 3-96 of the User's Manual and occurred during the assessment period of observation.

53: Regarding Section G4, when assessing Functional Limitations in Range of Motion, how are amputations coded?

A: Section G focuses on two areas of resident ability: (A) Range of Motion, and (B) Voluntary Movement. The coding scheme is the same for both items. If the resident has an amputation on one side of the body, code "1". If the amputation is bilateral, code "2". Refer to the User's Manual, pages 3-97 and 3-98.

54: How do you accurately assess cognitive status for an aphasic resident?

A: It is often difficult to accurately assess cognitive function, or how someone is able to think, remember, and make decisions about their daily lives, when they are unable to verbally communicate with you. It is particularly difficult when the areas of cognitive function you want to assess require some kind of verbal response from the resident (e.g., memory recall). It is certainly easier to perform an evaluation when you can converse with a resident and hear responses from them that give you clues to how the resident is able to think (judgement), if he understands his strengths and weaknesses (insight), whether or not he is repetitive (memory), or if he has difficulty finding the right words to tell you what he wants to say (aphasia).

To assess an aphasic resident it is very important that you hone your listening and observation skills to look for non-verbal cues to the person's abilities. For example, for someone who is unable to speak with you but seems to understand what you are saying (expressive aphasia), the assessor could ask the resident the necessary questions and then ask him to answer you with whatever non-verbal means he is able to use (e.g., writing the answer; showing you the way to his room; pointing to a calendar to show you what month/season it is). Observe the resident at different times of the day and in different types of activities for clues to their functional abilities. Solicit input from the observations of others who care for the resident.

In all cases code the cognitive items with answers that reflect your best clinical judgement, realizing the difficulty in assessing residents who are unable to communicate. Items B1, B4, B5, and B6 can be successfully coded without having to get verbal answers from the resident. Interdisciplinary collaboration will be helpful in conducting an accurate assessment. See pages 3-44 and 3-48 of the User's Manual for instructions.

55: Are gerichairs or merry walkers included in Section G5? How do you code these?

A: Merry walkers can be included in G5a because they are a type of walker. Gerichairs are not captured here because this section is looking at modes of locomotion that the resident is using. Gerichairs are considered a stationary vehicle.

56: In Section G6a, what if the resident spends all of his time in bed or is in a recliner chair for 22 hours a day <u>but</u> is out of his room in another part of the facility? Is the location of the bed or recliner a crucial point?

A: In this case, the location of the bed or recliner is the crucial point. Assess the resident's mode of transfer <u>in his/her own room</u>. If the resident is out of his room for most of the day, you would not check G6a. The User's Manual reference for this question in on page 3-99.

57: Section G6b assesses whether "Bed rails are used for bed mobility or transfer". In P4a, the item documents whether full bed rails are used in a section entitled "Devices and Restraints". Will this identify enablers as restraints on the HCFA 672?

A: Section P4 identifies whether full or partial side rails are used, but does not make a judgement regarding whether they are used as a restraint. When the siderails are used to assist in mobility and item G6b is also checked, then for the purpose of completing the HCFA 672 form, G6b minus P4a&b identifies restraints.

On the HCFA 672, a form used to document resident characteristics during a LTC facility survey, item F 104 is completed by the facility to identify the number of physically restrained residents in the facility at the time of the survey. The State survey team could use this as one piece of information in selecting a sample of residents for in-depth review during the survey. It offers a screening mechanism to determine the extent of restraint use within the facility. This information would need to be developed by the survey team as they investigate their concerns.

58: Regarding Section B1, "Comatose", providers with sub-acute units request a (further) definition of "no discernable consciousness". This would be for situations when there is no documented neurological diagnosis of coma or persistent vegetative state on admission; however, the resident, as assessed by the interdisciplinary team, has "no discernable signs of consciousness".

A: Coma is a pathological state in which neither arousal (wakefulness, alertness) nor awareness (cognition of self and environment) is present. The comatose person is unresponsive and cannot be aroused; he does not open his eyes, does not speak, and does not move his extremities on command or in response to noxious stimuli (e.g., pain).

Sometimes patients who were comatose for a period of time after an anoxic-ischemic injury (i.e., not enough oxygen to the brain), from a cardiac arrest, head trauma or massive stroke, regain wakefulness but have no evidence of any purposeful behavior or cognition. Their eyes are open and they seem to be awake. They may grunt, yawn, pick with their fingers and have random movements of their heads and extremities. A neurological exam shows that they have extensive damage to both cerebral hemispheres. This state is different from coma and if it continues is called a persistent vegetative state. Both coma and vegetative state have serious consequences in terms of long-term clinical outcomes and care needs.

Many other residents have severe impairments in cognition that are associated with late-stages of progressive neurological disorders such as Alzheimer's disease. Although such residents may be non-communicative, totally dependent on others for care and nourishment, and sleep a great deal of time, they are usually not comatose or in a persistent vegetative state as described above.

To prevent any resident from being mislabeled as such it is imperative that coding in MDS Item B1 reflect physician documentation of a diagnosis of either coma or persistent vegetative state.

59: Should intraocular lens implants (IOL's) be documented under Vision Patterns, Section D, or Disease Diagnoses, Section I? It's not a disease, as the cataract has been removed. Basically, it's an inactive diagnosis.

A: Section D of the original MDS was revised so that lens implants are no longer captured in Version 2.0. The presence of an intraocular lens implant should still be included in the resident's physical assessment and documented elsewhere in the resident's clinical record, for example: under ophthalmology.

60: Regarding Section G, ADLs, in interpreting toilet use, under what circumstances would it be appropriate to use code 8? Does toileting strictly refer to the resident being in the bathroom?

A: No, this item focuses on whether elimination occurs, rather than the process. The elimination may be in the toilet room, commode, in the bedroom on a bedpan or urinal. It includes transferring on/off the toilet, cleansing, changing pads, managing an ostomy or catheter and clothing adjustment.

The "8" code is rarely used in this section, as it would indicate that elimination did not occur. The User's Manual reference for this question is page 3-108 and 3-109.

61: If a resident displays a behavior prior to and after, but not once during the 7-day period of observation, would you still work the related RAPS?

A: If a behavior does not occur within the MDS observation period set by the assessment reference date in Section A3, do not code it on the MDS. The fact that the resident did not display a known behavior during the observation period does not mean it can be ignored. For episodes of behavior that occur outside the observation period, clinical judgment should be exercised regarding whether RAP review and care planning are clinically warranted and the type of documentation that is appropriate.

Questions on Items in MDS Sections H through R

62: How should Bladder Continence, item H1b, be coded for a resident who dribbles urine frequently and wears an incontinent pad, but changes the pad herself, and her underwear is never wet?

A: Bladder continence refers to control of urinary bladder function, which is distinct from the resident's ADL status and need for assistance during toileting. Proper coding of this item requires review of the number and frequency of incontinence episodes over the 14-day review period. With that information, code the continence level according to the 5 point scale in the User's Manual on pages 3-106 and 107.

63: On the Quarterly Review form in Section H2 - Bowel Elimination Pattern, why are there only two answer options: Fecal Impaction or None of the above?

A: Not all MDS items appear on the Quarterly Review form. In this case, the Quarterly Review was planned to look for sentinel events. Items a) Regular bowel elimination, b) Constipation, and c) Diarrhea, were not considered. In one year, one State reported deaths of five nursing home residents, with the cause of death linked directly to fecal impaction. In this case, "none of the above" is checked if fecal impaction did not occur during the assessment period of observation.

64: Regarding item H4, for a resident who had a catheter and was coded as continent on the last MDS, but 90 days later has had the catheter removed, is on a bladder retraining program but is leaking urine during the new observation period, is the MDS coded as "improved" or "deteriorated"?

A: Code as "deteriorated". The issue is performance. Refer to the explanation and examples in the User's Manual, beginning on page 3-105.

65: Regarding Item H4, Change in Urinary Continence: If a resident's condition has changed from dribbling urine without an indwelling catheter to dry with a catheter, would this be coded as "1", Improved?

A: Yes. According to the User's Manual on page 3-110, "Although one could perceive that [the resident] had deteriorated" because he now has a catheter for bladder control, remember that the MDS definition for bladder continence states "Control of bladder function with appliances (e.g., foley) or continence programs, if employed." The key issue in coding MDS items is "objective performance". In this case, the resident is continent and therefore coded as "improved," even though the catheter is the basis for the change in status.

66: Regarding Section I, item 1, all diseases are linked to an alpha character, in alphabetic order from a to rr. On the expanded Quarterly form, diagnoses are not in alphabetic order. Should the order on the form be changed to conform to the data dictionary?

A: No. Each item is associated with its respective label on both the full MDS and the expanded Quarterly Review form. The alphabetic order of the items is not as important as having consistent item labels.

67: Regarding HIV Confidentiality: Does staff need authorization to get information to complete I 2d? What about transmitting the information?

A: HCFA has treated the item for HIV infection the same as for other clinical diagnoses. Refer to the State regulations for guidance. Additional information regarding submission of this data element will be forthcoming with publication of HCFA's pending regulations on MDS automation. All such clinical information is considered confidential and protected as a part of the resident's clinical record.

68: Sensitive issues related to HIV infection and sexually transmitted diseases are documented on the MDS (I2d & I2h). Our State agency policy requires facilities within our State to omit documentation for these 2 items. What are we to do?

A: If a State has a policy that covers this, the State policy supersedes the MDS requirement.

69: Pneumonia and respiratory infections are both mentioned in Item I2. How do we work through this to code correctly?

A: Review the definitions on page 3-116 of the User's Manual. A key point according to the manual is that a "respiratory infection is any upper or lower (e.g., bronchitis) respiratory infection other than pneumonia". If the resident has only pneumonia, check only item I2e, rather than both I2e and I2f.

70: Are infections to be documented in Item I2 only if they have occurred in the past 7 days?

A: According to the directions for Section I, Disease Diagnoses, "Check only those diseases that have a relationship to current ADL status, cognitive status, mood and behavior status, medical treatments, nursing monitoring, or risk of death. (Do not list inactive diagnoses)." Therefore, if the resident has an infection that is currently active and impacts on one of the above areas, check the appropriate response. This category includes conditions that occurred prior to the past 7 days but are still actively treated. The exception is Item I2j, Urinary tract infection in last 30 days. If the resident had a urinary tract infection during this time frame, check Item I2j, even if the resident no longer received treatment or monitoring for the condition during the assessment period.

71: What information is entered on the MDS if staff are unable to obtain a resident's weight?

A: There may be circumstances under which a resident cannot be weighed, for example: extreme pain or immobility, risk of pathological fractures or extreme obesity. If, as a matter of professional judgement, a resident cannot be weighed, use the standard no-information code, which is either a "circled" dash or an "NA". Refer to the User's manual, page 2-24 for further information regarding coding when information is not available.

72: For Section K, are there any regulations or guidelines related to desirable weight gain or loss time frames? How much weight loss in what period of time is considered too fast?

A: There are no specific regulations that address the desirable weight and time frames for weight gain or weight loss. However, there is some general information in the interpretive guidelines and in the Nutritional RAP that may provide guidance in this area. The amount of weight gain or loss is reflective of individual differences. Guidelines related to acceptable parameters of weight gain and loss are addressed in the OBRA regulations at 42 CFR 483.25, nutrition (F325 and F 326) and 483.20(b)2(v), resident assessment nutritional status and requirements (F 272), which corresponds to the MDS Section K, Oral/Nutritional status.

The parameters for weight loss identified in the guidelines referenced above are:

1 month	5% significant	>5% severe
3 months	7.5% significant	>7.5% severe
6 months	10% significant	>10% severe

The measurement of weight is a guide in determining nutritional status. Therefore, the evaluation of the significance of weight gain or loss over a specific time frame is a crucial part of the assessment process. An adequate assessment should result in a "comprehensive care plan for each resident that includes measurable objectives and timetables to meet a resident's needs."

73: In Section K, is documentation required for 7 1/2% significant weight change in 90 days?

A: Yes. This change is recorded in K3a only when there is a minimum weight loss of 5% or more of total body mass over 30 days, or a 10% or greater loss over 180 days. In this example, scoring of K3a would depend on how much of the 7 1/2% weight loss occurred over the last 30 days. Documentation of the identification and evaluation of weight change is good clinical practice. The significance of the weight change for that resident should be reflected within that documentation.

74: Regarding item K2b, "weight", the entry field doesn't allow for fractions of a pound. How is this accounted for on the MDS? Also, how is a fraction of a pound handled when calculating weight change?

A: For purposes of completing item K2b on the MDS, round the resident's weight up to the next pound. Also round up to the next pound in calculating weight change.

75: Why are there two weight change questions on the MDS? Are questions K3a and b the same?

A: Item K3a captures weight loss; K3b captures weight gain.

76: We use hypodermoclysis and subcutaneous ports in hydration therapy. Should we code these nutritional approaches in Item K5a, Parenteral/IV?

A: Yes. Although it is not defined in the User's Manual, the term parenteral therapy means 'introduction of a substance (especially nutritive material) into the body by means other than the intestinal tract (e.g., subcutaneous, intravenous).' If the resident receives fluids via these modalities, also code Item K6a and K6b which refer to the caloric and fluid intake the resident received in the last 7 days.

77: How is the presence of a gastrostomy coded?

A: Code a gastrostomy tube at item K5b, under Nutritional Approaches. A gastrostomy tube would meet the definition for Feeding Tube, "any type of tube that can deliver food/nutritional substance/fluids/medications directly into the gastrointestinal system". Refer to the User's Manual, page 3-130.

Also refer to page 3-149 regarding Section P1f, (special treatments, procedures, and programs) response f for "ostomy care." This item focuses on the care and treatment a resident with an ostomy receives.

78: Regarding Section M, "Skin Condition": Since the response holds only a single digit, what is the appropriate code for a resident having more than 9 pressure ulcers? If the resident has more than 9 areas, how would you know the exact number of pressure areas?

A: Your particular question only applies if there are more than 9 ulcers at any one stage. If so, use code 9 for nine or more. Refer to the coding instructions in the User's Manual on page 3-135.

The MDS response regarding the number of ulcers is determined by physical examination of the resident. Staff should not rely solely on the MDS for information concerning pressure ulcers. The number and stages of ulcers could change shortly after the MDS is completed, and the MDS, in itself, does not include enough information to support the on-going care and evaluation of pressure ulcers.. Documentation of clinical information pertaining to the number, size, description, care and the resident's response to treatment of pressure ulcers should be maintained in the resident's clinical record and updated on an on-going basis.

79: Are ankle problems to be included in Section M6, "Foot Problems and Care"?

A: No. The ankle is the joint between the ankle and the foot, and is not included here.

If you are dressing the foot as well as the ankle, code the foot issues in M6 and code the ankle issues in M5h and M5i.

80. Regarding item M1, "Ulcers", how should a pressure ulcer that is eschared, necrotic or blistered be staged?

A: Code it as stage IV in terms of using the MDS scale. However, HCFA acknowledges that the NPUAP has recently published guidelines for pressure ulcer staging, and will be investigating this area in the future.

81: Regarding MDS item M6d, "Nails/Calluses trimmed during the last 90 days", and the guideline in the User's Manual on page 3-140 that includes trimming by a nurse or any health professional, including a podiatrist, is a CNA considered a "health professional" for the purpose of coding this item?

A: No. The item is intended to capture licensed professional time.

82: Current literature on staging pressure ulcers suggests that stage 4 ulcers which are healing cannot be characterized as stage 3, stage 2, and stage 1, as they are healing. The alternate approach is to identify the ulcer as a healing stage 4 ulcer. Consultants and providers are very upset that they have spent the past year training personnel how to stage ulcers in this manner, but the MDS encourages them use a reverse staging system. Can we have resolution? For example, is a healing Stage 3 Pressure Ulcer coded as a 3 or 2?

A: Code it as a 3. For the MDS Version 2.0, code the ulcer in terms of what you see (i.e., visible tissue). That is, the MDS should be coded the way it was in the original version. Currently, there is no uniform nomenclature or scoring system approved for coding a healing pressure ulcer. In the clinical record, describe the appearance of the healing ulcer (i.e., presence of granulation tissue, size, depth, color, and so forth).

83: Is time spent involved in independent, unstructured leisure activity, (for example: watching favorite soap operas, talking on the phone, knitting), to be included in "average time involved in activities"?

A: Yes. Include time spent in pursuing independent activities, (e.g., watering plants, reading, letter-writing); social contacts (e.g., visits, phone calls) with family, other residents, staff, and volunteers; recreational pursuits in a group, one-on-one or on an individual basis; and involvement in therapeutic recreation. Refer to the User's Manual, page 3-141. Keep in mind that the definition of "activity pursuits" refers to any activity other than ADLs that a resident pursues in order to enhance a sense of well-being. Efforts should be made to provide activities suited to the resident's preferences and capabilities.

84: Section N, item 2 is not clear; does this mean while awake or involved in activities?

A: Item N2 refers to the amount of "free time" a resident has while awake and is not involved in receiving nursing care, treatments, or engaged in ADL activities, and could therefore be involved in activity pursuits and therapeutic recreation of their choice. This item has a 7-day observation period, which should give an accurate indication of the resident's activity involvement pattern. Refer to the User's Manual, page 3-141.

85: Regarding item N2, "Average Time Involved in Activities", is it accurate to say that cognitively impaired residents would likely be coded as having little or no involvement (based on available time), since they are lacking the ability to consciously "pursue" their interests?

A: No. Many cognitively impaired persons continue to "pursue" their interests and also develop new interests. Activities must be tailored to their cognitive abilities. Record the amount of time the person spends in structured and non-structured activities. Refer to pages 3-140 to 3-142 of the User's Manual, which includes a broad definition of activity pursuits.

86: Where would you record a preference for activities such as trivia games, intellectual groups or party-type activities?

A: If the activity is predominantly a social-type activity then record it under N4k. If the activity is more "game-like" in nature, then record it under N4a. The MDS does not provide a separate item to document resident's preference for every possible type of activity. Coding decisions should be based upon the predominant overall nature of the activity. Refer to the User's Manual, page 3-142.

87: Define Activity "pursuits" vs: "programs", and how the assessment guidelines distinguish between what the resident prefers, and what the facility offers.

A: N4 refers to resident activity preferences (adapted to the resident's current abilities). N5 determines if the resident is interested in activities that are either not offered, or are offered but not available to the resident. Refer to the User's Manual, pages 3-142 & 143.

88: Regarding item N2, "Average Time Involved in Activities", is time spent eating to be included in the calculation of time available for activities? In other words, is dining considered an activity?

A: Although dining is a social experience for some residents, and at times, meals may be planned around certain events or occasions, eating is not to be counted as an activity. Available time for activities refers to free time when the resident was awake and was not involved in receiving nursing care, treatments, or engaged in ADL activities (including eating) and could have been involved in activity pursuits and Therapeutic Recreation. Refer to the User's Manual, page 3-141.

89: Regarding MDS items N3 and N4, when the resident is marginally responsive and family is not available, what is the most appropriate method of gathering information concerning "Activity Pursuit Pattern"?

A: Explore other possible sources of information, such as a responsible party that admitted the resident into the facility, or a surrogate decision maker who might know the resident's preferences. Is there any useful information in records that precede admission to the facility, such as hospital, community or home care records? If all resources are exhausted and you still do not have information, code the responses as information not available, (see the User's Manual page 2-24). Also, as noted in the User's Manual on page 3-143, observe the resident in current activities. If the resident appears content during an activity (e.g., smiling, clapping during a music program), check the item on the form.

90: If a resident receives more than one type of insulin, is each type recorded in MDS item O1?

A: Yes. For example, Lente, Humulin, and Regular are different types of insulin and are considered different medications.

91: Is Sustacal or any nutritional supplement considered a medication as it relates to MDS Section O?

A: Section O is designed to capture data concerning the use of over-the-counter and prescription medication. The User's Manual, on page 3-145, expands the definition of medications to include topical preparations, ointments, creams used in wound care (e.g., Elase), eye drops, vitamins, and suppositories. Although the pharmacy sometimes supplies such items, Sustacal is not counted as a mediation for coding in Section O. Vitamins should be counted (as noted above). The Sustacal could be recorded in Section K5, provided it fits the definitions.

92: In Section O, Medications: Why doesn't a hypnotic drug trigger the Psychotropic Drug Use RAP?

A: Hypnotic drug use does not add any discriminating ability in terms of identifying residents who warrant additional assessment.

93: In Section O1, "Number of Medications", are B12 injections that are given once per month, but outside of the assessment period included (as are the long acting antipsychotics illustrated in the User's Manual)?

A: Yes. If the resident received an injection of Vitamin B12 prior to the observation period, code in Section O1. Vitamin B12 maintains a blood level, as do long acting antipsychotics.

94: Where should we code suppositories administered as part of a continence/bowel program?

A: Record suppositories in Item O1, Number of Medications. For facilities in States using Section U, also record in Section U.

95: Are suppositories, enemas, fleets, and glycerin to be included in Item O1, Number of Medications?

A: Of this list, only suppositories are to be coded in Item O1.

96: In Section O3, "Injections", would this include B12 injections given once per month but outside of the observation period?

A: No. In O3, code only the injections administered during the observation period.

97: Regarding item O4, should over-the-counter sleeping medications be coded as hypnotic even though they are not pharmacologically classified as hypnotic drugs?

A: No.

98: Regarding item O4, one facility has a resident receiving Serax, classified as an anxiolitic drug, specifically for sleep. Should this drug be coded as a hypnotic because of its intended use?

A: No. Although in practice Oxazepam (Serax) may be used as a hypnotic, it is classified as an antianxiety (anxiolitic) agent in Appendix E of the User's Manual, and should be coded as such. Code the MDS according to the drug's pharmacological classification, not how it is used. This enables monitoring of side effects associated with the drug.

99 Regarding item P4e, "Chair Prevents Rising", the User's Manual, page 3-158 includes as an example a chair with a lapboard that locks. Is a chair with a lapboard that does not lock also considered a "chair prevents rising"?

A: A chair with an unlocked lapboard could be included as a chair prevents rising if the resident cannot easily remove the lapboard. It is also considered a restraint if the chair prevents rising for the resident who ordinarily could rise. If the resident can remove the lapboard and can rise from the chair, do not code P4e.

100: In Section P, Intake and Output, would this include daily I and O for residents receiving tube feeding or short-term IV fluids?

A: Yes. Intake and output includes "all" fluids the resident received and/or excreted for at least three consecutive shifts during the 14-day period of observation. Refer to the User's Manual, page 3-149.

101: Regarding Section P1, item a, r, "Training in skills required to return to the community", does this training include that provided as part of Occupational Therapy, Physical Therapy, and Speech Therapy?

A: Yes.

102: In Section P1f: Does "Ostomy" refer to any and all ostomies (except tracheostomy) that require nursing assistance for care, e.g.: gastrostomies as well as colostomies, urostomies, etc?

A: Yes. The User's Manual reference is on page 3-149.

103: In Section P1 - Is whirlpool included in Physical Therapy services?

A: If whirlpool is specifically ordered by the Physician to be done under the supervision of the Physical Therapist, it is included in that service.

104: Regarding Section P 2, "Evaluation by a licensed mental health specialist", please define "psychiatric social worker". Our State does not have a definition of this term in our practice guidelines.

A: Each State licenses independent providers of mental health services who can provide care in the facility, at home, office or clinic. The term "psychiatric social worker," (synonymous with clinical social worker) refers to someone with training in clinical mental health practice who is qualified to practice as a psychotherapist. Depending on State licensure requirements, a psychiatric/clinical social worker functions as an independent practitioner or under consultation, usually to a psychiatrist.

105: Should we define psychiatric nurse credentials? Can this include LVN/LPN? And what about credentials for Psychiatric Technician?

A: Psychiatric nurses usually have a Master's degree and/or certification from the American Nurses Association as a psychiatric specialist. Psychiatric Technicians do not fall under this category.

106: How is MDS item P2b, "Evaluation by a licensed mental health specialist in the last 90 days", coded in States where mental health workers are not required to be licensed?

A: If your State doesn't license a certain category of therapists, then do not count it at item P2b.

107: Regarding Item P1b, if one Physical Therapist has a group of 5 residents in an activity, does each resident get the full value of the therapist's time, or is that time shared among members of the group?

A: Generally, in a group larger than 4 residents, the residents are receiving supportive services, not treatments, unless there are at least 2 staff persons with the group. For the most part, the therapy services section assumes individualized treatment and the category does not include services received as part of a group of more than 4 residents per supervising helper (as stated in the Nursing Rehabilitation section on page 3-154 of the User's Manual). If, however, the group has four or fewer residents per supervising therapist (or assistant), give each resident the full time value spent in the therapy session. For example, if a therapist worked with three residents for 45 minutes on training to return to the community, each resident received 45 minutes of therapy. Remember, code for the resident's time, not for the therapist's time.

Also, the service must meet all of the following criteria to be coded in the therapy section:

- The service must be ordered by a physician.
- The therapy intervention must be based on a qualified therapist's evaluation and plan of care as documented in the resident's record.
- An appropriate licensed or certified individual must provide or directly supervise the therapeutic service and coordinate the intervention with nursing services.

108: When looking at time for PT, OT or Speech, do we consider direct resident contact time only? For example, if you set a resident up for a treatment, is the entire time of the treatment counted or only the start/stop time required by the professional?

A: The MDS 2.0 measures the resident's characteristics and services received. The amounts of time reported in Section P1b must be the "resident's time in treatment," not the time and effort of the staff to produce and document the treatment. The resident's treatment time starts when he begins the first treatment activity or task and ends when he finishes with the last apparatus and the treatment is ended. Set-up time is also included. In some cases, the resident will be able to perform part of the treatment tasks with supervision, once set up appropriately. Time supervising the resident is a part of total treatment time. For example, as the last treatment task of the day, a resident uses an exercise bicycle for 10 minutes. It may take the therapist 2 minutes to set the resident up on the apparatus. This therapist or assistant under the supervision of a PT may then leave the resident to help another resident in the same exercise room. However, the therapist still has eye contact with the resident and is providing supervision, verbal encouragement and direction to the resident on the bicycle. Therefore, if it took 2 minutes to set the resident up with the cycling apparatus, the resident was supervised during two 5-minute cycling periods; one 2-minute rest between the exercise periods; and took 1 minute to get out of the apparatus, the total cycling activity is 15 minutes. Include in this example that the resident did three additional treatment activities totaling 45 minutes before beginning to cycle. The total time reported on the MDS is 60 minutes. The key is that the resident was receiving treatment the entire time and had the physical presence of a therapist in the room, supervising the entire treatment process.

109: Does therapy provided by Recreation and Art therapists count as Psychological Therapy in answering item P1be?

A: No. Psychological therapy is provided by a licensed mental health professional, such as a psychiatrist, psychologist, psychiatric nurse or psychiatric social worker. Refer to the User's Manual, page 3-151.

110: Regarding MDS item P1bd, "Respiratory Therapy" and the guidelines in the User's Manual on page 3-151, ...[therapy] provided by a qualified professional, (i.e., trained nurse, respiratory therapist); what is the definition of a "trained nurse"?

A: "Trained Nurse" refers to a nurse who received specific training on the administration of respiratory treatments and procedures. This training may have been provided at the facility during a previous work experience or as part of an academic program. Nurses may not necessarily learn these procedures as part of formal Nursing training.

111: Do breathing treatments given by a nurse count as a respiratory treatment?

A: Respiratory therapy can include coughing, deep breathing, heated nebulizers, aerosol treatments, mechanical ventilation, etc., which must be provided by a qualified professional (i.e. trained nurse, respiratory therapist). Refer to the User's Manual, page 3-151.

112: When a resident talks to a nurse about emotional problems, does it count as Psychological Therapy in answering item P1be?

A: No. Although this is helpful to the resident, and is a part of good nursing practice, this item is intended to capture Psychological Therapy time, which is specifically provided by a licensed mental health professional. If the conversation occurred as part of a structured therapy session, and the nurse was a psychiatric nurse, it could be coded as Psychological Therapy. Refer to the User's Manual, page 3-151.

113: When a psychiatrist conducts an evaluation, how and where is it coded?

A: The assessment of a mood or behavior disorder, or other mental health problem by a psychiatrist is identified on the MDS in Section P, item 2b (evaluation by a licensed mental health specialist in the last 90 days). Additionally, if the visit occurred in the 14-day period of observation, a psychiatrist's visit is coded in item P7, Physician Visits.

114: What is the difference between a qualified therapist's evaluation (such as Occupational, Physical, or Respiratory Therapist), and a psychiatrist's evaluation in terms of MDS coding?

A: A therapist's (OT, PT, ST) initial evaluation would not be coded on the MDS. However, evaluations done as part of the treatment process would be included in treatment time. A psychiatric evaluation would be checked in Section P2b, if conducted within 90 days prior to the Assessment Reference Date. An evaluation by a psychologist, psychiatric nurse or psychiatric social worker would be checked in P2b.

115: Our facility has Physical Therapists evaluating the residents on a weekly basis. Can the Therapist's evaluation of the resident's ROM be substituted for an evaluation by a licensed nurse, for the purpose of completing Section P3?

A: Section P3 addresses Range of Motion exercises provided as part of nursing rehabilitation restorative care. The definition specifically states that it does not include procedures or techniques carried out by or under the direction of qualified therapists, as identified in item P1b. Periodic evaluation of ROM, unless done as a part of a treatment program, does not count.

116: Regarding P3a, b and c, "Nursing Rehabilitation/Restorative Care", if in the same shift a resident is provided 11 minutes of Passive ROM, 11 minutes of Active ROM, and a splint is applied, which takes 5 minutes, can the total of 27 minutes be combined in a single MDS response?

A: No. Passive ROM, Active ROM and splint/brace assistance time must all be coded separately, in time blocks of 15 minutes or more. For example, in order to check item P3a, 15 or more minutes of Passive ROM must have been provided in each of the last 7 days. The 15 minutes of time in a day may be totaled across 24 hours (e.g., 10 minutes on day shift plus 5 minutes in the evening). However, 15-minute time increments cannot be obtained by combining P3a, b and c. Refer to page 3-155 of the User's Manual.

117: Regarding MDS items P3a & b, the guidelines on page 3-154 include a definition of Active Range of Motion, but not of Passive Range of Motion. At some time, will a definition of Passive be added? What is the definition of Passive Range of Motion to be used in completing these MDS items?

A: Passive Range of Motion exercise - The care giver moves the body part around a fixed point or joint through the resident's available range of motion. The resident provides no assistance. Code under P3a.

118: Regarding MDS item P1b, does the therapist have to complete and sign off for this section, or can the RN Coordinator complete it after obtaining information from therapy?

A: This item may be completed directly by the therapist, or the therapist may document this information elsewhere in the record or otherwise share this information with another staff member (such as the RN Coordinator), who then documents this information on the MDS. If the RN Coordinator documents the information on the MDS, she must make sure that the therapist understands and uses the MDS concept of treatment time. Federal regulations offer facilities a great deal of flexibility in how the RAI assessment is completed and documented, requiring only that the RAI assessment must be conducted or coordinated with the appropriate participation of health professionals. Facilities have flexibility in determining who should participate in the assessment process as long as it is accurately conducted. Refer to the User's Manual, page 2-16.

119: Regarding Section P, if a small group (4 residents or less) participate in an activity consisting of the resident's applying make-up, and which conducted by a member of the activity staff under the restorative nursing program with goals, objectives and documentation of progress, could it be included in Section P3g, (grooming)?

A: Yes. Refer to the User's Manual, page 3-153 for the definition of Rehabilitation/Restorative Care, and page 3-154 for the list of criteria that (all) must be met in order to be included in P3. According to the criteria, other (non-nursing) staff or volunteers may be assigned to work with specific residents, under licensed nurse supervision.

120: Some restraint-specific assessment forms duplicate information collected on the MDS. Must a restraint assessment be done in addition to the MDS?

A: In response to this specific question, the assessment for restraint use could be documented in the record in a non-standardized manner or it could be conducted using a specific form to guide the assessment. The facility may choose whatever format they like, but as the RAI is already required, it makes sense to integrate the forms and thereby minimize unnecessary duplication. If physical restraints are triggered on the Trigger Legend, proceed to the Physical Restraint RAP. Medical symptoms warranting restraint use (chemical or physical) must be reflected in the clinical record. In most instances, it is expected that the facility should engage in a systematic and gradual process toward reducing restraints simultaneous with restorative/rehabilitative care. Refer to 42 CFR 483.13 (a).

121: If a resident has used a gerichair for over a year without adverse effect, do we need to continue to care plan for restraints?

A: Care planning is an ongoing process which requires the interdisciplinary team to develop, implement and evaluate individualized interventions, treatments and therapies for a resident. A resident's need for an intervention may or may not change over time. This determination can only be made through assessment, reassessment, and evaluation.

122: Regarding item P4, "Devices and Restraints", should the facility code this section regardless of whether the device/restraint is an enabler?

A: Yes. If bed rails are used for mobility aids, refer to G6b on page 3-99 in the User's Manual. Please write this cross-reference guide in your User's Manual on page 3-158.

123: Regarding item P4, "Devices and Restraints", are facilities to code only those restraints or devices that staff consider to be restraints?

A: No. Code <u>all</u> restraints and devices <u>that are used</u>. Use the same logic applied throughout the MDS for "objective performance." In this case, a particular device is being used by the resident; the item does not ask the assessor to evaluate why the device is being used.

124: In Section P4, are side rails coded as a restraint even if they're ordered at the resident's request, and the resident could call to have them released?

A: Yes. Depending on the frequency of their use, siderails would be coded as 0, 1 or 2. In this section, objectively code any device or restraint that was used during the last 7 days.

125: How are facilities in which the call light system and bed control mechanisms are contained within the bed rail to code Section P4, "Devices and Restraints"? Residents in these types of beds generally have the bed rails up. However, the railing may be up to allow the resident to adjust the bed or use the call light. How would this be coded if the resident had full side rails up daily?

A: Section P4, "Devices and Restraints", assesses the objective presence of devices and restraints. A resident who is in a bed with full side rails up on a daily basis is coded in P4a as "2". Also refer to the Question & Answer regarding G6b "Bed rails used for bed mobility and transfer''.

126: Regarding item P4e (chair prevents rising), for a resident with a J-tube, who is unable to voluntarily move and is positioned in a gerichair-chair on a daily basis, is the geri-chair coded as a restraint?

A: Assess the objective presence of devices and restraints listed on the MDS. In this case, the resident is in a chair that prevents rising on a daily basis. Code P4e as a "2". Once coded, staff should assess why they are using the gerichair and its impact on resident functioning. The device may actually be an enabler, rather than a restraint, but the care planning needs will be similar (e.g., skin, toileting, fluids, etc.).

127: We were informed that a merry walker was not considered a restraint on a particular resident. Is this a judgment call, or is a merry walker always considered a restraint?

A: Merry walkers can be very helpful mobility devices for some residents. For others however, (e.g. for residents who wander), merry walkers may be a restraint. Staff should code merry walkers in G5a (walker) as well as P4e (chair that prevents rising). Staff would then assess necessity during a review of the Restraint RAP. This logic is similar to that used for bed rails in terms of whether they are considered as enablers or restraints.

128: Exactly how should 3/4 siderails (up x2) be coded?

A: Full bed rails are defined as "one or more rails along both sides of the bed that block three-quarters to the whole length of the mattress". Code for full bed rails. Refer to page 3-158 of the User's Manual. When the siderails are used to assist in mobility and item G6b is also checked, then for the purpose of completing the HCFA 672 form, G6b minus P4 a & b identifies restraints.

129: Item P4 addresses devices and restraints, however, all items refer to restraints. Where do we address assistive/rehabilitation device usage?

A: In Section K5g, "plate guard, stabilized built-up utensil, etc.". Transfer aids, such as a slide board, trapeze, cane, walker or brace are found under G6e.

130: How should item P5 be coded for a resident who has a 23 hour hospital stay and is not admitted? Also regarding P5, in counting hospital overnight stays in the last 90 days, does that include hospital stays in the 90 days preceding admission to the NF?

A: Code item P5 only if the resident is admitted, regardless of length of time away from the facility. If the resident is a new admission to the facility, this item includes hospital admissions during the 90-day period prior to admission to the NF. Refer to the User's Manual, pages 3-159 & 160.

131: Regarding item P7, "Physician Visits", in addition to the physician types listed in the User's Manual, can the facility count visits made by "Medicine Men"?

A: No.

132: Is it appropriate for therapists to include documentation time in completing items in Section P?

A: No. The MDS 2.0 measures the resident's characteristics and services received. It is not a tool to report "staff effort." The amounts of time reported in Section P1b must be the "resident's" time in treatment. These amounts do not measure the time or the number of staff used to provide the service. This is clearly stated in the User's Manual on page 3-151, "the time should include only the actual treatment time, (not time waiting or writing reports)." The NHCMQ Demonstration has conducted two staff time studies. The 1990 study only collected direct and indirect time. The one in 1995 collected all on duty time of rehabilitation staff including direct (treatment, education and evaluation time), indirect resident specific time (documentation, conferences about individual residents, etc.) and resident non specific therapist time (in-service, travel, administration, supervision of staff, etc.). This information will be used to be sure that non treatment time of therapists, assistants and therapy aides is appropriately accounted for in the payment rates.

133: We're dealing with the issue of whose time to include for therapy. Under what circumstances would time spent by a Rehab Aide be captured as therapy time in Section P1b.?

A: First, note that the MDS 2.0 measures the resident's characteristics and services received. It is not a tool to report "staff effort." The amounts of time reported in Section P1b must be the "resident's" time in treatment. Regarding Physical and Occupational Therapies, Aides cannot independently provide a skilled service, therefore, if there is not a licensed person supervising the Aide, it should not be counted as therapy. Speech Therapy does not currently recognize an Assistant or an Aide as providing "treatment services". Occupational and Physical Therapies credential Assistants and do allow Aides to be supervised by either licensed staff (including contractors), but both Occupational and Physical Therapies, in their professional standards, require that Aides receive intense supervision and therefore, an unsupervised service provided by a licensed Aide should probably be included under Nursing Rehabilitation/Restorative Care in Section P3, rather than under Therapies in P1b. Even when included in Section P3, the Aide providing the service should be supervised.

134: Regarding Section P9, " Abnormal Lab Values", there is no longer a place to code that no lab work was done. Should this be coded as "8" (did not occur) to show that no lab work was done?

A: Enter "0" if there was no abnormal laboratory value noted or if no lab work was done. The "8" code is only for use in Section G.

135: Providers question why lab tests done during hospitalizations, prior to nursing home admissions, are not coded?

A: The MDS is designed to track activity primarily during the nursing home stay, which is used to calculate the resident's case-mix score.

136: Does the discharge potential and discharge plan (Section Q), suffice as the facility's discharge potential evaluation and discharge plan when the resident is not a candidate for discharge?

A: Section Q provides data on discharge potential. Depending on the resident's clinical status and circumstances, additional assessment to determine why the resident is not a candidate for discharge at this time and what plan can be implemented to improve discharge potential may be warranted.

Questions on Items in MDS Sections T and U

137: In the User's Manual, Section T, page 3-169, should "skip to item 3" be "skip to item 2", as noted on the MDS form?

A: Yes. Directions for Section T are correct on the MDS form. The User's Manual, page 3-169 is incorrect, and should read skip to item 2.

138: Regarding Section T, if PT or OT is performed outside the building, (i.e., the facility contracts with an outside vendor for therapy), is the therapy time captured on the MDS?

A: Yes, as long as the staff providing the therapy meet the qualifiers. See SOM Transmittal #272, p. R-64, "The therapy treatment may occur either inside or outside the facility."

139: Regarding MDS item T2b, at some time, will HCFA consider allowing a response for walking less than a minute?

A: This is a special case-mix question for purposes of evaluating residents' progress and making continuing treatment decisions. The reliability and usefulness of this group of items will be evaluated during the demonstration. The results of the evaluation will determine future use.

140: Regarding the second qualifier in item T2, "Physical therapy was ordered for the resident involving gait training (T2b)", is the reference to T2b correct?

A: No. In this area on the MDS form, T2b should be replaced with T1b. You may also wish to make the corresponding change in the User's Manual, on page 3-171. A corrected transitional copy of the form is included with this document and will be formally published by HCFA in a new State Operations Manual.

141: Are services coded in Section P also coded in Section T, or are the Sections mutually exclusive?

A: Code "ordered therapy" in both Sections P and T. The services are not mutually exclusive. Services (OT, PT, and Speech/Language Pathology) coded in Section P as provided should be included in the Section T estimation of ordered treatment time. An algorithm will be developed using items both in Sections P and T for use in a case-mix prospective payment system (PPS). This matter is currently under review by case-mix staff, with further clarification expected when therapy payment is added to the demonstration PPS rate.

142: For facilities using MDS Sections T and U, how often do these sections need to be completed?

A: Sections T and U are required to be completed, if included in the State's RAI, for all Full assessments (Initial Admission, Significant Change, and Annual Assessments). Some States may also require facilities to complete these sections for each Quarterly review. The reference for this question is found in the User's Manual on page 3-1 and page 3-168.

143: Regarding Section U: Are medications taken outside the facility (i.e., at a dialysis center) coded on the MDS?

A: Code only medications on the physician's orders at the facility. If a facility medication order is carried out off premises, (e.g., a dose administered at a dialysis center), that should be included in Section U. As part of communication of care, the facility should probably be aware (e.g., via report) of medication administered at the Dialysis Center without a physician's order on the resident's record at the facility, but there is no item on the MDS to capture this information. Otherwise, dialysis itself is captured in P1 ab.

144: Regarding Section U: Some NDC codes only have 8 digits, not 9. How does this affect entering the codes on the MDS?

A: There should be 9 digits in an NDC code. Check or re-check the source of an 8 digit NDC code to see if a zero might have been dropped. Begin recording the code in the leftmost box on the MDS. Many NDC codes begin with one or more zeros. The zeros are important. Do not omit them. Some NDC codes have 11 digits. In this case, disregard the last 2 digits, (they are package size codes). Refer to the User's Manual, page 3-184.

145: Regarding Section U: If the pharmacy sends a medication for a resident sometimes by brand name and sometimes by generic name (same medication and dose, different NDC), which NDC is coded on the MDS?

A: Code the NDC for the medication that was administered during the observation period. If during the observation period, both the generic and the brand name medications were administered (under the same order), it's up to the facility to decide which to code. For example, the facility may decide to routinely code the generic in such instances. Whatever the decision, it should be carried out consistently. Do not code both, as it would give the appearance of a double order of the same medication. Refer to the User's Manual, page 3-184.

146: Regarding Section U: How is NDC coded when a medication dosage involves 2 separate drug strengths (i.e., with different NDC codes)?

A: If a medication dosage involves 2 separate NDC codes, (e.g., for a physician's order of Coumadin 3 mg., the pharmacy sends (1) 1 mg and (1) 2 mg tablet), code only the NDC for the highest dose. Record the ordered dose, (in this example, 3 mg), in column 1 of Section U.

147: If an oral medication is crushed and administered via G-tube, is the route of administration coded as oral or enteral tube?

A: Use code 9, enteral tube. A note of caution: some oral medications should not be crushed.

148: How are stat doses recorded in Section U?

A: Code as 1 in the PRN column. Refer to the User's Manual page 3-183.

149: Sections T and U are required for Case Mix Demonstration States. Can other States elect to require Sections T and U for facilities in the State?

A: Yes. A request for an alternate instrument for the State should be sent to HCFA, indicating those sections or items the State desires to add to the core MDS (e.g., the State may create a Section S, specify the use of Sections T or U, and add items found in the State RAI to the Quarterly review).

150: Are OTC (over-the-counter) medications to be included in Section U?

A: Yes. All medications received by the resident, including OTC's, should be ordered by the physician and included in Section U. Refer to the NDC List of Common Drugs available from demonstration State project directors, and the World Wide Web site, under the supplemental directory for NDC -- 0296.ZIP.

151: Is it acceptable for a pharmacy printout of Section U information to be attached to the MDS in lieu of completing Section U? If so, what are the specifications for coding/review/signature?

A: A pharmacy printout is acceptable. It is the responsibility of the nurse doing the nursing portions of the MDS to review and verify or correct information, and sign the document. In verifying the accuracy of the report, pay particular attention to PRN medications given or not given in the last 7 days. Medication information needs to be included in data entry for States that submit MDS data electronically. Record specifications for Sections T and U have been developed and published by HCFA. The report itself should be included with the MDS in the resident's active record.

152: Regarding item U5, "PRN-n", are staff to code the total number of doses given in the last 7 days, or the number of days the PRN medication was given one or more times?

A: Record the total number of doses, in the last 7 days, that the PRN medication was given. The corresponding change should also be made in the instructions for #5, PRN-n, in Section U of the MDS form. Refer to the User's Manual, page 1-14.

153: In Section U, page 3-177 of the User's Manual (the last paragraph in the "Definitions" section) reads "...these persons must certify its accuracy with their signature in Section R5". Is this correct?

A: No. In this sentence "R5" <u>should be "R2"</u>.

154: The calculated number of minutes of therapy time in the example in the User's Manual on page 3-169 seems incorrect. Please clarify.

A: There was an error. The corrections in this response are in **bold** type. The last sentence of the first paragraph of the example <u>should read</u> "Within the 15 days from the resident's admission date (Thursday), the resident will receive 8 days of physical therapy (**480** minutes) and 4 days of speech therapy (240 minutes for a total of **720** minutes in the fifteen days." <u>Also</u>, the bolded sentences at the bottom of this page <u>should read</u> "Enter "8" in 1c..." and "Enter "720" in 1d".

155: Regarding Section T, in the example on page 3-170 of the User's Manual, the bolded sentences at the bottom begin with "Enter "6" in 2c" and "Enter "360" in 2d". Is this correct?

A: No. Corrections are in **bold** type. These sentences <u>should read</u> "Enter "6" in **1**c" and "Enter "360" in **1**d".

Questions Regarding RAPs, Triggers and RAP Documentation

156: Does HCFA have or provide software for facility validation of software trigger logic, (i.e., to check the trigger logic of software purchased from a vendor)?

A: Test files have been developed, which can be imported into the vendor's software, to ensure that triggers have been correctly programmed. This information is available on HCFA's World Wide Web site.

157: Please review the Briggs Trigger Legend format, in comparison to the Trigger Legend in the User's Manual, and comment.

A: The Briggs format is somewhat modified. There are several small changes that do not appear to change the triggering rules.

158: On the RAP Summary form, the directions are to describe complications and risk factors. What is the difference?

A: A risk factor increases the chance of having a negative outcome, or complication. For example, compromised bed mobility increases the risk of a pressure ulcer. In this example, compromised bed mobility is the specific risk factor, and the pressure ulcer is the complication. RAP guidelines may contain cues regarding risk factors and complications associated with the RAP condition.

159: Please give an example of a description of factors that must be considered in developing individualized care plan interventions, as requested on the RAP Summary form.

A: Refer to the RAI User's Manual, pages 4-19 through 4-34, for a detailed case example.

160: Are the RAPs a required component of the RAI process?

A: Yes. Additional assessment is required for each clinical condition (i.e., RAP that triggers). Any triggered RAP must be reviewed as part of the RAI Federal requirements governing the process.

161: On an annual assessment, if a resident triggers the same RAP(s) that triggered on the last comprehensive assessment, is it a requirement to complete the RAP protocol(s) again?

A: Because the same RAP may trigger for a different reason, or for the same reason at a different intensity, or for a reason based on an item not included in the trigger complex prior to MDS 2.0, it's a good idea to review the RAP again. Also keep in mind that even if the RAP triggers for the same reason, (no difference in MDS responses), there may be a new or changed related event identified during RAP review, that might call for a revision to the resident's plan of care. The interdisciplinary team determines when a problem or potential problem needs to be addressed in the Care Plan. Refer to User's Manual, page 4-16.

162: When will the new updated RAPs be available?

A: We anticipate the first release of revised RAPs in mid 1997.

163: Must all four factors described on page 4-5 of the User's Manual be present in RAP assessment documentation?

A: Generally yes. RAP assessment documentation should usually describe the nature of the condition and may include presence or lack of objective data and subjective complaints, complications and risk factors that affect the staff's decision to proceed to care planning, factors that must be considered in developing individualized care plan interventions, and need for referrals or further evaluation by appropriate health professionals. However, documentation should be tailored to the condition of the resident. Depending upon the resident's status, RAP documentation does not need to be highly detailed or exhaustive.

164: On the RAP Summary form, the signature at B3 of the "Person Completing the Care Planning Decision" is associated with the date at B4. Is the date at B4 the date when it is decided what to include in the care plan <u>or</u> the date the care plan is completed? And what is to be accomplished by the date at B2?

A: On the RAP Summary form, VB2 is the date that the RN Coordinator certifies that the RAPs have been completed. This date is considered the date of completion for the RAI (i.e., the date used to determine compliance with Federal time frames for assessment and the date that drives future due dates for when the RAI needs to be completed). VB4 is the date on which a staff member completes the care planning decision column, which is done after the care plan is completed. The User's Manual reference for this question is on page 4-18.

165: Is there a format, other than the RAP, to make brief, concise, written commentary to support MDS responses?

A: Documentation systems are largely a matter of facility policy and general practice standards, provided State and Federal requirements are met. Facilities have complete flexibility in determining how to organize their clinical records. Supportive documentation may be kept, for example, in additional assessment worksheets, flow charts, progress notes, the care plan, profile of care, attendance records, or in documentation from outside agencies, such as hospital discharge summaries, lab reports, consultant reports, etc. Facilities may also handwrite information related to MDS items directly on the MDS. The MDS itself is a primary source for describing resident function and in itself may be a primary location for information in the facility. Not every assessment item calls for supportive documentation.

166: On the RAP Summary form, question 4 says to "indicate whether a new care plan, care plan revision, or continuation of current care plan is necessary to address the problem(s) identified in your assessment". In completing column b on the form, how can the type (new, revision or continuation) be indicated?

A: It is not necessary to indicate the type. Simply check the column if the identified problem is addressed in the care plan.

167: Regarding the RAP Summary form: can the signature lines at VB1 and VB3 be signed by the same person?

A: Yes, provided that person actually completed both functions. It is not a requirement that the same person complete both.

168: Pertaining to documentation supporting RAP decision-making, and RAP Assessment documentation (as noted by location and date on the RAP Summary form), is there a requirement to write a RAP Summary note?

A: No. It is not necessary to summarize all information related to the RAP in one location. Documentation of the RAP findings and decision-making process may appear anywhere in the resident's record. It can be written in flowsheets, progress notes, in the care plan, in a RAP summary narrative, or on a RAP questionnaire, etc. However, the requirement is that you document information from the resident's assessment and staff's decision making about care. This should already be an easily accessible part of the medical record, in which case a summary note may be redundant. Ask yourself this question: "If I was a newly hired care giver for this resident, will I be able to find and understand the assessment and decision making process?" If the answer is yes, then you should feel secure that your documentation is complete. If you answer no, consider pulling together key information or "filling in the gaps" in a short note. No matter where the information is recorded, use the "Location and Date of RAP Assessment Documentation" column on the RAP Summary form to note where the RAP review and decision-making documentation can be found in the resident's record, and the date of the information. Also indicate in the column "Care Plan Decision" if the triggered problem is addressed in the care plan. Refer to the User's Manual, pages 4-10 through 4-18 for information concerning decision-making and documentation of the RAP findings, examples of assessment documentation using the RAP guidelines as a framework, and a Q & A section on frequently asked questions concerning RAP documentation.

169: In the example in the User's Manual on page 4-32, the Visual Function RAP is not checked as triggered, but in the example on page 4-27, D1 = 1. Should the Visual Function RAP have been checked in this example?

A: Yes. The Visual Function RAP triggered in this example, and should have been checked on the example RAP Summary form on page 4-32.

170: Why is the Visual Function RAP <u>not</u> triggered when D1 = 4? (Reference the User's Manual, page C-18).

A: Potential for visual improvement is not indicated if D1 = 4.

171: Please further explain the difference between ADL Rehabilitation triggers A and B.

A: Refer to the ADL RAP information in the User's Manual, beginning on page C-22. "The two MDS trigger categories (A and B) suggest the types of residents for whom special care interventions may be most important. Such residents may have either the need and potential to improve (Rehabilitation) or the need for services to prevent decline (Maintenance)". If a resident triggers the ADL RAP, they will trigger ADL category A, B or both, as determined by the responses to MDS items linked with each category.

If category A is triggered, a rehabilitation/restorative plan of care is suggested. If category B is triggered, a plan of care designed to maintain function/avoid complications is suggested.

For residents who trigger both ADL categories A and B, category B takes precedence in the RAP review. A resident whose MDS indicates B4 = 3 (No ability to make decisions) is not a rehabilitation candidate, but rather an individual whose care plan would be designed to maintain function.

172: Is the ADL Supplement required when completing the ADL RAP?

A: The ADL supplement was designed to be a worksheet that may be of benefit to facility staff, but it is not required. The ADL Supplement was designed to help care planners to focus on ADL areas that might be improved, and may be particularly useful where rehabilitation goals are envisioned. Part 1 of the Supplement also helps to identify risk factors. Refer to the User's Manual, page C-25.

173: Regarding the Urinary Incontinence and Indwelling Catheter RAP (see the User's Manual page C-31) under "Abnormal Lab Values", are the examples of "tests that should have been done within the last 60 days" requirements or guidelines?

A: Use the test results if the tests were done within 60 days. Tests older than 60 days have no utility. The lab tests mentioned in the RAP may be appropriate to include in evaluating causal factors associated with incontinence. They are guidelines and should only be ordered if appropriate based on the specific resident's condition. This is determined based on the clinical judgment of the physician/health care provider responsible for ordering the laboratory tests.

174: What is the clinical/social rationale for item F1d, "Establishes own goals", to trigger the Psychosocial Well-Being RAP?

A: F1d identifies an area of strength for the resident, which may have implications for planning care to maximize resident functioning and quality of life.

175: The Behavioral Symptoms RAP trigger "Resists Care", (E4eA) is noted in the User's Manual, but does not appear in the SOM Transmittal #272. Which is correct?

A: The User's Manual is correct. See page C-43, which indicates "Resists Care, E4eA = 1,2,3" triggers the Behavioral Symptoms RAP. This was inadvertently omitted from page R-118 of the State Operation Manual (SOM), Transmittal No. 272. Change pages will be issued in a future SOM and also published on HCFA's World Wide Web site for Version 2.0.

176: Why does the combination of items N1a and N2 trigger the Activities RAP?

A: This combination of MDS responses has predictive value suggestive of possible overstimulation in activities. Further assessment is therefore warranted. For example, the resident may be so involved in activities that he becomes too tired to eat. On the other hand, a high degree of involvement in activities may be used in a therapeutic manner by a resident who is depressed.

177: Regarding item N1, (see the User's Manual, page C-50), why is the Activities RAP triggered if just N1a, "morning" is checked?

A: Note that N1a alone does not trigger the RAP; rather, it must be present in combination with N2 = 0. Analysis of MDS data sets demonstrated that the "Morning", item N1a, was highly predictive (i.e., that this item was able to identify a high percentage of residents warranting additional assessment and care planning in this area). Triggers in Version 2.0 were studied to determine which triggers contributed most significantly to the identification of problems warranting care plans. Trigger items with low predictive validity were eliminated.

178: Please clarify the differences between Activities RAP triggers A and B, and how evaluation of the care plans would differ.

A: The Activities RAP triggers A and B point to very different treatment strategies. Trigger A identifies the need to evaluate expanded care/activity involvement when current involvement levels are low or new activity options are desired by the resident. Trigger B identifies the need to evaluate how to manage, and possibly reduce, activity patterns when involvement in activities is high and consistent throughout all waking hours of the day.

179: In Section O, Medications: Antidepressant (04b) and antianxiety (04c) medications both trigger the Falls RAP, but antipsychotic (04a) medication does not. However, when reviewing the Falls RAP, under the external risk factors, anti-psychotics are included. Should anti-psychotic medication trigger the Falls RAP?

A: Antipsychotic medications were not included in the Falls RAP for Version 2.0 because there is no predictive power gained by adding this group of medications.

180: Why does the Dental Care RAP trigger for residents who are edentulous and do not have or use dentures, and who receive daily mouth care?

A: For the Dental Care RAP, a follow-up review is required when one or more of the six conditions or oral hygiene problems are present. It is not self-evident that this three-item combination would not be appropriate for follow-up. For example, has there been a review for why dentures are not used? As noted in the User's Manual on page C-73, does the resident have the cognitive ability and motivation to wear dentures?

181: Are the Briggs modules by themselves sufficient evidence that the RAP protocols were used?

A: No. Briggs checklists may be used, but simply checking the boxes on the forms does not provide adequate, descriptive documentation regarding the resident's status as is required by the SOM transmittal #272. Analytic documentation should include risk/contributing factors, symptomatology, work-up and treatment, discussion of medication (if pertinent), and any resident/family involvement in the decision-making process. This may be written directly on the Briggs form if desired by the facility. See examples of RAP documentation in Chapter 4 of the User's Manual.

Questions Regarding Significant Change, Significant Correction of Prior Assessment, Signature and Dating, Admissions of Less than 14 Days and Other Policy Issues

Significant Change

182: Is it necessary to complete a new RAI (MDS and RAPs) if the resident develops only one problem listed under the definition of significant change?

A: Generally no, as the guidelines for significant change included in the User's Manual on page 2-9 and 2-10 indicate, a significant change reassessment is appropriate if there are either two or more areas of decline or two or more areas of improvement. If there is only one change, however, staff may still decide that the resident would benefit from a comprehensive reassessment.

183: Please address the following situation regarding significant change: A resident who has a 5% weight loss in 30 days and is not on a weight change plan begins to regain weight during the 14 day assessment period. Do we need to continue with the significant change, especially if the care plan already includes the problem, potential for weight loss?

A: First, a 5% weight loss in 30 days does not generally require a significant change reassessment in unless it is accompanied by a second area of decline from the list on page 2-9 of the User's Manual. Second, as the resident has started to regain the weight (and assuming the appropriate care plan interventions are in place), it is probably sufficient to continue to monitor the resident's nutritional status and weight gain, but delay conducting the comprehensive RAI reassessment unless it appears that the resident would benefit from an immediate reassessment and holistic revision of the care plan. Note that this answer assumes that the care plan has already been modified to actively treat the weight loss as opposed to continuing with the original problem, "potential for weight loss". This situation should be documented in the resident's clinical record along with the plan for subsequent monitoring. However, each resident situation is unique and the interdisciplinary treatment team must make the decision as to whether the resident will benefit from an RAI. Refer to the User's Manual, page 2-8.

184: Can the Assessment Reference Date (item A3a) be the date the resident was admitted to the facility?

A: Yes. The date at A3a can be any date from admission until the 14th day following admission. When the admission date is used as the Assessment Reference Date, the assessment is based on information from an observation period that precedes the resident's stay (e.g., hospital records). Refer to the User's Manual, page 3-29.

185: Is it a requirement to complete a Significant Change Assessment if, as a result of a hip fracture, the only change is in the ADL areas?

A: No, if the only change is in the area of ADLs. However, other changes (such as the resident receiving more support, incontinence or depression) often accompany a hip fracture. Given that the hip fracture often has a major effect on the resident and impacts on more than one area of the resident's health status, a significant change reassessment is often warranted. Refer to the User's Manual, pages 2-8 through 2-12 for guidelines concerning Significant Change.

186: Do staff have 14 days to decide if changes in the resident's status constitute a Significant Change? Once it is decided that a Significant Change occurred, do staff have 14 days to complete the Significant Change Assessment?

A: A Significant Change Assessment is not required in a case where the resident's condition is expected to return to baseline within a short period of time, such as one to two weeks. If the condition does not return to baseline, the assessment should be completed as soon as needed to provide appropriate care to the individual, but in no case less than 14 days after the determination was made that the Significant Change occurred. Refer to pages 2-8 through 2-12 of the User's Manual for guidelines concerning Significant Change.

187: Some providers are interpreting that Significant Change Assessments require two or more areas (as listed in the User's Manual) of decline before a new full assessment is to be done. For example, this interpretation would mean that a resident would require both a significant weight change and development of a pressure ulcer before a new assessment is required. The State Agency interpretation is that any change that impacts two or more areas of a resident's health status would trigger a new MDS. A pressure sore, for example, impacts multiple areas of health status: skin condition, nutrition/hydration, special treatments, more aggressive nursing care, mobility, psychosocial well being, etc. Which interpretation is correct?

A: The provider's interpretation is correct. A Significant Change assessment is appropriate if there is a consistent pattern of changes in two or more areas of decline or two or more areas of improvement from the MDS item categories listed on pages 2-9 and 2-10 of the User's Manual. These categories were identified by an empirical analysis of MDS data sets. A "Significant change" is defined as a major change in the resident's status that:

1. Is not self-limiting
2. Impacts on more than one area of the resident's health status; and
3. Requires interdisciplinary review or revision of the care plan.

Please note per the User's Manual that the lists of MDS item categories for Significant Change Assessment are not exhaustive. In fact, there may be other areas of decline or improvement that have such a profound impact on the resident and his or her needs for care that they would also appear to warrant a comprehensive reassessment.

188: If a resident develops a Stage II Pressure Ulcer and it heals in 10 days, is this a significant change?

A: Generally no. The facility will need to note the resident's condition in the clinical record and implement necessary clinical interventions. However, if the change in the resident is self-limiting and improves within two weeks, a significant change RAI would not be necessary. In this case, care plan changes such as interventions to prevent the recurrence of a pressure ulcer would probably be appropriate. Review the conditions of significant change on pages 2-8 through 2-12 of the User's Manual.

189: Does an unplanned weight loss of 5% in 30 days trigger a Significant Change Assessment, if that is the only change?

A: Generally no, although it would be expected that the facility would note the resident's condition in the clinical record and implement necessary clinical interventions. In this case, a discreet assessment in the area of nutritional status may provide evidence of the extent of the problem, as well as information on which to base appropriate changes in the resident's care plan that will result in weight gain. However, if the problem persists or worsens, a comprehensive RAI reassessment may be clinically indicated. Review the criteria for significant change on pages 2-8 through 2-12 of the User's Manual.

190: If a resident has one area of decline <u>and</u> one area of improvement, do you need to complete a Significant Change Assessment?

A: No, a Significant Change Assessment is appropriate if there is a consistent pattern of changes in <u>two</u> or more areas of decline or two or more areas of improvement.

191: Is a Significant Change Assessment required when the only change in status is a weight loss of more than 10%? And in 3 months, at the time of the next scheduled assessment, if the resident did not re-gain or still has the 10% weight loss, is a second Significant Change Assessment required?

A: The answer is "No" for both questions, although the facility would be expected to assess and care plan for the weight loss, if it was not planned. If the weight loss continued on the subsequent assessment, it would probably be appropriate for the facility to indicate why the desired change had not occurred and to modify the existing care plan. For detailed information concerning guidelines for Significant Change, refer to the User's Manual, pages 2-8 through 2-12.

192: Are Quarterly assessments required when someone has had a Significant Change within the quarter?

A: In most States, a Significant Change in Status Assessment re-starts the assessment calendar for the individual resident. The next assessment due, (provided there has not been another Significant Change) is a Quarterly assessment conducted within 3 months of the Significant Change. Refer to the User's Manual, page 3-11, paragraph 5. If a Significant Change in Status is identified in the process of completing a Quarterly Assessment, code the assessment "3", Significant Change in Status, and complete a full assessment. Do not code this as a Quarterly review.

Please check with your State if you are unsure. For payment system purposes, in some States, a Significant Change assessment does not re-start the assessment calendar, or change the date the next Quarterly Assessment would be due.

Significant Correction of Prior Assessment

193: How is it handled when an MDS has been scored by two different staff members from one assessment to the next, and due to a variance in interpreting how to score the assessment, it looks like a Significant Change has occurred, when it has not.

A: Complete a Significant Correction of Prior Assessment, (A8a=4). Reassess the resident by completing a new MDS and RAP Summary form, and revise the care plan if appropriate. Adherence to item definitions and instructions, as well as the requirements for completion of the assessment (e.g., interview direct care staff across all 3 shifts), should result in high rates of inter-rater reliability for MDS items. Variance in staff scoring the same resident may indicate a need for staff education on how to complete the MDS. Refer to the User's Manual, page 3-11.

194: If you find the last full assessment was wrong during the quarterly review, do you code quarterly review or significant change?

A: Code Section AA8 "S" for quarterly review on the Basic Assessment Tracking form which is completed along with the Quarterly Review assessment. However, if the quarterly review is not yet complete and staff decide to conduct a full reassessment, the quarterly review need not be completed. If inaccuracies are identified in the last full assessment, determine if those inaccuracies are such that a comprehensive reassessment is appropriate. Refer to the User's Manual, pages 2-26 and 2-27 for guidelines concerning when a Significant Correction Assessment is appropriate. If facility staff determine that a reassessment is necessary, initiate a full assessment and code the full assessment form Section A, item 8 (Reasons for Assessment) as a "4", significant correction of prior full assessment. This signifies that the resident's status is significantly different from the previous assessment as opposed to the resident having experienced a significant change in status. This process will identify your initiation of the required quarterly review assessment and your identification of significant inaccuracies requiring a reassessment.

195: Can a Significant Correction of Prior Assessment be performed on a Quarterly review, or only on a Full Assessment?

A: A Significant Correction of Prior Assessment may be necessary for a Quarterly Review assessment and a new Reason for Assessment (record type) has been created to allow for this. In the near future, HCFA will publish a revised MDS form and record specifications as well as information regarding the anticipated effective date. It will be available to software vendors on HCFA's World Wide Web site. On the revised form, Items AA8a4 and A8a4 will be relabeled "Significant correction of prior full assessment," and new Items, AA8a10 and A8a10 will be added, and labeled "Significant correction of prior Quarterly assessment." Change pages to the SOM will also be published. The change will not be formally required until the SOM is re-written.

Signature and Dating

196: Is it a requirement that the data entry person sign the MDS?

A: A specific MDS package may identify the MDS data entry person, but there is no HCFA requirement to do so. The MDS data record submitted to the State does not include such information.

197: May the facility staff use a signature stamp on the forms?

A: The use of signature stamps is allowed. The State Operation Manual Transmittal No. 274, survey protocol, F386, has the following guidance to surveyors on this topic: "When rubber stamp signatures are authorized by the facility's management, the individual whose signature the stamp represents shall place in the administrative offices of the facility a signed statement to the effect that he/she is the only one who has the rubber stamp and uses it. A list of computer codes and written signatures must be readily available and maintained under adequate supervision." The State and facility may have additional policies or regulations that apply.

198: A facility utilizes a signature sign-in form for conferences where care planning and MDS forms are completed. May this type of signature and date form replace the signature and date on the MDS 2.0 form?

A: The text of the regulation CFR 42 483.20(c)(1)(ii) states that "Each assessment must be conducted or coordinated by a registered nurse who **signs** and certifies the completion of the assessment". Further, CFR 42 483.20(c)(2) states that "Each individual who completes a portion of the assessment must **sign** and certify the accuracy of that portion of the assessment."

For a facility to use a signature sign-in form, the facility would need to have a written policy that explains how the sign-in process and format are used. It would have to provide attestation by the registered nurse regarding the completion of the assessment, and for each individual, who must certify the accuracy of the portion of the assessment that they completed. The State may have additional regulations that apply.

199: Is it true that there can be no more than 7 days between the date at A3a and the date at R2?

A: No. Note that A3a and R2 are independent of each other. A3a can be as early as the day of admission (i.e., it sets the endpoint of a common period of observation). The period of observation may be over long before the "forms" are actually completed, which is signified by the date R2b.

200: Please clarify the dating conventions for the Assessment Reference Date (A3a), the MDS Assessment Completion Date (R2), and the dates on the RAP Summary form at VB2 and VB4.

A: The Assessment Reference Date (A3a), signifies the end of the observation period for all assessment items. For example, for an MDS item with a 7-day period of observation, assessment information is collected for 7 days prior to and ending at the date at A3a; for a 14 day assessment item, the observation period is the 14 days prior to and ending at the date at A3a. A3a is the common date for which all observation periods end.

The Assessment Reference Date can be no later than 14 days after admission. A3a and R2 are independent of each other. The period of time between A3a and R2 is the time during which staff actually complete the MDS form. This activity is completed by the date at R2, which can be no later than 14 days after admission. It is allowable under the statute for the Assessment Reference Date (A3a) to be the same as the MDS Assessment Completion Date (R2). It may be more practical, although it is not a federal requirement, to leave some time between the dates at A3a and R2.

It would not make sense for the dates at R2 to precede the date at A3a, as this would indicate that the MDS form was completed before the observation period has ended. In this case, the MDS form would have been completed before all observations were to have been completed. Remember that the date at R2b is the date on which the RN Coordinator is certifying the MDS as being complete, which is a statutory responsibility. Signatures and dates at R2c-h indicate that other staff members have accurately completed particular sections of the MDS. It makes sense, therefore, that the date at R2b should be no earlier than the latest date at R2c-h. In any event, dates at R2b-h can be no later than 14 days after admission. RAP review must be complete no later than 14 days following admission. If the MDS is completed (dated at R2b) earlier than the 14th day after admission, staff still have until the 14th day to complete the RAP portion of the assessment.

The date at VB2 on the RAP Summary form indicates that the RN Coordinator is certifying that the RAP review is completed. The date at VB2 can be no later than the 14th day after admission. The date at VB2 signifies completion of the RAI and can be used to determine the due dates of subsequent assessments.

The date at VB4 is the date that the care planning information required in column (b) of the RAP Summary form is completed. This column provides information on final care planning decisions for all RAP clinical conditions and may be completed by any professional staff member (i.e., it does not need to be completed by the RN Coordinator). It is completed after the interdisciplinary team has met and developed or revised the resident's care plan, incorporating the findings from that particular assessment. The date at VB4 can be no later than 7 days after the date at VB2, as the care plan must be completed within 7 days of RAI (MDS and RAPs) completion per Federal regulation. Refer to the User's Manual, pages 2-17 & 18, 2-28 & 29, and 3-29.

201: Is 12:00 midnight, at the end of the Assessment Reference Date (the date at A3), the last of the observation period? Or is 12:00 midnight, at the beginning of the Assessment Reference Date, the last of the observation period?

A: Observe across all three shifts, (24 hours per day) for the full observation period, (i.e.,: 7 days, 14 days, etc... as determined by the observation time periods noted at the MDS item). Allow for the full observation period to be sure to capture any events occurring in the appropriate time frame. HCFA has no requirement that the observation "clock" start or end at midnight.

202: Is it necessary to have the dietitian sign the MDS if they did not complete any portion?

A: No. The reference for this response is page 2-17 of the User's Manual, under "Certifying Accuracy and Completeness". Each individual team member who completes a portion of the assessment must sign and certify its accuracy. Team members should not sign the MDS if they did not complete any portion.

203: When the RN Coordinator completes sections of the MDS, does the Coordinator need to indicate those sections and sign under "other signatures" in Section R, or can it be assumed that the RN Coordinator who signs at R2a and dates R2b is the person who completed any sections not signed for by anyone else?

A: It is assumed that the RN Coordinator completed any portions of the MDS that have not been designated by other staff. The RN Coordinator must sign at ADa and R2. The RN Coordinator signs at ADa when the Face Sheet portion is complete, and signs at R2a to certify that the MDS is complete. Refer to the User's Manual, page 3-167. Federal regulations at 42 CFR 483.20 (c)(1) and (2) require each individual who completes a portion of the assessment to sign and certify its accuracy. If the RN Coordinator also completed sections of the MDS, signature at R2a is sufficient. If the RN completing the MDS sections is not the Coordinator, that RN signs under R2c-h, and the Coordinator signs at R2a.

204: Please confirm that the day of admission counts as day 0, not as day 1. There are conflicting examples in the User's Manual.

A: The day of admission is counted as day 0 under Federal policy. The example shown on page 2-6 is clear and consistent with Federal interpretation of the OBRA '87 requirement. The example on page 3-30 is incorrect. In this example, day 7 following an admission on 8/20/94 would be 8/27/94, and day 14 would be 9/3/94.

Counting the day of admission as day 0 allows the maximum flexibility in terms of time to complete the RAI. For case-mix/reimbursement purposes, however, some States require that the day of admission be counted as day 1.

Admissions of less than 14 Days

205: If a resident enters the facility and does not stay at least 7 days, is it necessary to begin an MDS?

A: No. The MDS/RAI does not need to be completed, either in part or in entirety, unless the resident has been in the facility 14 days or longer. Refer to the User's Manual, page 2-4.

206: If an individual is hospitalized for several days during the initial 14 days of the NF stay, is the MDS still due on day 14, or when would it be due? For example, if the resident is hospitalized day 2 thru day 12, and returns on day 13.

A: The facility would have 14 days after "readmission" to the facility to complete the RAI. Refer to the User's Manual, page 2-7.

207: What subset of information must be completed on short-term respite admissions, when a resident expires or is discharged prior to day 14?

A: Currently, there is no required subset of information. Once HCFA's automation requirements are effective, facilities will be required to complete the Discharge Tracking form. See page 3-2 of the User's Manual.

208: Must an MDS be completed for a respite stay of less than 14 days?

A: No. Keep in mind, however, that there should be a process in place to identify the resident's needs and to initiate a plan of care to meet those needs upon or shortly after admission. Refer to the User's Manual, page 2-6.

209: If a resident is discharged on the 14th day, would the facility still be required to complete the entire MDS?

A: No. Refer to the User's Manual, page 2-6. Keep in mind, however, that evidence of assessment and care planning to meet the resident's needs should be in place, and have been initiated on or shortly after admission. Once computerization requirements are effective, facilities will be required to complete a discharge tracking form for all residents admitted to the facility regardless of length of stay.

Other Policy Issues

210: What is the date of HCFA's final version of the MDS 2.0?

A: The current version is dated 10/18/94N. However, HCFA has a commitment to continue to refine the instrument to reflect state-of-the-art practice standards and assessment methodologies, and accommodate the changing needs of the nursing home population. In that regard, there will not be a "final" version. The transitional MDS that contains minor changes as noted in this document (and on the World Wide Web site) will be dated 10/18/94H. Information regarding the anticipated effective date of 10/18/94H is pending.

211: Is there a requirement to have additional assessments in place that substantiate information documented on the MDS?

A: No. From a Federal perspective, the MDS is considered a primary source document, as it is part of the clinical record. However, some States require documentation that validates MDS coding as the MDS is used to derive payment. A different but related question is whether the MDS and RAPs alone provide a comprehensive assessment as is required by Federal regulations. Neither the MDS or RAPs covers every conceivable area that may be pertinent to a resident's needs and care. Such areas must nevertheless be addressed in the resident's clinical record and on the care plan. There is not a Federal requirement specifying the format of such documentation, only that it be a part of the resident's clinical record. Such information can be maintained, for example, in progress notes, or on flow sheets. Documentation systems and the order and format of information in the clinical record is generally a matter of facility policy. Refer to the User's Manual Section 4.9, pages 4-18 through 4-23.

212: Is it necessary to reassess on an annual basis the need for a feeding tube for patients who require this intervention? Also, would a goal for a tube fed resident be to eventually have them back on a solid diet?

A: The answer to both questions is yes. If the Feeding Tube RAP is triggered, reassessment is required at least yearly (i.e., with each annual assessment) and perhaps more frequently, if clinically warranted. Refer to the RAP, beginning on page C-62 of the User's Manual and note that restoration to normal feeding should remain the goal throughout the treatment program. Comprehensive reassessment and evaluation allows the interdisciplinary treatment team to determine if this is an achievable goal. For some residents, this may not be realistic. For others, it might be a suitable long-term goal, where an intermittent short term goal, (i.e., to tolerate thickened fluids p.o.) might be more appropriate. Note the guidance provided on page 4-16 of the User's Manual (regarding the extent of reassessment and documentation required for subsequent reassessments after a comprehensive evaluation (i.e., for a neurological swallowing deficit) has been conducted.

213: Is there a requirement to document on the resident's plan of care the number of bed days used?

A: No. There is not a Federal requirement that bed days be documented on the plan of care. Check with your State regarding whether there is an existing State code, rule or regulation.

214: When does the 15 month requirement for MDS 2.0 record keeping start? Do we have to keep 15 month's worth of records on computer files?

A: Per the State Operations Manual (SOM) Transmittal #272, with the implementation of Version 2.0, facilities are required to have 15 months of assessment data in the resident's active clinical record. This includes all MDS forms, RAP Summary forms and Quarterly Assessment forms as required during the previous 15 month period. For the 15 months immediately following MDS 2.0 implementation, facilities will have a combination of MDS 2.0 and MDS version 1 information in the active records. Refer to the User's Manual, page 2-18. Note that this time period was decreased from the 24-month period required by SOM Transmittal #241.

RAI information completed 15 months ago or longer may be thinned from the active record and stored in the medical records department, provided the information is easily retrievable if requested by clinical staff or State Agency surveyors. The **exception** is that Face Sheet information (Section AB, AC, and AD) must be maintained in the active record until the resident is permanently discharged. If the resident returns to the facility following a discharge (i.e., a situation in which the record has been closed), the facility should copy the original and place it in the resident's new record. The above also applies to facilities that maintain an electronic clinical record, **except** that a hard copy of the RAI need not be maintained if the entire clinical record is stored electronically, and the additional conditions on page 2-19 of the User's Manual are met.

215: Is it required that staff members write on the Interdisciplinary Care Plan when goals are met and approaches are changed, if the changes are already documented in progress notes?

A: Yes, the care plan should be revised on an on-going basis to reflect changes in the resident and the care the resident is receiving. The care plan is an interdisciplinary communication tool. Review 42 CFR 483.20 (d), Comprehensive Care Plans. There is a Federal requirement that the comprehensive care plan include measurable objectives and time frames, and must describe the services that are to be furnished to attain or maintain the resident's highest practicable physical, mental, and psychosocial well-being. The care plan must be periodically reviewed and revised, and the services provided or arranged must be in accordance with each resident's written plan of care. Refer to the RAI User's Manual, pages 2-27 through 29 regarding the linkage of MDS and RAPs to the formulation of the care plan, and refer to the SOM Transmittal # 274, (F Tag 279), "The results of the assessment are used to develop, review and revise the resident's comprehensive plan of care".

216: How long do facilities have to update all residents to the MDS 2.0 after the January 1, 1996 implementation date? Will the 2.0 assessment be phased in according to the resident's annual assessment schedule?

A: As of the State's implementation date, the next MDS due for each resident, regardless of reason for assessment, (and whether it is a Quarterly or Full assessment), is done using the appropriate MDS 2.0 form. In this manner, all residents in the facility will have a Quarterly or Full assessment using Version 2.0 within 3 months of the implementation date. All subsequent assessments are also done using the MDS 2.0 form. For Quarterly Assessments, be sure to use the Quarterly Assessment form specified by your State. State RAIs may also include Sections S, T and U. Note: Not all States implemented Version 2.0 as of January 1, 1996. If you have questions, check with your State.

217: Is it okay for a resident or family member to complete sections of the MDS?

A: No. Refer to the User's Manual, page 2-16. Facility staff are required to include the resident and family in the assessment and care planning process, but this means that they are key sources of information for assessment data, not that the resident or family should be involved in completing the "forms" themselves. It is the facility's responsibility to complete the assessment and ensure that all participants in the assessment process have the requisite knowledge to complete an accurate and comprehensive assessment. A facility may assign responsibility for completing the RAI to a number of qualified staff members who are generally licensed professionals. The MDS was developed to be completed by professional staff members. It was not designed for self-reporting of information.

218: While the User's Manual states that it is not "required to assess a resident if he/she is readmitted" (page 2-12), can the facility elect to complete a full comprehensive RAI on any readmission, even if it is after a temporary absence?

A: Certainly, and many facilities have adopted such policy. However, it is not a Federal requirement.

219. After receiving approval from HCFA for the MDS instrument or alternate instrument specified by the State, some States are making further additions or changes to the instrument. Please advise.

A: HCFA is aware of this situation and is in the process of following up with individual States. Per the SOM Transmittal #272, all States are required to notify HCFA of their intent to adopt HCFA's RAI or request approval of an alternate instrument. States are then required to implement the instrument that HCFA has approved for use by all long term care facilities within the State. States may not subsequently change the State RAI unless approval has been granted in writing by HCFA.

Questions on MDS Quarterly

220: Regarding item A4a of the Quarterly and Annual Assessment, if the resident has not been hospitalized, is the item left blank?

A: Yes. For both the Full and Quarterly Assessments, if the resident has not been hospitalized in the past 90 days, leave this item blank. The User's Manual reference for this question is on page 3-31.

221: On the Quarterly Assessment, how do you set the date at item A3?

A:The date is set by the RN Coordinator in the same way as for the admission and annual assessments. This Assessment Reference Date is the last day of resident observation for the current quarterly assessment. This date sets the designated endpoint of the observation period, and all MDS items refer back in time from this point. Refer to the User's Manual, page 3-29. There is not a specific requirement for the date at A3 for a Quarterly Assessment. Data specifications on timing edits are based on the date at R2b.

A Quarterly Assessment must be completed in each 3 month period, in-between Full Assessments (i.e., annual or significant change). Refer to User's Manual, page 2-13.

222: For a resident whose annual review comes due in the middle of 1996, which Quarterly Assessment form is to be used?

A: Regardless of whether the last full assessment was completed using version 2.0, use the Quarterly Assessment Form for Version 2.0 for all quarterly reviews completed after the State's version 2.0 implementation date. For most States, this was January 1, 1996. Check with your State to find out whether the standard or the expanded Quarterly Assessment form was specified for use by the facilities in the State.

223: On page B-14, Section I1., Diseases: z., quadriplegia is out of order on the RUG III Quarterly Assessment Form. In Section I3b, the decimal point is missing on the ICD-9 code.

A: These items are noted and changes will be released on the World Wide Web site soon. A copy of the transitional MDS form is included with this document.

224: When completing a Quarterly Assessment, what are the requirements regarding holding a care conference?

A: The Quarterly MDS offers an opportunity to review the resident's status and progress but there are no Federal requirements that mandate the interdisciplinary team have a face-to-face meeting for this purpose. The facility determines how to approach updating the care plan, as indicated, based on the current assessment. Refer to the User's Manual, page 2-13 for the intent of the statement "based on the Quarterly Assessment, the resident's care plan is revised if necessary".

225: Is RAP Summary documentation required for Quarterly Assessments?

A: RAP review is only required for full assessments. Refer to the User's Manual, pages 4-16 through 4-18, for guidelines concerning RAP documentation. Certain vendor's MDS forms label trigger items on the form. For a Quarterly Assessment, this should not be construed as a requirement to complete RAPs.

226: In completing a Quarterly Assessment, is it required to complete a "full, comprehensive assessment", including RAPs and triggers, or just the subset of MDS items on the Quarterly assessment?

A: Though the Quarterly assessment requirement varies from State to State, HCFA has specified a subset of key MDS items that make up the Quarterly Review under Federal requirements. The Quarterly Review is used to track the resident's status between comprehensive assessments, and to ensure monitoring of critical indicators of the gradual onset of significant changes in the resident's status.

Each State's RAI includes HCFA's Quarterly Review items at a minimum. However, States may add items from the core MDS, their Section S, or Sections T or U. They may even require the "MDS" portion of their RAI (i.e., everything except the RAPs) be completed each quarter. One popular alternative, particularly for States that are using the MDS to support payment systems, is HCFA's optional RUG III Quarterly Review form, found on pages B-13 through B-15 of the User's Manual. If you are unsure, check with your State RAI Coordinator (listed in Appendix A of the User's Manual) to determine what is required in your State.

227: Does a request need to be made to HCFA to use the optional 3 page Quarterly?

A: Yes. The State determines the need to add items to the MDS or Quarterly Review form and requests approval from HCFA to specify an alternate instrument for use by all facilities in the State.

228: If the State specifies the standard Quarterly instrument, can a facility opt to use the expanded (RUG III) version? (Note: the SOM refers to the standard quarterly and calls for using all and only that information).

A: A facility is required to use whatever Quarterly Review instrument has been specified by their State. However, facilities have the prerogative of adding items to the core MDS or Quarterly Review, provided that they are capable of separating this information and reproducing the State-specified RAI. Contact your State's RAI Coordinator (listed in Appendix A of the User's Manual) if you have questions.

MDS Automation

229: Are facilities required to complete the Basic Assessment Tracking Form prior to implementation of the Data Automation Requirement?

A: Yes, a copy of the Basic Assessment Tracking form must accompany each Full or Quarterly Assessment that is completed. Refer to page 3-1 of the User's Manual.

230: Section AA, item 8 on the Basic Assessment Tracking form, Section A, item 8 on the Full assessment, and Section AA, item 8 on the Reentry Tracking form all refer to the same 2 digit field on HCFA's MDS 2.0 record layout/data dictionary. Also, the record specifications indicate all assessment items except those on the Reentry Tracking form [Section AA, items 1-9 and Section A, items 4a, 4b (this is not on the full form), and 6] are blank on record type R (Reentry).

Since all Reason for Assessment references apply to the same 2 digit field, it is impossible to enter both an "09" and an "03" as the reason for assessment in the transmission record. Also, the processing of record type R's will only look to the limited number of responses contained on the Reentry Tracking form.

A: Once a resident is "discharged" from the system (i.e., a Discharge Tracking form is completed, signified by use of "06", "07", or "08" as the reason for the assessment), a Reentry Tracking form must be completed on the resident's "reentry" to the facility. If a significant change in status has occurred, the facility then must complete a comprehensive assessment (i.e., the MDS and RAPs). In this case "03" is entered as the Reason for the Assessment. Each "assessment" process requires a separate "transaction", which is indicated by the corresponding record type code.

231: Do facilities entering MDS data into a computer have 7 days from MDS completion (date at R2b) to make changes/corrections as are necessary to pass the edit process?

A: It's more advantageous for facilities to use 7 days from the date at VB2. Technically, the correct date to use to calculate when the electronic record must be locked is VB2. See the User's Manual pages 2-25 and 2-26.

232: Would the date at R2b plus 7 days be the most logical date to trigger an automatic lock? Would this also apply to Quarterly MDS's?

A: The date to trigger an automatic lock is seven days after VB2 for all full assessments (i.e., those for which RAPs are required). Use R2b to calculate the automatic lock date for all Quarterly assessments.

233: Regarding Chapter 2-18, "Electronic vs: Clinical Record", does this pertain to "paperless" facilities? If a facility is not completely automated and doesn't have the entire clinical record stored in the computer, do they have to have a paper MDS? RAI? If the MDS alone is in the computer, is a hard copy required?

A: The answer to each of the questions is yes. Refer to the User's Manual, pages 2-18 and 2-19.

234: The RAI Manual indicates that a check mark must be used in certain fields. HCFA's Web site indicates that a capital X may be used in lieu of the check mark when processing the MDS in the computer. Is the capital X still an acceptable symbol for the check mark?

A: Yes.

235: When will all States be required to submit MDS data electronically? (When will HCFA's ADP requirement be in effect?)

A: HCFA anticipates the MDS automation requirements will become effective in mid 1997, after publication of final regulations related to the RAI.

236: Will HCFA place vendors on mailing lists for immediate notification regarding RAI updates/information?

A: Due to the large number of software vendors and limited internal resources, HCFA is unable to maintain a mailing list or mail information directly to software vendors. To provide vendors with the most up-to-date information in a timely manner, HCFA established an MDS 2.0 World Wide Web site at the University of Wisconsin. The e-mail address for the World Wide Web primary information source is:

http://linear.chsra.wisc.edu/mds_info.htm

and the Internet e-mail account for technical questions is:

www.chsra.wisc.edu/mds_info.htm

237: Is the CFR information available on-line for outside queries?

A: The Code of Federal Regulations is available on CD ROM.

238: Is there an acuity tool available that matches the MDS 2.0?

A: A case-mix classification system, RUGs III, is available and is being used by many States to support Medicaid payment systems. It is also being evaluated for potential use as a prospective payment system for Medicare. It is available on HCFA's World Wide Web site.

239: Nurses are using MDS data to do Quality Assurance Studies. They put data into the computer on a weekly basis, without locking it in. Can they do this?

A: Provided it doesn't interfere with State and Federal requirements pertaining to MDS implementation and electronic submission. Not all vendors provide this capability. Refer to HCFA's policy on Expectations for Facility Automation.

240: Will HCFA be recommending software that meets HCFA specifications?

A: HCFA's policy on Expectations for Facility Automation addresses what function MDS software programs will have to perform. However, HCFA cannot recommend specific software products or give guidance to the industry on whether specific products meet the HCFA specifications.

241: What is the requirement for the arrangement of the MDS when printed from a computer?

A: Basically, it should be formatted like the HCFA MDS. Refer to the SOM Transmittal #272, 4145.5, Variations in Formatting the State-Specified RAI. "States are encouraged to permit some flexibility in form design (for example: print type, color, shading, or integrated triggers) or through use of a computer-generated printout of the RAI. HCFA's approval is not required for you to permit such formatting variations. However, you must assure that any RAI form or printout in the resident's record accurately and completely represents your RAI as approved by HCFA, in accordance with 42 CFR 483.20 (b). That is, it includes all and only the items on your instrument with the exact wording and in the same sequence". If a manually completed MDS form is not placed in the clinical record for a resident, then a computer printout of the MDS must either be produced and placed in the clinical record or must be produced on demand (i.e., of a staff member or State Agency surveyor). This printout must be a replica of the paper MDS form, with all items in similar positions and on the same pages as the paper form.

242: If the MDS is computerized, will the new Quarterly Assessment information update the old MDS, so that when the new MDS is run, it will automatically be updated?

A: Each individual record must be "locked" per HCFA's policy on Expectations for Facility Automation. Locked records cannot automatically be copied to form the basis for subsequent assessments without the assessor verifying that each individual item response is accurate for the new assessment record.

243: For MDS data entered into a computer real-time by the assessor, is there a requirement for an additional item-by-item entry into the computer to confirm the accuracy of each response?

A: When completed real-time, the Assessor is responsible for reviewing each item for each required assessment, discharge or reentry. How this is accomplished is a matter of facility policy. Physical confirmation is not required. Visual review is adequate.

Questions Regarding the RAI Process and Survey

244: Is it possible to be on a medication, e.g., a diuretic or pain medication, without a diagnosis?

A: A resident should not be on a drug without a valid reason, e.g., symptomatology that justifies the use of the drug. Refer to the CFR 483.25 (l) (1) regarding "Unnecessary Drugs - General". Each resident's drug regimen must be free from unnecessary drugs. An unnecessary drug is defined as a drug used without adequate indications for its use. Guidance to Surveyors calls for surveyors to allow the facility the opportunity to provide a rationale for the use of the drug(s), and the facility may not justify the use of a drug solely on the basis of a doctor's order. F tag 329 includes the following note: "The unnecessary drug criterion of "adequate indications for use" does not simply mean that the physician's order must include a reason for using the drug (although such order writing is encouraged). It means that the resident lacks a valid clinical reason for use of the drug as evidenced by the survey team's evaluation of some, but not necessarily all, of the following: resident assessment, plan of care, reports of significant change, progress notes, laboratory reports, professional consults, drug orders, observation and interview of the resident, and other information.

245: A particular state agency is mandating that only narrative documentation can be used for RAP review documentation, and is giving deficiencies if any other format is used. Please comment.

A: The guidelines found in the SOM Transmittal #272 address the content, but not the format of RAP review documentation. Indeed, in Chapter 4 of the User's Manual, it is clear from both the text and documentation examples that facilities have a great deal of flexibility in how this documentation is done. Citing facilities for failing to use a narrative format cannot be supported under the Federal requirements. Rather, HCFA provides guidance on key documentation issues as outlined in SOM #272, and in the examples of appropriate documentation in Chapter 4 of the User's Manual. If it is not clear that a facility's documentation provides this information, surveyors should ask facility staff to provide such evidence.

246: Now that the enforcement regulation refers to each resident, if assessment or RAP documentation information is inadequate, is it appropriate to cite 272 even if there is only an occurrence for one individual?

A: It's difficult to provide precise guidance on what constitutes an inadequate assessment. Generally speaking, this decision should be based on whether the resident received appropriate care to meet his medical, nursing, mental and psychosocial needs that are identified in the comprehensive assessment. As stated in the regulations at CFR 483.20, the comprehensive assessment provides the foundation for the development of a care plan that meets these needs. If the facility did not accurately identify and care plan for the resident's needs because of an inadequate assessment, this could be cited as a deficiency.

247: Regarding the balance test, item G3, sometimes residents are unwilling to participate, despite instruction and support. Will surveyors accept that the resident declined to participate? Should staff document extensively that the resident declined to participate?

A: In approaching a resident for a balance test, staff should provide privacy and an explanation. The resident may, of course, decline the test but the facility should attempt to determine why the resident is refusing. Since this would affect the MDS response, it seems worthy of a short notation which may be written directly on the MDS form. Surveyors will accept individual residents declining to participate, but will probably be suspicious if an untoward number of residents decline participation in this test.

248: Are Activity Department staff required to write monthly or quarterly progress notes?

A: There is a Federal requirement for progress notes, but there is not a Federal regulation regarding the frequency of progress notes for any discipline. Refer to CFR 483.75 (l) (1), Clinical Records, which requires the facility to maintain clinical records on each resident in accordance with accepted professional standards and practices that are (i) complete, (ii) accurately documented, (iii) readily accessible, and (iv) systematically organized. See also F Tag 514. As a practical matter, progress notes should facilitate interdisciplinary team communication and coordination of care. Review your State codes, rules and regulations, professional practice standards and facility policy.

249: Regarding RAP documentation: How much documentation is enough? For example, if a resident is incontinent and most documentation is present, but there is no note re: family involvement in the care plan, should the survey team cite this?

A: Not necessarily. Refer to the examples of resident assessment documentation in the User's Manual on pages 4-11. The main issue is whether facility staff have documented key findings regarding the resident's status and associated implications for care. If the family is particularly involved in the resident's care or concerned about the incontinence problem, then it may be appropriate for some reference to the family appear in facility documentation. However, surveyors should not expect to see references to family involvement for each triggered RAP or care plan problem.

Index--RAI Version 2.0 Manual

Springer Publishing Company

The Licensing Exam Review Guide in Nursing Home Administration

Third Edition

James E. Allen, PhD, MSPH, CNHA

Serving as the key companion to James Allen's **Nursing Home Administration,** this highly successful and useful new edition has been updated to reflect the changes in the domains of practice for nursing home administrators. It contains 1,000 test questions (and answers) and reviews key concepts to be mastered by candidates for the licensing exam.

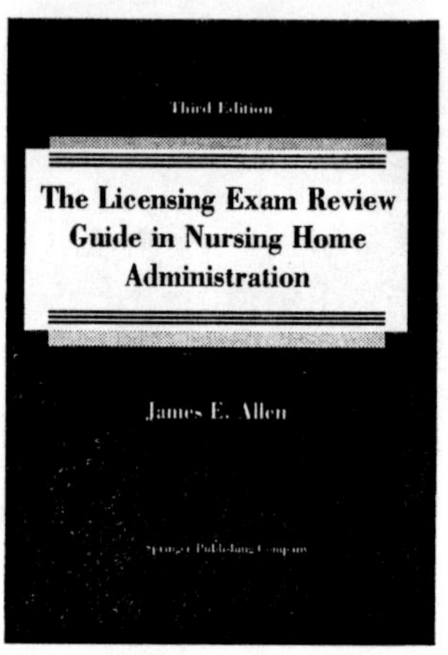

Contents: Uses of This Study Guide • Management, Governance, Leadership • Personnel • Finance • Environment / Federal Requirements • Nursing: Resident/Patient Care • Answer Key

1997 208pp 0-8261-5922-2 softcover

Nursing Home Federal Requirements and Guidelines to Surveyors, Third Edition

James E. Allen, PhD, MSPH, CNHA

In a highly accessible and user-friendly format, this updated and retitled third edition contains new information that is especially useful for nursing home administrators as well as educators and professionals preparing for licensure. It presents the latest federal guidelines and procedures used by federal surveyors in certifying facilities for participation in Medicare and Medicaid. These policies present a quality assurance program which the federal Health Care Financing Administration require that nursing facilities utilize.

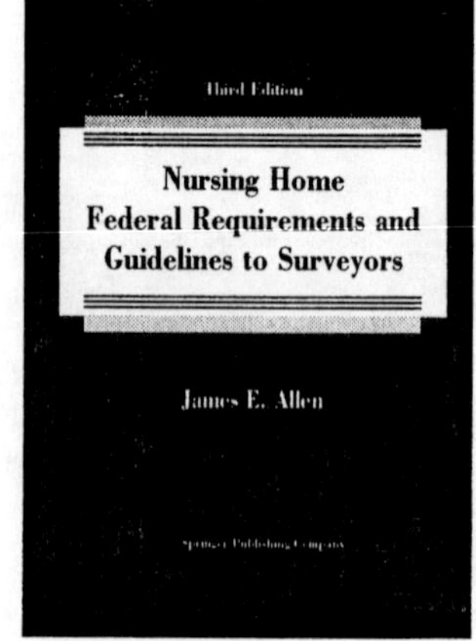

Contents: Basis and Scope • Definitions • Resident Rights • Admission, Transfer, and Discharge Rights • Resident Behavior and Facility Practices • Quality of Life • Resident Assessment • Quality of Care • Nursing Services • Dietary Services • Physician Services • Specialized Rehabilitative Services • Dental Services • Pharmacy Services • Infection Control • Physical Environment • Administration

1997 312pp 0-8261-8122-8 softcover

536 Broadway, New York, NY 10012-3955 • (212) 431-4370 • Fax (212) 941-7842